The Shadow Welfare State

The Shadow Welfare State

Labor, Business, and the Politics
of Health Care in the United States

MARIE GOTTSCHALK

ILR Press

an imprint of *Cornell University Press*

ITHACA AND LONDON

First published 2000 by Cornell University Press

First printing, Cornell Paperbacks, 2000

Printed in the United States of America

Library of Congress Cataloging-in-Publication Data
Gottschalk, Marie.
    The shadow welfare state : labor, business, and the politics of
    health care in the United States / Marie Gottschalk.
        p. cm.
    Includes bibliographical references and index.
    ISBN 0-8014-3745-8 (cloth) — ISBN 0-8014-8648-3 (paper)
    1. Labor unions and health insurance—United States.
    2. Public welfare—United States. 3. Insurance, Health—
    Government policy—United States. I. Title.
    RA412.2 .G68 2000
    331.25'5—dc21   99–088449

Cornell University Press strives to use environmentally responsible suppliers and materials to the fullest extent possible in the
publishing of its books. Such materials include vegetable-based,
low-VOC inks and acid-free papers that are recycled, totally
chlorine-free, or partly composed of nonwood fibers. Books that
bear the logo of the FSC (Forest Stewardship Council) use paper
taken from forests that have been inspected and certified as
meeting the highest standards for environmental and social
responsibility. For further information, visit our website at
www.cornellpress.cornell.edu.

Cloth printing   10   9   8   7   6   5   4   3   2   1
Paperback printing   10   9   8   7   6   5   4   3   2   1

Contents

Preface

This project has disparate origins, some that I can only appreciate as I come to the end of a long journey and ask, how did I end up here? The route seems so obvious as I look back. But it would be disingenuous to say that I knew all along where I was going and why.

In the 1980s, I was an eyewitness to the first wave of economic reforms in China after the Cultural Revolution. Deng Xiaoping and his supporters set out on a long march to smash the iron rice bowl and rewrite the terms of employment for hundreds of millions of Chinese. The so-called reformers sought, among other things, to dispense with lifetime guarantees of job security and greatly reduce state subsidies for housing, medical care, and other key pieces of the public safety net. At the university I was teaching at in the ancient city of Xian in northwest China, the authorities also struggled, with mixed success, to figure out how to build an incentive structure into university education so that the more "productive" professors and teachers would somehow be rewarded for their efforts.

These attempts to rewrite the terms of employment and to change people's expectations about what they are entitled to by virtue of their employment had pervasive political and economic consequences at the local, provincial, and national level. I took a keen interest in these consequences during my two-year stay in China and subsequently. Return visits and newsy letters from friends and former students in China helped keep me apprised of how these macro-level political and economic developments affected everyday life in the People's Republic.

When I returned to the United States, the country was beginning to dig itself out of the worst recession of the postwar years. Employed as a journalist and an editor over the next several years, I noticed that a quieter revolution was under way to rewrite the terms of employment and to reconfigure the social safety net in this country. Even though the economy was roaring once again by the mid-1980s, many workers in the United States were told to shoulder more of the costs of their health care, to make do with part-time and temporary jobs, to accept smaller pensions, and to labor under the threat of being "downsized" at a moment's notice. Anger, anxiety, and insecurity characterized the work lives of many people I knew, including coworkers, friends, and family members, most of whom were told to make do with less. While political scientists focused on the efforts by the Reagan administration and its successors to roll back the public safety net, the private-sector safety net was quietly under siege.

Given all the hostility and insecurity I witnessed in the workplace and the enormous gains that corporations made as wages stagnated, I began to wonder why organized labor was not more successful in defending the porcelain rice bowl that labor, business, and the state had forged in the United States after World War II. The stock answer about how U.S. labor unions were politically enfeebled because of a dwindling membership base was unconvincing and seemed too circular an explanation. As the debate over health-care reform heated up in the early 1990s, I also wondered whether the optimism was justified among analysts and labor officials that business was prepared to be a constructive partner with labor and the state to resolve the pressing problems of escalating health-care costs and the growing number of the uninsured. Furthermore, I was perplexed by organized labor's decision to stick by a private-sector solution for health-care reform. Labor remained committed to an employer-mandate solution even though the bond between employer and employee was disintegrating in the United States, so much so that the very definition of what constitutes an employee was up for grabs.

For these reasons, I decided to use health-care reform as a window to explore larger questions related to the politics of economic restructuring in the United States. This book addresses several important but largely neglected areas in the field of American politics and public policy, including: the private face of the U. S. welfare state; labor's continued, evolving, and multifarious role in shaping contemporary social policy; the ways in which health-care reform is inextricably bound up with larger questions related to the U.S. political economy; and the likelihood that a durable rather than a sporadic coalition of organized labor and other groups will congeal to challenge the rightward thrust in social and economic policy in the United States.

I have accumulated a number of personal and intellectual debts along the way. I am beholden to David Mayhew, Stephen Skowronek, and Rogers Smith of Yale for their thoughtful, constructive criticism at each step of this project and for letting me write the dissertation I wanted to write. David Cameron's critical eye, optimism, and frank and levelheaded advice were invaluable from start to finish. One could not ask for more in a dissertation committee chairman. I am grateful to Walter LaFeber for initially showing me how much history has to teach us about contemporary politics and for his ongoing support and encouragement long after I was his student at Cornell.

Cathy Cohen, Daniel Cornfield, William Foltz, Victoria Hattam, Elise Jaffe, David Montgomery, Sherle Schwenninger, Kathy Thelen, and my classmates in the 1994–95 prospectus seminar at Yale University helped me define and refine the project at a time when it was just a glimmer in my eye. Alan Draper, Ted Liazos, Charles Lindblom, Mark Peterson, Ted Marmor, and Adolph Reed interceded at key junctures and helped move the project along. Cathie Jo Martin deserves special thanks for her active involvement in the evolution of this project over the years.

I am particularly indebted to James Morone and the other anonymous reviewers of the book manuscript. Their insightful, engaged, and constructive criticisms were invaluable.

Yale University generously bankrolled my initial studies and research. My new home at the University of Pennsylvania has provided critical research support and a congenial and stimulating environment. I have been blessed with talented and attentive research assistants at Penn. I especially thank Allan Alicuben and Joanne Lee for their help. Eric Lomazoff's persistence and formidable research skills helped immeasurably to make the completion of this project a smooth one.

I am much obliged to the dozens of representatives of labor, business, and public-interest groups who found time in their busy schedules to have a thoughtful conversation with me about health care and related issues. I want to thank in particular Robert McGarrah of AFSCME for letting me examine his personal files on health-care reform, and Keir Jorgensen of UNITE for granting permission to use the ACTWU archives at Cornell University.

My research was facilitated (and made much more enjoyable) by many talented and dedicated librarians and archivists. I especially thank Richard Horn, Bernard Roger, and Jeannie Solensky of Yale University's Social Science Library, Stuart M. Basefsky at the Industrial and Labor Relations Library at Cornell University, Hope Nisly at the Labor-Management Documentation Center at Cornell University, Mike Smith and Walter Gulley at the Walter P. Reuther Library at Wayne State University, Lee Sayrs at the George Meany Memorial Archives, and Marjorie G. McNinch at the Hagley Museum and Library.

Frances Benson of Cornell University Press shepherded the project along with good cheer and sound advice. I am grateful to Robin Anderson and Melissa Nelson for deftly guiding the copyediting of the book.

Chapter 7 is based on "The Missing Millions: Organized Labor, Business, and the Defeat of Clinton's Health Security Act," *The Journal of Health Politics, Policy, and Law* 24, no. 3 (June 1999): 489–529. Portions of chapter 3 originally appeared in "The Elusive Quest for Universal Health Care: Organized Labor and the Institutional Straightjacket of the Private Welfare State," *Journal of Policy History* 11, no. 4 (1999): 367–98, copyright 1999 by the Pennsylvania State University Press and were reproduced with permission.

Members of my family are still not clear what this project is all about, but I am beholden to them all the same. The discussions and debates I have had with them at holiday gatherings over the years and the struggles they have faced in the workplace had a deep effect on my choice of subjects and on the final shape of this project. Thanks to them, my interest in political science continued to develop in tandem with my interest in real world concerns. Finally, my love and thanks to Atul for everything—and then some.

MARIE GOTTSCHALK

Philadelphia

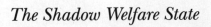

The Shadow Welfare State

CHAPTER 1

Introduction

Labor, Business, and the Shadow Welfare State

The U.S. welfare state is a peculiar institution that is not well understood. The United States is widely considered a "welfare laggard" because it developed a welfare state much later than other industrialized countries, spends comparatively less on social welfare, and lacks universal social programs like national health insurance. Although explanations for why the United States is a welfare laggard vary, a central factor commonly held is the relative weakness of organized labor in this country. This book seeks to revise this perspective on the U.S. welfare state, by focusing especially on the development of the private welfare state and labor's actual role in making health policy.

The fact is, the United States has quite an extensive but generally overlooked welfare state that is anchored in the private sector but backed by government policy. Consequently, the private sector is a key political battlefield where business, labor, the state, and employees hotly contest the contours of social welfare provision in the United States. This recognition of the central importance of the private face of the U.S. welfare state in the development of social policy calls into question the view that the welfare state has successfully withstood conservative attacks and attempts to dismantle it. More importantly, it also casts doubt on the widespread assumption that organized labor in the United States is so politically enfeebled by its shrinking membership base that it can be largely ignored when analyzing contemporary social policy.

Organized labor, a central architect of the private welfare state, remains a pivotal player in the politics of health policy. For example, in the late 1980s and early 1990s, national health insurance returned briefly to the political limelight with renewed calls for the creation of a single-payer healthcare system in the United States.[1] Unions, which were longtime and out-

1

spoken proponents of national health insurance, did not warmly embrace the single-payer solution. Instead, many unions favored proposals that perpetuated the employment-based system of health benefits rooted in the private welfare state. Their stance fundamentally shaped the contours of the debate over health policy at the time.

Labor's tepid and hesitant response to this new push for national health insurance must be understood within the larger historical context of the development of the private welfare state. The private welfare state of job-based benefits developed since World War II to impede the efforts of organized labor to secure universal and affordable health care in the United States. Put differently, specific institutions and ideas associated with the private welfare state molded how labor defined its policy interests and political strategies. They impeded the quest by organized labor for universal health care. To understand the political terrain of health policy in the postwar United States and specifically setbacks by labor, it is important to grasp the subtleties of the changing institutional context and the interplay between institutions and ideas.

The institutions of the private welfare state, that patchwork of employment-linked social benefits sometimes called the "shadow welfare state,"[2] became an institutional straightjacket for organized labor. Over time these institutions helped to reorient labor's interests, worldview, and political strategies about health policy, leading many unions to prefer private-sector solutions over public-sector ones. The institutional context thus brought the interests of the national leadership of organized labor more closely in line with those of large employers and commercial insurers, who eschewed any kind of public-sector or state-led solution to achieve universal health care. They also aggravated divisions within and between organized labor and public-interest groups over health policy, which made assembling an effective political coalition on behalf of universal health care that much harder even as the size of the country's health-care tab and its uninsured population continued to escalate.

The story of labor's twists, turns, and about-faces on health-care issues in the postwar era is an interesting and neglected one. The aim here is to do more than restore organized labor to its once prominent position in discussions of U.S. social policy. This book also uses organized labor as a lens to examine broader analytical questions concerning the expansion and retrenchment of the U.S. welfare state and the interaction of institutions, ideas, and interests in the formulation of social policy.

THE SHADOW WELFARE STATE

Studies of postwar development of social policy in the United States and other advanced industrialized countries tend to focus too narrowly on the activities of the state and ignore private-sector developments. Yet many social protections flow through the private sector, so much so that employment-based benefits often function as "de facto social policy," especially in the United States.[3] Furthermore, the state penetrates private-sector activities, blurring the line between where the public-sector safety net ends and the private-sector net begins. Employment status and employer policies and practices profoundly shape pension, health care, disability, unemployment, and many other social welfare benefits. In turn, specific government policies shape these private-sector activities. Tax codes permit employers to deduct the cost of employee benefits, and Social Security establishes the minimum age of eligibility for state-sponsored retirement benefits. Thus the United States has a peculiar employment-based welfare system that is neither wholly private or public. Only by considering the complex interplay of the private- and public-sector safety nets can we begin to develop a full picture of what drives expansion and retrenchment of social welfare provision in the United States and labor's role therein.

Many scholars give short shrift to organized labor and the private welfare state when dissecting the politics of contemporary social policy.[4] For example, Paul D. Pierson contends that organized labor, which may have been critical to the early development of the welfare state, is less relevant to retrenchment politics today because of its shrinking membership base and the emergence of new interest groups, including the aged and disabled, that are dependent on the state for various social provisions. He views these new groups as the welfare state's most ardent defenders and persuasively argues that the thicket of interest groups that grew up around the "public" welfare state may be its best defense against any major retrenchment.[5]

As argued here, this jungle of interest groups may be poorly suited or situated to forestall a retrenchment of the "private" welfare state on which so many people in the United States depend for health insurance and other social provisions. Many of the same groups that act as the major bulwark against retrenchment of the public welfare state, notably organized labor, also may represent a considerable obstacle to any major expansion of that welfare state to compensate for the retrenchment of the private welfare state, such as establishing national health insurance and eliminating the employment-based system of medical benefits.

Once private-sector developments are factored in, it becomes more difficult to sustain Pierson's claim that "the welfare state remains the most resilient aspect of the postwar economy."[6] Indeed, the last two decades were transformative for the welfare state in the United States. Even though health care in the United States consumes a greater percentage of the country's gross national product (GNP) than other advanced industrialized countries, a growing proportion of the U.S. population cannot access adequate medical care.[7] For more than a decade now, "an average of a million Americans a year have either lost their health insurance or failed to obtain insurance for which they became eligible." By the late 1990s, an estimated 44.3 million Americans, more than 16 percent of the U.S. population, had no health-insurance coverage.[8] A closer examination of the specific social welfare benefits that flow through the private sector reveals that a significant retrenchment is under way. Since the early 1980s, a shrinking proportion of people in the United States has received medical insurance and other health benefits through their employers, and those who do must shoulder more and more of the cost burden. Since President Clinton took office in 1993, the uninsured population has grown by more than 4.5 million.[9]

Social welfare provision in the private sector is undergoing a deep qualitative change. Many employers no longer provide a "defined benefit," such as basic health insurance when an employee retires. Instead, more employers are putting aside a "defined contribution"—a fixed amount of money that may or may not cover the cost of a specific social welfare need, such as comprehensive health-care coverage.

LABOR AND THE PRIVATE WELFARE STATE

A key architect of the private welfare state in the United States, organized labor remains a pivotal defender of a peculiar system of social welfare provision, which has had important consequences for social policy. Analysts of contemporary health-care politics dismiss the significance of organized labor, viewing U.S. labor unions as too politically enfeebled by their dwindling membership base to shape health-care politics and policy in any meaningful way. They have said little about the specific role of organized labor in the most recent quests for universal health care. In a similar vein, many labor officials and union staff members attribute labor's latest political setbacks on health-care reform and other issues primarily to membership woes. Yet organized labor's capacity for political action depends on many factors besides the size of its rank and file. Although labor's ranks thinned considerably since the 1950s, on other fronts unions acquired new political resources in recent years that complicate any simple picture of inexorable political decline. These resources include a swelling number of activist union retirees, important favorable shifts in public opinion regarding unions, labor's formidable financial resources, and closer institutional and financial ties between organized labor and the upper-level of the Democratic Party.

Labor's relative ineffectiveness on the health-care issue is not merely a consequence of its contracting membership base. Also inadequate are the other factors that are historically invoked to explain why unions are politically enfeebled in the United States, notably the absence of a labor party or a disciplined left-of-center party that has strong ties to labor and can navigate the racial shoals of U.S. politics. Although certainly important, those factors focus more attention on labor's weakness and inaction and less on what labor actually did and why. Organized labor's political activities, especially its dogged embrace of private-sector solutions in the health-care debate, were self-defeating and demand a more direct explanation. Analysts also need to consider the specifics of the internal politics of organized labor and not treat unions as merely "passive, monolithic objects of change."[10]

The story of organized labor's role in making health policy in the post-war era is complex. It is more than a simple tale of unions charging Don Quixote–like into the fray with dwindling membership and sparse resources, only to be crushed again by opponents better organized, better financed, and better connected to the political establishment. As Douglas A. Fraser, the former president of the United Auto Workers (UAW), reminds us, "The strength and influence of the labor movement" is not based on size and resources alone. "It is also dependent on the agenda, the sense of commitment and the manner in which the labor movement allocates resources."[11] Labor's political strategies, in turn, are influenced by the specific institutional context that entangles unions.

The term "institution" refers to two kinds of institutions. The first type is those formal organizations and procedures that determine "who gets what, when and how" for a society, thus circumscribing political choice and political behavior.[12] Chapters 3 and 7 focus on three such formal institutions that organized labor, together with large employers and insurers, helped to create and perpetuate. These three institutions decisively molded the incentives and political behavior of labor and other groups. The system of Taft-Hartley health, welfare, and pension plans was established under the Labor-Management Relations Act of 1947, better known as the Taft-Hartley Act. These plans became a major source of health, pension, and other benefits for tens of millions of U.S. citizens. The second institution is the Employee Retirement Income Security Act (ERISA) of 1974, which set up federal standards for pensions. Then considered a major victory for employees and a major defeat for business, this landmark pension legislation ironically helped to undermine the quest for universal health care. The third and final institutional pillar is the experience-rated, health-insurance market in which insurance policies are priced based on the health experience of a particular group rather than of the whole community.

The Taft-Hartley funds, ERISA, and the practice of experience rating profoundly shaped the development of the U.S. welfare state in the postwar decades. It is important to clarify the historical development of these three institutions to illuminate their dramatic and pervasive effect on the contours of the health-care system and the politics of health policy. These institutions evolved with far-reaching and often unintended consequences. They helped cement the commitment of large employers and unions to what is by now a quasi-feudal system of health-care delivery rooted in one's employment status. As a consequence, organized labor found itself implicitly or explicitly siding with large employers and insurers or sitting mute on the sidelines during some of the major skirmishes over health policy leading to the war against the Health Security Act introduced by the Clinton administration in 1993.

Chapter 5 looks more closely at a second type of institution, one characterized by "stable, recurring and valued patterns of behavior" rather than by formal organizations and procedures.[13] In spite of vast shifts in the U.S. political economy, many of the leaders of organized labor held fast to a pattern of labor-management relations institutionalized in the 1950s. It was premised on the belief that business and labor leaders shared many interests and could work out any differences through semi-private, elite-level discussions facilitated by political actors. This enduring faith in the quasi-corporatist possibilities for harmonious labor-management relations cast a spell over much of organized labor through the 1980s, a decade in which business went on the offensive against labor to a degree not matched since the all-out assault on unions in the 1920s and 1930s. This entrenched pattern of labor-management relations led unions to seek what turned out to be an elusive alliance with business on the health-care reform question.

An interest in institutions per se is nothing new in discussions of why the United States is unable to develop, enact, and implement comprehensive social policies except under very special circumstances.[14] A number of scholars concerned specifically with the politics of health policy in the United States have been keenly interested in institutions.[15] Sven Steinmo and Jon Watts contend that the fragmented and federated set of U.S. political institutions is biased against comprehensive national health insurance.[16] Their analysis does not answer why proposals for comprehensive health-care reform go down to defeat time and time again, as evidenced most recently by the 1993–94 debacle, while other pieces of major legislation such as the North American Free-Trade Agreement (NAFTA) persevere in the face of virulent opposition and the same fragmented and federated set of political institutions. In short, what is so exceptional about health care? The health-care issue is exceptional because the institutions of the private welfare state compound the fragmentation of public institutions. These institutions of the shadow welfare state impede efforts to forge a winning coalition anchored by organized labor.

The institutional context is central to many recent studies of the politics of organized labor and the welfare state in Western Europe and Canada.[17] In discussions of the politics of organized labor in the United States, however, the institutional context is more peripheral.[18] Several analysts have ably demonstrated how the fragmented institutional environment in the United States stymied efforts by segments of business to mobilize on behalf of some version of comprehensive health-care reform in the 1980s and the early 1990s.[19] Few considered how the institutional context affected organized labor's political capacity to mobilize on behalf of universal health care. Scholars who take an interest in institutions and the politics of organized labor tend to focus on the distinctive political structures and public institutions of the United States—such as the weak and undisciplined party system—not on how the particular institutions of the private welfare state might affect labor's political fortunes in public policy.[20]

The handful of scholars who are interested in labor, health policy, and the private welfare state tend to concentrate on much earlier periods and then extrapolate to the present. Alan Derickson and Beth Stevens convincingly show the central role organized labor played in the turn toward private-sector, employment-based solutions for medical coverage in the 1940s and 1950s as unions embraced collectively bargained health benefits after the campaign for national health insurance sputtered. This shift subsequently posed formidable obstacles to achieving universal health care over the long run.[21] Yet the line between the institutional developments of the 1940s and 1950s and the contemporary failure to achieve universal health care in the United States is not a straight and predictable one. Such extrapolations from the immediate postwar years to the present fail to explain the twists and turns over time, and fail to identify the mechanisms that perpetuate certain policy preferences.

One notable exception to this tendency to extrapolate from the immediate postwar years to the present is Sanford Jacoby's *Modern Manors*.[22] Jacoby contends that leading nonunion firms reinvented welfare capitalism in the decades after the Depression by creating a new kind of private-sector safety net. They consciously structured job-based health and other benefits to stem the spread of unionization and blunt the edge of public demands for national health insurance and other expansions of the public safety net. As such, the benefit packages of nonunion firms became a major piece of the institutional straightjacket that constricts the possibility of national health insurance and contributes to the persistence of great inequities in health care. This book complements Jacoby's work, focusing on other important features of the institutional straightjacket of the private welfare state and the major role that organized labor played in their construction and maintenance.

THE IDEA OF AN EMPLOYER MANDATE

While the institutional contours of the private welfare state are important, they did not singlehandedly determine the policy path organized labor would set out on and whether it would succeed or fail in its pursuit of universal health care. It is important to also consider the "fumbling efforts" that political actors make in "deciphering their environment,"[23] and the key role that ideas—even a single policy idea—play in this process. Ideas serve as an important prism through which political actors decipher their environment. Like institutions, they can cause individuals or groups to re-think their interests, shift their political strategies, and establish new alliances.

Instead of embracing national health insurance in the 1980s and 1990s, much of organized labor's leadership supported an alternative approach for comprehensive health-care reform that was based on employers paying a portion of their employees' health-insurance premiums. This employer-mandate solution left the private welfare state of job-based benefits largely intact and allowed the commercial health insurers to continue doing busi-ness as usual. At the time, labor unions assiduously courted employers only to discover that they had overestimated business support for comprehen-sive health-care reform based on an employer mandate. Unions, which have played a critical part in the passage of a number of major pieces of so-cial welfare legislation, notably Medicare and Social Security, failed to put together a winning coalition in favor of an employer mandate. Instead, they found themselves divided and on the defensive as they struggled to prevent any further erosion of the private-sector safety net of the U.S. wel-fare state.

This book attempts to explain why organized labor held fast to the idea of an employer mandate despite a drastically changing economic and political environment and examines the wider political consequences of that choice. In doing so, it demonstrates how an idea that was initially adopted because of political expediency took on a life of its own "separate from the context within which it arose."[24] In short, the idea of an employer mandate had a life of its own long before the Clinton administration embraced it and prior to the spread of the anti-government ideas that were the leit-motif of the Reagan era. This idea became embedded in labor's worldview, one that inched closer to business's worldview and was even at odds with the case or-ganized labor was trying to make in other policy realms. The employer-man-date idea played a critical role in defining the strategies and coalitions around which the health-care debate would be waged in the early 1990s. It may have reduced the likelihood that labor could put together an alternate winning coalition to promote universal health care in the United States.

Ideas take on a life of their own when there is a "fit" between the idea and the environment into which it emerges. "Carriers"—individuals or groups who adopt an idea and make others receptive to it—help create that fit.[25] They use all the resources at their command to convince others that the idea they advocate meshes with the existing environment and can solve, or is relevant to, the problem at hand. Carriers, like any political actor, present a selective picture of the political and economic situation. In the case of the employer mandate, labor, as an important carrier, attempted to show how this idea, while a departure from its longstanding commitment to national health insurance, in other ways fit neatly with the existing environment.

A good fit is not merely a function of the carrier's political imagination, skills, and resources. It depends on two other factors. First, objective reality sets limits on the carrier's license to interpret. The institutional context also influences why certain ideas take root. In this instance, the institutions of the private welfare state, together with labor's longstanding modes of discourse about labor-management relations, provided hospitable soil for the employer-mandate idea to flourish. This book highlights the role of ideas in shaping health policy in conjunction with the role of institutional factors. Indeed, the employer-mandate idea and the institutions of the private welfare state were mutually reinforcing, and both, in turn, molded labor's political choices and behavior.

Organized labor's commitment to the idea of a health-care reform solution based on an employer mandate had far-reaching political consequences. Unions traveled an enormous political distance between the early 1970s when they held the torch for national health insurance, and the late 1970s when they wholeheartedly embraced an alternative that perpetuated the link between employment status and health benefits. By the late 1970s labor came to accept the premise that the federal budget deficit was the most important domestic problem facing the United States. In this era of fiscal belt-tightening, an employer mandate appeared irresistible for two central reasons: it expanded the welfare state through private, not public, means and seemed to build upon and ratify the existing system of job-based benefits. Organized labor latched onto a social policy solution arguably in tune with the political tenor of the times as some leading Democrats, notably Sen. Edward M. Kennedy (D-Mass.), came to view proposals for national health insurance as politically unfeasible.

Organized labor endorsed an employer mandate without seriously considering the wider question of the suitability of such a solution given the enormous transformations taking place in the U.S. economy as employers sought to create a more flexible labor market. Over time, labor embraced a solution increasingly out of sync with the economic realities that more and more Americans faced in the workplace in an era of large-scale economic restructuring in which even the definition of what constitutes an "employee" became a highly contested issue. Paradoxically, as the bond between employer and employee frayed with the rise of the contingent workforce, organized labor's commitment to the private welfare state of job-based social benefits became more intense. The national leadership of organized labor was less willing to battle for national health-insurance proposals that would greatly reduce or eliminate the role of commercial insurers in health care and sever the connection between employment status and health benefits once and for all.

From the 1970s onward, health policy and employment policy moved in contradictory directions. Labor's attachment to an employer-mandate formula grew even as employers' attachment to their employees, as traditionally understood, attenuated. In pressing for an employer mandate, labor argued that most employers already provided health benefits; therefore, an employer mandate was a moderate solution. In doing so, labor unwittingly helped draw public attention away from the enormous transformations in the labor market and employer culpability in these changes as companies rapidly shred health benefits and other core pieces of the private-sector safety net. Unions also downplayed the huge gaps and inequities on which the private welfare state was built. Labor, trapped by ideas adopted earlier, helped minimize the vulnerability of the institution of employment-based benefits to shifting political and economic winds. In other words, labor failed to create its own understanding of how to pursue its interests.

In the 1980s and 1990s, a social movement or reform coalition pushing more radical proposals for health-care reform—such as national health insurance—never congealed. The political conditions seemed promising enough for a movement to emerge, given the economic dislocations associated with an employer quest for greater labor-market flexibility. After all, workers faced a radically new economic environment with the downsizing of the labor force, the retrenchment of the private-sector safety net, growing income inequality, and a burgeoning contingent workforce.

There are numerous reasons why a social movement or powerful reform coalition did not emerge around these issues and why the health-care reform question failed to galvanize one.[26] One central reason was the role of organized labor. With its attempts over the years to woo the business community, culminating in what it thought to be a business-friendly legislative solution, organized labor helped lay the political groundwork for the Clinton administration's Health Security Act and how the White House attempted to sell it. Business ultimately dominated the health-care debate because the whole health-care problem was defined, with the help of organized labor, in ways that favored the economic worldview of business.[27] By serving as an important carrier of the employer-mandate idea, organized labor ended up legitimizing a highly selective understanding of the U.S. political economy, one generally uncritical of the role of corporations in the restructuring of the U.S. economy. This view was ultimately at odds with the

explain
why labor acting
seemingly against its
interest.

case labor was trying to make in other policy areas, notably in the 1993 battle over NAFTA.

This book does not contend that the idea of an employer mandate and the institutions of the private welfare state mortally wounded Clinton's Health Security Act. Nor do I mean to imply or suggest that had organized labor solidly embraced an alternative idea, such as a single-payer health-care system, that this alternative would have become law. The aim is to demonstrate how the employer-mandate idea and the institutions of the private welfare state posed major obstacles to developing a winning political strategy and coalition that could secure universal health care over the long term. All these factors made it more difficult for labor to lead rather than follow in the debate over health policy and reinforced organized labor's tendency to defer to the leadership of the Democratic Party on social policy questions. The institutional and ideological logic of the private welfare state subverted labor's stated quest for universal health care. This focus on organized labor's mistakes in the latest health-care debate should in no way minimize the fact that labor faced formidable opponents who could muster enormous resources, financial and otherwise, to shape the fate of comprehensive health-care reform. Nonetheless, labor's own failures were significant and are worthy of serious study.

opponent

Given organized labor's historical role in negotiating and defending the U.S. welfare state, and the ways in which benefits in the unionized sector helped to set the standard for nonunion employers up until recently (when the pattern reversed), the activities of labor unions remain critical to any discussion of social welfare provision in the United States. We need to understand why—or why not—certain segments of organized labor have—or have not—forged meaningful political alliances with other interest groups to mobilize for an expansion of the welfare state in a political climate dominated by calls for retrenchment. By understanding how the private welfare state of job-based benefits developed over time, one can make better sense of the shifting interest-group alliances and the ways in which the institutional context has conditioned organized labor's interests and political strategies.

Organized labor's lukewarm response to the renewed calls for national health insurance in the late 1980s and early 1990s was not merely the consequence of the ideological tenor of the times as the drumbeat of balanced federal budgets and market-led solutions continued to drown out the ideals of the New Deal and Great Society.[28] While the re-calibration of the American political spectrum to the right beginning in the late 1970s is important, it does not explain why private-sector solutions trumped public-sector ones time and again in discussions of health policy, nor why organized labor was a willing contributor to this ideological drift. Moreover, it does not explain the persistence of significant inequities in health care, and why labor was so politically ineffective at addressing these inequities. It is important to understand how the U.S. welfare state developed in the years prior to the Reagan revolution to facilitate organized labor's continued embrace of private-sector solutions and its lukewarm stance toward proposals for national health insurance in recent years.

One final caveat is in order. This book should not be read as a treatise on behalf of the single-payer option. It seeks to explain why labor remained wedded to the private welfare state and to the idea of an employer mandate and was either incapable or unwilling to explore alternatives despite drastic changes in the U.S. political economy. As for any detailed assessment of the pros and cons of the single-payer option, that is left to others.

ORGANIZATION OF THE BOOK

The term "labor," just like the term "business," can obscure interesting shifts in interests and ideology that occur within a broad category.[29] While variations in the national character of labor movements between one country and the next have long been a subject of scholarly inquiry, analysts only recently refocused attention on important differences within a single country. This book analyzes the similarities and differences between major unions as well as tensions within the AFL-CIO over health policy, and the interactions between labor, business, and the state on the issue of universal health care. This close examination of organized labor's stance on health-care reform illustrates striking differences in political and economic goals within the same labor movement. These internal divisions within organized labor over health-care reform are more complex than is commonly understood. They cannot be neatly summed up as the primordial struggle between the "business unionists," who aim to get the best deal for their card-carrying members, and the "social unionists," who are oriented to the needs of union members and workers and society more broadly.

This study focuses on those unions, corporations, business organizations, and public-interest groups that have been particularly active on the health-care issue. It is primarily concerned with political activities surrounding health policy at the national level. Developments at the national level have had important ramifications for unions and health policy at the state and local level. While this analysis will touch on some of the political developments at the subnational level, they are not a central concern.[30]

This book concentrates on the activities of several pivotal unions, including the Service Employees International Union (SEIU), the American Federation of State, County and Municipal Employees (AFSCME), the building and construction trades, the UAW, the United Steelworkers of America (USWA), and the Oil, Chemical, and Atomic Workers (OCAW). It draws on a mixture of primary and secondary materials, including the archival collections of the AFL-CIO, individual unions, and the Committee for National Health Insurance (CNHI), a labor-funded organization prominent in health-care issues in the 1970s and early 1980s. It also is based on a close reading of the labor press, including periodicals published by individual unions and the labor federation, convention proceedings, and public statements by prominent labor officials. It draws on about three dozen semi-structured interviews with labor and business representatives, Congressional staff members, and staff members of public-interest groups. Nearly all of these interviews were conducted in person and usually lasted at least one hour.

My account of the views and activities of the business sector with respect to health policy is based on these interviews, the publications and policy statements of major business organizations, and the public remarks of leading business executives and spokespersons. This book also relies on the business press, academic journals geared to business and management affairs, and accounts of business and health policy in the popular press. It relies less on business archives because these generally are off limits to scholars, especially for the contemporary period. However, the archival collections of the U.S. Chamber of Commerce, the National Association of Manufacturers (NAM), and the Conference Board at the Hagley Library in Wilmington, Del., were useful in filling out earlier periods. Some labor archives, notably the collections at the Walter P. Reuther Library in Detroit, proved surprisingly helpful in teasing out the elusive business side of the political equation. They provide an illuminating glimpse into the political activities of business that often remains shrouded because individual corporations, unlike many labor unions, seldom open their company files to outside researchers, even many years after the fact.[31]

This book is organized into seven chapters in addition to this introductory one. Chapter 2 begins with a discussion of the importance of the private welfare state and how it is generally ignored in social policy discussions. It then explores why, when the private welfare state came into view, analysts concentrated on the activities of the business sector. Meanwhile organized labor was largely ignored because it was mistakenly considered to be too weak to have any political significance.

Chapter 3 begins with a brief discussion of the early history of organized labor and the spread of job-based health-care benefits. Next, it examines the development of three institutional pillars of the private welfare state that were key in molding labor's interests and political behavior: the Taft-Hartley funds, ERISA, and the experience-rated health-insurance market.

It shows how the Taft-Hartley health and welfare funds, originally intended to be a stopgap measure in the provision of social welfare for union members, eventually helped anchor a number of unions to the private welfare state. It then demonstrates how ERISA and the development of a health-insurance market based on experience rating further bolstered labor's commitment to the private welfare state.

Chapter 4 analyzes how and why organized labor abandoned its commitment to national health insurance, and, in a major policy shift during the Carter administration, endorsed the idea of an employer-mandate solution for health-care reform. It focuses on two questions: why did this idea become politically significant—and politically attractive—in the first place, and how did this idea take on a life of its own?

Chapter 5 focuses on the interactions of labor and business over health policy from the late 1970s to the late 1980s. It examines in particular the widespread belief among labor leaders—and many health policy analysts—that big business was prepared to be a constructive and reliable partner in comprehensive health-care reform. It discusses why labor fundamentally misread sentiment in the business community, whose support for a comprehensive health-care solution that labor could live with turned out to be ephemeral. Both institutional factors and labor's misjudgments were at work. As mentioned earlier, organized labor cleaved to a view of labor-management relations that was institutionalized in the 1950s and put great stock in American-style corporatism. A series of misjudgments on the part of organized labor buttressed this institutional legacy as labor leaders mistakenly assumed that the sympathetic mutterings of Chrysler's Lee Iacocca and a handful of other leading business executives somehow represented Fortune 500 sentiment overall on the health-care reform question. Chapter 5 concludes with a discussion of the brief and aborted attempt by some unions in the late 1970s and early 1980s, notably the UAW, to stake out a political path more independent of business and the Democratic Party.

Chapter 6 dissects and critically evaluates three core assumptions about the U.S. political economy on which labor staked its health-care strategy from the late 1970s onward. These assumptions eventually were embedded in how President Clinton's Health Security Act was developed and sold to the public. The first is the idea that an employer-mandate formula was built upon the well-established institution of job-based health benefits, and thus was not a radical or new solution. The second assumption is a belief that business bore the brunt of the costs of the private welfare state and, in particular, the increasingly heavy burden of escalating health-care costs. The third and final assumption is that skyrocketing medical costs imperiled the competitiveness of U.S. firms in the global marketplace and were the root cause of many of the economic woes for the U.S. worker.

Chapter 6 shows how labor leaders, in developing their stance on health-care reform, failed to appreciate the fragility of the private-sector safety net that emerged after World War II and how the campaign waged by U.S. firms to be leaner and meaner to face supposedly tougher economic competition from abroad threatened to shred it entirely. Much of organized labor treated as fact highly contested claims about the U.S. political economy—notably that escalating health-care costs hurt the competitiveness of U.S. workers and were a primary cause of a stagnant or declining standard of living. In doing so, organized labor conceded important political and intellectual ground to business in several critical areas related to the competitiveness issue, as well as broader economic and social questions.

Chapter 7 examines a number of these tensions and assumptions about health care, the U.S. political economy, the role of business, and how they played themselves out in the 1993–94 struggle over health policy at the start of the Clinton administration. It attempts to explain why labor, which played a critical role in the passage of other major pieces of social legislation, not only failed to put together a winning strategy and coalition, but also found itself divided and on the defensive most of the time.

The final chapter addresses the broader analytical themes raised by this book, notably the intricate relationship between institutions, ideas, and interests in formulating social policy; the desirability of expanding our conception of what constitutes the welfare state to include the activities of the private sector; and the importance of embedding discussions of health policy within a deeper understanding of the U.S. political economy. It also briefly speculates about what the denouement of Clinton's Health Security Act bodes for the future of health policy, organized labor, and the contours of the private welfare state.

CHAPTER 2

The Missing Millions

The "Exceptional" Politics of Organized Labor and the U.S. Welfare State

The private-sector safety net, the result of decades of negotiations and confrontations between labor and management in the United States, is an integral part of the U.S. welfare state. Yet analysts of the welfare state usually focus on state activities, largely ignoring private-sector developments. Direct government spending on social welfare provision is a central concern while social welfare provided through the private sector, notably job-based employee benefits, is not.

The sharp distinction analysts make between public- and private-sector activities is an artificial one, especially in the United States. The term "welfare state" is highly misleading because it obscures how a vast array of both public- and private-sector actors, incentives, and initiatives shape the provision of social welfare.[1] Such an exclusive focus on the public sector slights the significant part that unions have played in the development, expansion, and retrenchment of social welfare provision in the United States. Organized labor's advances and setbacks at the bargaining table, in the courts, and in Congress and state legislatures fundamentally have shaped both the private-sector safety net and the public provision of social protection in the United States.

It may be more illuminating to understand social welfare provision as the product of the interaction between the public and private sectors; referred to here as the public and private welfare states. Scholars who take a more comprehensive view of the welfare state highlight the importance of private-sector developments and public-sector activities, such as tax expenditures, that have an important but indirect bearing on social provision in the private sector. As these analysts "cast a wider net and redefine the welfare state to include previously ignored or under-emphasized phenomena," certain non-state actors feature more prominently in social welfare analyses.[2] For example, rising complaints from employers about the growing cost burden of employee health benefits helped rivet national attention on the corporate contribution to the private welfare state. However, the heightened interest in the past two decades over how business shapes the private welfare state and the politics of social welfare was not matched by an upswing of interest in another key private-sector actor, organized labor.

The omission of labor is surprising in several respects. For over a century, labor has been instrumental in the development of the U.S. health-care system. It established some of the first prepaid group practices and health maintenance organizations (HMOs), was the leading voice for national health insurance until the 1970s, and was decisive in the passage of Medicare.[3] The employment-based system of health benefits in the United States today is largely the product of a collective-bargaining regime established during and immediately after World War II.[4] By the 1980s, health benefits were a major arena of labor-management strife in the United States. Cuts in medical benefits were the prime factor in nearly four out of five strikes by the late 1980s. In 1990, health benefits were cited as a major issue for almost 70 percent of workers on strike who were "permanently replaced" by their employers.[5] The neglect of labor in discussions of contemporary health policy also is surprising because labor has been instrumental in shaping a number of major social programs, including Social Security and the Great Society.[6] Some scholars even credit labor with the creation of modern liberalism and the expansion of democracy in the United States.[7] Moreover, organized labor has been the primary defender of the interests of workers, the poor, and the disadvantaged.[8] Except for a passing reference to a dying dinosaur or some such creature, union members are the missing millions in most analyses of contemporary social policy in the United States.

Wedded to a constricted view of what constitutes the welfare state, scholars of social welfare render both the private welfare state and organized labor invisible. The longstanding tendency to view the United States as a "labor laggard" relative to Canada and Western Europe further bolsters this tendency to ignore organized labor in discussions of the politics of social welfare provision. Organized labor remains invisible in part because U.S. unions lack the two ingredients thought essential for the expansion of social welfare programs in Canada and Europe: a labor party or a disciplined left-of-center party with strong ties to labor, and a densely unionized workforce.[9]

Most analysts of contemporary U.S. health policy treat organized labor as little more than a minor player. After a ritualistic recitation of the latest figures on labor's shrinking membership base, they generally dismiss the political significance of organized labor to focus on other political actors, such as physicians and the corporate sector.[10] For a long time, physicians were considered the central protagonists in the health-care drama, able to block national health insurance time and again because of their formidable political power.[11] From this grew the belief in the need for a comparably powerful interest group to break the choke hold medical providers were said to have on health policy in the United States. By the 1980s, business was a probable candidate.

This chapter examines how and why the private welfare state, or shadow welfare state, is largely ignored in most analyses of contemporary social policy. It is argued that when the private welfare state came into view, analysts and policy-makers focused almost exclusively on the business sector. Business was seen as a central figure in the debate over health policy, which fueled expectations that the corporate sector would pave the way toward universal and affordable medical care in the United States. This optimism persisted despite evidence that universal or near-universal health-care systems took root in Western Europe, Canada, and Hawaii largely in spite of business, not because of business.

Most analysts dismiss organized labor in the United States as too weak to have political significance. This chapter argues instead that unions, enmeshed as they are in the workings of the private welfare state, remain a pivotal player in the politics of social welfare, especially contemporary health policy, in the United States. Furthermore, unions have acquired new political resources in recent years that complicate any simple picture that equates dwindling membership with political irrelevance. This chapter takes a more nuanced look at organized labor's relative strengths and weaknesses and treats the size of labor's membership base as a crude barometer by which to measure labor's political strength. The general discussion in this chapter of labor, business, and the private welfare state sets the stage for a more detailed discussion in subsequent chapters of the institutions of the private welfare state in the United States and the role that labor and other actors played in shaping contemporary health policy.

THE SHADOW WELFARE STATE

Studies of the origins of the modern welfare state generally consider the influence of both public- and private-sector activities on its early development.[12] But examinations of the postwar development of social welfare policy in the United States and other advanced industrialized countries usually focus more narrowly on activities of the state and largely ignore the private sector. Scholars of the contemporary welfare state have tended to focus on aspects of how the state channels income transfers to provide certain social protections like health care, retirement income, and disability payments. Concerned primarily with direct government spending on social welfare, scholars generally neglect indirect tools, such as tax expenditures, that the government wields to shape social policy. In focusing so intently on public-sector activities, analysts generally ignore the private welfare state, which is more fragmented, less visible, and "inhabit[s] a legal no-man's land."[13] This tendency to classify a benefit as private or public based on what kind of agency delivers the benefit to a household is misleading because "the interplay of a range of public and private institutions is often implicated in the decisions to make that delivery, and in its financing."[14]

Growing concern in recent years about the possible retrenchment of the welfare state prompted some scholars to take a more encompassing view of specific state activities that should be considered in weighing the fate of the welfare state. Paul D. Pierson, for example, examines items usually not considered integral to discussions of social policy—notably defense spending and fiscal policy—in his work on the comparative retrenchment of the welfare state in the United States and Great Britain.[15] In a similar vein, other scholars have shown how redistribution issues associated with reducing state allocations for social welfare represent a contest over dollars and cents and a battle about which groups can make legitimate political claims against the state.[16] Pierson and these other scholars convincingly demonstrate that the welfare state is more than the sum of the government's direct expenditures on various social provisions. In one important respect, however, their analyses are highly conventional. They all address, almost exclusively, the public-sector provision of social protection and ignore the vast array of social protections that flow through the private sector.

This rigid and somewhat artificial distinction between the public and private sectors is an outgrowth of several intellectual traditions. First, until recently the linear model of welfare state development held enormous sway.[17] This model assumes that over time the state takes over more and more of the obligations of social provision from the private sector. This steady transformation of private provision to public provision is assumed to go in one direction only; hence there is little concern about the flow back from the public sector to the private sector. Most attention is riveted on the public arena where all major action is assumed to occur.

Second, a more expansive understanding of the welfare state was slow to take root because of the ways the disciplines of industrial relations and political science developed. In short, there is little interaction between the two.[18] The discipline of industrial relations focuses on what goes on in the workplace, in particular how workers seek to modify the market through collective bargaining over wages, benefits, and working conditions. Political scientists, on the other hand, are interested primarily in what happens outside the workplace. In the social welfare arena, their main interest is how the state uses non-market channels to provide money, goods, and services to compensate for negative effects of the market on society. Political scientists view social policy as the public sector intervening outside the market. Accordingly, states make social policy, individual firms do not.[19]

The gap between these two intellectual traditions is especially pronounced in the United States because of the widespread and abiding belief that postwar labor-management relations were largely consensual in this country. Beginning in the 1950s, the belief grew that the strains intrinsic to the process of industrialization were tamed in the United States with minimal intervention from the state. This perspective, closely identified with John Dunlop of Harvard University, posits that a mature system of industrial relations emerged in the postwar years as labor and management learned to govern themselves through an agreed upon set of rules while the state sat by as a generally passive referee.[20] Since conflict was believed to be minimal and state intervention limited, the politics of the workplace were of little interest to political scientists. Consequently, the workplace and labor-management relations became the domain of specialists in industrial relations who were primarily interested in how market forces shape the relative power of labor and management at the bargaining table. These specialists were concerned with collective bargaining and market conditions. They generally neglected the political aspects of labor-management relations, notably the importance of government policies and political power in determining who wins and why.[21]

This is not to say that studies of labor-management relations at the firm level were entirely unconcerned with political questions or that industrial relations specialists were the only ones to take an interest in what happened in the workplace. A rich literature in sociology and history, inspired by Harry Braverman and Reinhard Bendix, portrays the workplace as a highly contested political arena. Yet this literature mostly focuses on the enterprise-level politics of the relationship between managers and workers; specifically on how managers use the tools of bureaucracy, technology, ideology, and scientific management to maintain control over their workers on the job, and how employees resist that control.[22] It does not delve into broader political questions, like how the battles between labor and management over the private-sector safety net at the firm or sector level shaped the contours of postwar social policy in the United States.

This failure to make private-sector developments a central component of any discussion of the welfare state is a particularly serious oversight in the case of the United States. Workers in the United States depend far more on the private sector for social protection than employees in other advanced industrialized countries. Nearly 60 percent of all U.S. health-care expenditures are private compared to an average of 20 percent in other advanced industrialized countries.[23] In Sweden barely 4 percent of all social protection benefits (health care, disability insurance, pensions, etc.) flows through the private sector. In the United States, the figure stands at 23 percent, more than twice the national average for the countries of Western Europe.[24] An additional 10 percent of employee welfare benefits in the United States are in the form of government employee welfare benefits. Thus about one-third of all social benefits in the United States are negotiated "as part of the labor contract rather than through the political channels of the welfare state."[25]

A few scholars of U.S. social policy take a more encompassing view of what constitutes the welfare state. Private-sector developments are central to their analyses, as are indirect government tools, such as loans, loan guarantees, and tax expenditures.[26] In the case of health policy, a growing interest in the role of private-sector actors in providing social welfare has focused since the 1980s on the potentially pivotal role of business in health-care reform. Corporations themselves helped focus national attention on the shadow welfare state as they complained loudly about how the escalating cost of providing employee health benefits took a big chunk out of their bottom line. During the 1970s, the business press was filled with articles about the rising cost of employee health benefits and about what individual firms did on their own to contain health-care costs. In 1976, the Council on Wage and Price Stability issued a major policy statement imploring the business sector to be more active in controlling health costs. In the late 1970s, the efforts by many businesses to start their own HMOs as a way to contain costs received widespread attention.[27]

By the mid-1980s, earlier optimism that firms could stem the escalating cost of health care through unilateral internal changes (such as enrolling their employees in HMOs and requiring second opinions in surgery cases) dissipated. As a consequence, business executives shifted their sights from the individual firm to the wider public policy arena. During this period, many businesses formed coalitions at the local, state, and national levels to focus on health policy issues. Confidence grew that the coalitions could stem rising medical costs.[28] By the late 1980s, there were about 180 coalitions nationwide.[29] Activities of Washington-based coalitions like the Washington Business Group on Health (WBGH), comprised of nearly 200 leading U.S. corporations, bolstered the view that business was prepared, in the words of its president Willis B. Goldbeck, to be the "dominant change agent" in health policy.[30] Around this time, some business executives used dire language to describe their concerns about escalating health-care costs. Thomas R. Burke, a former official in the Reagan administration, likened the cost of medical care to a "plague spreading out over corporate America."[31] And Robert E. Mercer, the retired chairman of Goodyear Tire and Rubber Co., emphatically told *The New York Times*, "I never thought I would be in favor of a government health policy, but there are certain things the government must do."[32]

As a consequence of these activities by the business sector, a number of analysts and policy-makers suggested that the business community, especially the Fortune 500, might hold the key to comprehensive health-care reform. They indicated that corporations at last appeared ready to work with the government to pave the way for a satisfactory comprehensive solution.[33] Sociologist Paul Starr foreshadowed some of this new thinking about business and health policy when he predicted in 1982 that a concern for the escalating costs of employee health benefits would push business to become a more active player in the politics of health policy, thereby neutralizing the medical profession's political domination of health policy.[34] His prediction about the potential importance of the private sector in shaping health policy was generally compatible with the growing belief in the Reagan years about the virtues of the private sector and the vices of the government.

THE COMPARATIVE POLITICS OF BUSINESS AND UNIVERSAL HEALTH CARE

The persistent faith that business would somehow unlock the door to universal, affordable health care in the United States was surprising for several reasons. First, poll data indicated great ambivalence and differences of opinion among business executives about government-led health-care solutions and how serious an issue rising medical costs were thought to be.[35] Earlier enthusiasm was waning for what business involvement in health policy could accomplish at the state level as much heralded reform efforts stalled or were reversed in Massachusetts and other states.[36] Most importantly, this faith in business flew in the face of the experience of other countries. While analysts may disagree about precisely why universal and near-universal health care took root in Europe and Canada, they concur that business was at best a passive player and at worst an obstructionist force.

It is not the intention here to get sidetracked into a lengthy debate about U.S. exceptionalism in health politics—nor to go over well-trod ground about whether the United States belongs analytically in the company of other advanced industrialized countries in discussions of social policy and other issues. Certainly the U.S. health-care system is exceptional in some respects, most notably in the extensive roles business and labor play in administering the private welfare state. My main point here is that few analysts attempted to carefully explore whether the political origins of national health insurance in other countries were relevant to later political struggles to achieve universal health care in the United States.

In general, universal health care came about in other countries in spite of business, not because of business. For example, in the late 19th century Bismarck extended social protections, notably the Health Security Act of 1888, primarily because of pressure from below. Fearful of popular uprisings at home in the aftermath of the Paris Commune of 1871 and the Depression of 1873, the German chancellor bestowed certain social protections so as "to prevent having to grant enlarged political rights." He—not the business class—provided the ideological justification for granting social rights to citizens. By tying citizens closer to the paternalistic state, Bismarck aimed to weaken the attraction of the rival Social Democrats.[37]

In the case of Great Britain, it is also hard to discern a major role for business in establishing the National Health Insurance Plan of 1911 and later the National Health Service shortly after World War II. The country's extensive and powerful "friendly societies," some of which dated back to the 18th century, were far more significant in establishing universal health care.[38] The societies were able to shape the specifics of the National Health Insurance Plan because of their sizable membership, substantial legitimacy, and the vital political connections cultivated over their long history. Widespread public alarm about the inadequacies of the British health-care system also helped the measure along.[39] Public dissatisfaction with Britain's medical services persisted during the inter-war years and crystallized during World War II. The Labour Party, together with state officials and leading policy intellectuals (notably members of the Socialist Medical Association), were decisive in shaping the measures that created Britain's National Health Service following the war, again without much input from business.[40]

The direct experience with state solutions and the massive dislocations during the two world wars were critical to establishing a national health service after the Second World War. It appears that national health insurance did not come about in Great Britain because business was organized and mobilized to participate in social policy questions. Rather, it was established because the British public was better situated to press the government to respond to its needs due to the existence of the powerful friendly societies and because the medical profession was divided.[41] In England, the friendly societies forcefully represented the public on health issues before World War I, as did the unions and Labour Party during and after World War II. By contrast, the U.S. public is comparatively unorganized and incapable of steering health policy in a direction that serves the broader needs of society.[42]

Although there is no ironclad consensus on why national health insurance took root in Canada, by most accounts business played only a negligible role.[43] The most exhaustive study of the Canadian case by Malcolm G. Taylor focuses on the importance of the social-democratic Cooperative Commonwealth Federation (CCF) in Saskatchewan.[44] Taylor underscores two other factors that paved the way for truly universal medical care in Canada: decisive political leadership and the unwavering and uncompromising support of organized labor.[45] From the start, health care was central to the CCF's agenda. In the "Regina Manifesto," which the CCF adopted at its founding in 1933 and served as its platform until the late 1950s, the party explicitly called for the socialization of health services. In 1946, two years after it became the first social-democratic government to come to power in Canada, the CCF enacted the country's first universal and compulsory hospital insurance program. It broadened the program in 1959 to include physician services and weathered a contentious strike by doctors to implement the new measures. The CCF's initial experiments with universal coverage in Saskatchewan had a decisive influence on the timing and course of development of national health insurance in Canada, according to Taylor. The measures prompted other provinces to create hospital insurance programs and put pressure on the federal government and the Canadian Medical Association to develop a national solution. In 1957, Ottawa enacted the Hospital Insurance and Diagnostic Services Act, which instituted universal hospital coverage across Canada.

Even though its electoral performance failed to improve during the 1950s (it hovered around 10 percent of the national vote), and the Conservatives mocked the party for its "obsession" with health insurance, the CCF did not back down on universally-based and progressively funded national health insurance. Notably, despite the CCF's failure to expand its electoral base, organized labor did not vacillate about the universal approach. It elevated health insurance to a more prominent place in its social reform agenda and stepped up pressure on the government.

In her comparative account of the development of health insurance in Canada and the United States, Antonia Maioni accords even more significance than Taylor to the ties between Canadian unions and the CCF.[46] She argues that organized labor in Canada was instrumental in establishing national health insurance even though it shared some of the same apparent weaknesses that vexed labor in the United States, notably deep divisions between its craft and industrial unions and membership levels in the 1950s that were low relative to many European countries.[47] Like the CCF, organized labor in Canada consistently supported a universal health-care program based on a progressive system of taxes. During the national debate over various health-care reform proposals in the late 1950s and early 1960s, the Canadian Labour Congress rejected outright any solution that entailed merely tinkering with the existing insurance system. It also stridently rejected the premise that the private sector on its own could fulfill the medical needs of Canadians.[48]

This pressure on the national government to expand the insurance program to include outpatient services intensified after CCF leader Tommy Douglas left the premiership of Saskatchewan to head the New Democratic Party (NDP) formed in 1961 out of the CCF and an alliance with the Canadian Labour Congress. In its founding platform, the New Democratic Party reaffirmed the party's support for social policy reform and put comprehensive health insurance at the top of its list. After 1961, Canadian labor intensified its campaign on behalf of national health insurance and, together with the NDP, put critical pressure on the minority Liberal government, which was returned to power in 1963.[49] This new social-democratic party prodded the Liberal Party to make good on the commitment made to national health insurance in its party platform more than four decades earlier.[50] Dependent on outside support for his minority Liberal government, Premier Lester Pearson pushed for passage of the National Medical Act in 1966, which expanded coverage to include outpatient services and physicians' fees. In short, business does not figure much in Maioni's account of the development of national health insurance in Canada. While other accounts place varying stress on the importance of working-class agitation and crucial alliances forged with Canadian farmers in explaining the establishment of national health insurance, they treat business as a minor actor in the drama that established universal care in Canada.[51]

Similarly, business was not a critical player in establishing near-universal health care in Hawaii, the only state that requires employers to provide health insurance for employees. Analysts attribute the emergence of near-universal health insurance coverage in Hawaii to several other factors: a plantation and immigrant economy that engendered efficient production of health services; the enormous political transformations in the state shortly after World War II; and an insurance market overwhelmingly dominated by two providers.[52]

Most analysts and advocates fail to consider in any serious and sustained way whether the political origins of national health insurance in other advanced industrialized countries could shed light on how to achieve universal access to affordable, high-quality care in the United States.[53] In according business a special place in the debate over health-care reform while dismissing labor as just too weak to matter in any significant way, analyses of the U.S. case take a highly selective view of developments abroad. They trumpet the potential of U.S. corporations to break the stalemate in health policy, despite ample evidence from abroad and Hawaii that business interests were largely inconsequential in establishing state-sanctioned social protections. Studies of the politics of health policy elsewhere indicate that medical providers, the business sector, and other "conservative political forces" fiercely opposed universal health care.[54] Furthermore, they demonstrate the importance of labor and other non-business actors in securing universal health care. By contrast, analysts of the U.S. case treated organized labor as largely inconsequential in the politics of health care because, after all, the United States is a "labor laggard" compared to other advanced industrialized countries. Yet this characterization of the United States as a "labor laggard" is highly simplistic.

THE UNITED STATES AS A "LABOR LAGGARD"

The United States is considered a labor laggard because, relative to Canada and Western Europe, it lacks a labor movement strong enough to pull the political arena in a significantly more proworker direction.[55] This view attributing labor's political successes primarily to strong and self-conscious labor organizations mobilized against recalcitrant employers is being challenged from a number of directions. Some scholars contend that traditional or conventional measures of union power, such as membership levels and the degree of centralization, do not on their own "appear to explain relative union success," especially in the turbulent economic and political environment since the 1980s.[56]

Scholars working primarily on the comparative politics of organized labor in Western Europe recently singled out a range of other political and institutional factors to account for the varied political fortunes of organized labor in different countries.[57] In the U.S. context, organized labor's membership base continues to be the main yardstick by which its political clout is measured. It is as if establishing the fact of labor's dwindling base is enough to explain its electoral and legislative setbacks and dismiss the need for any systematic study of U.S. labor unions as diverse and important political actors.[58] The central issue is to account for the membership decline and explain what might reverse it.[59]

In the wake of the latest failed attempt to achieve universal health care, labor leaders reached much the same conclusion. Many explain the failure of health-care reform in the early 1990s in two parts. The immediate blame goes to the Clinton administration for its ineptness. The more fundamental cause, according to union officials, is labor's weakness relative to the "moneyed interests," a weakness they attribute to labor's thinning ranks. Not surprisingly, "organize the unorganized" was the mantra of delegates to the biennial convention of the AFL-CIO held in October 1995, a year after the death of Clinton's Health Security Act.[60] Although the greater attention that the federation pays to labor's dwindling base is long overdue, it is wrong to identify labor's shrinking membership as the central reason for its setbacks in the health-care debate and its political ineffectiveness in general. Although labor's ranks have thinned considerably since the 1950s, unions in the United States have made potentially important gains in other areas.

The Membership Yardstick

That union membership in the United States plummeted from more than one-third of the workforce in the 1950s to barely 14 percent today—or just over 16 million members—is significant.[61] The drop is even more perilous if one leaves out the public sector and considers just the private workforce. Today barely 10 percent of the private sector is unionized—a figure comparable to the one on the eve of the Depression in 1929.[62] In most other industrialized countries, union membership remained reasonably constant over the last two decades or so, averaging about 45 percent of the employed workforce as of the late 1980s.[63] Though nearly all unions lost some ground since the 1970s, union density declined substantially in just a handful of advanced industrialized countries. The United States, France, and Japan saw significant drops in the 1970s and 1980s, while Ireland, the United Kingdom, and the Netherlands experienced sizable drops in the 1980s.[64]

The connection between union density, political mobilization, and political success is neither a simple nor a direct one in the United States, or elsewhere. For example, in France only about 10 percent of the workforce is unionized. Yet unions together with students carried out nearly a month-long series of strikes and demonstrations across the country in late 1995 that forced the Juppé government to reverse its austerity policies. Similarly, despite a small and declining membership, Spanish unions in the 1980s demonstrated a remarkable capacity for general worker mobilization, as did the ideologically splintered and organizationally weak Italian unions.[65]

Historically the relationship between union density and political activism is not a direct one in the United States either. The desire to form legally recognized unions set off a wave of political activism in the mid-1930s at a time when labor's ranks were anorexic in the wake of the "open shop" campaign and other anti-labor measures of the 1920s and early 1930s. Union membership peaked in the United States in the mid-1950s, with AFL-CIO unions representing 40 percent of the private-sector labor force at that time.[66] Despite record membership levels, U.S. labor unions generally were considered weak and quiescent in the 1950s.[67] Two of labor's most notorious legislative setbacks—passage of the Taft-Hartley Act in 1947 and the

Landrum-Griffin Act in 1959—occurred when its membership rolls were flush. The Landrum-Griffin Act was enacted despite the influx of a record number of liberal legislators into Congress after the 1958 elections.[68]

For all the talk of membership decline, the AFL-CIO, with its 13 million members, arguably remains the largest organization in the United States committed to defending the rights of working people. The membership rolls and resources of the major unions dwarf those of many major public-interest groups. For example, much was made in recent years of the size of the Christian Coalition and that organization's central importance in shifting U.S. politics to the right. As of 1993, its dues-paying members (450,000) and affiliated activists (300,000) totaled less than the combined active and retiree membership of just one union, the United Auto Workers.[69]

Concerns about labor's thinning ranks overshadowed a number of potentially more favorable developments for organized labor. First, retired unionists are a force to reckon with in local, state, and national politics in the United States. Over the last two decades, unions attempted to revitalize their retiree roots by establishing retiree chapters in local unions and creating new retiree councils. Many retirees first became politically active during the early 1980s in response to the Reagan administration's assaults on Social Security. Organized labor's retirees became significant political players in states like Nevada, Florida, and Arizona that are home to large retirement communities. Even though the United Auto Workers represents only a handful of workplaces in Nevada, for instance, it is a major player in state politics because thousands of retired UAW members live there and team up with senior citizen groups and progressive organizations. In 1986, Democrat Harry Reid credited UAW retirees in Nevada with helping him win the U.S. Senate seat of outgoing Republican Paul Laxalt and returning the state government to the Democrats.[70]

In another favorable development, by the late 1980s public opinion shifted significantly in favor of unions. In a 1988 Gallup poll, 61 percent of the public approved of unions, up from 55 percent in 1979 and 1981, the two lowest years for the American labor movement since the surveys began. Among 18- to 24-year-olds, the approval figure was 67 percent, which rivals the 65 percent or more approval rating among the general population throughout much of the postwar period and comes close to the high point of 70 percent in 1965.[71] A 1987 *Business Week* poll found that 61 percent of the public nationwide believes unions serve as a good check on big business, and 79 percent think unions are positive forces for working people, fighting for such things as improved health programs, better unemployment benefits, and a higher minimum wage.[72] Other negative perceptions of unions held in the early 1980s are less prevalent today. For instance, opposition to union membership fell sharply, as demonstrated most starkly by an upsurge in physicians interested in forming or joining unions.[73] Furthermore, the public is much more likely to sympathize with strikers and against companies during labor strife and less inclined to blame unions for inflation. One of the most dramatic examples of this shift in public opinion in favor of labor is a widely publicized Gallup poll conducted during the 1997 United Parcel Service (UPS) strike that found Americans backed the striking teamsters in the dispute by a two-to-one margin.[74]

Financial resources are another indicator of union strength—or potential strength. Despite a marked drop in membership, the financial resources available to unions remain virtually unaltered. Unions in the private sector softened the blow of falling membership by increasing fees, dues, and fines. Despite the loss of millions of members, union wealth (after adjusting for inflation) holds steady. Between 1979 and 1993, the total assets and wealth of the 28 major private-sector unions in the United States, as measured on a per-member basis, "actually increased by a significant amount."[75] As of 1993, these unions had $2.2 billion in total assets.[76] Furthermore, overall financial capacity to weather a strike or finance other major job actions has improved for most unions.[77] Similarly, labor's campaign war chest has not dwindled despite its waning membership. Eighteen of the 28 major private-sector unions "actually raised more PAC money in real terms in 1994 than in 1980."[78] Between 1979 and mid-1994, labor's political action committees (PACs) contributed over $239 million.[79]

The Democratic Party is increasingly dependent on labor money. Soon after he became chairman of the party in 1981, Charles Manatt offered organized labor unprecedented representation on the Democratic National Committee and Committee on Rules. In return, labor provided enormous financial support. In 1983 it gave $2.5 million to the DNC, or about one-third of the committee's annual budget.[80] The labor movement bestows substantial sums of "soft money" (contributions that are exempt from the limits and restrictions of federal campaign law) on the Democratic Party. In the early 1990s, organized labor accounted for slightly over 12 percent of the total "soft money" received by the Democrats, and its PACs contributed $40 million, on average, to Congressional elections in each campaign cycle. Almost all the PAC money went to Democratic candidates.[81] The Democrats became even more dependent on labor PAC money after business contributions dried up following the 1994 Republican takeover of Congress. By 1996, contributions from labor PACs comprised 48 percent of all PAC donations to House Democrats, up from 33 percent in 1992.[82]

Since the 1980s, unions have strengthened their institutional ties to the Democratic Party. In 1981, Douglas A. Fraser, president of the United Auto Workers, served as cochair of the Hunt Commission, which restructured the Democratic Party's nominating process to shore up the influence of party officeholders and union officials in the presidential nominating process.[83] As a result, labor was well represented at the Democratic national convention in the 1980s and 1990s. In 1996, 28 percent of the delegates and alternates to the convention were members of the AFL-CIO or the National Education Association, one of two leading teachers' unions.[84] Labor fortified its ties not only to party officials but also to leading officeholders. Coordination and cooperation between organized labor and Congressional Democrats increased dramatically during the second half of the 1980s, especially in the House, as a close alliance between labor and the Democrats was consolidated, thanks in large part to the efforts of House Speaker Jim Wright (D-Tex.). The contacts between the Speaker's staff and labor lobbyists were so extensive that the latter "became, in effect, an arm of the Democratic leadership."[85] Around this time, labor's lobbying capacity also expanded dramatically as the AFL-CIO and individual unions invested more heavily in lobbyists, enlarged their research departments, and developed a grass-roots lobbying network.[86]

Labor unions remain among the few organizations with power to reach straight into the pockets of their members as they channel dues directly from members' paychecks to union coffers. In the months prior to the November 1996 election, the AFL-CIO levied a one-year surtax on each of the federation's 78 unions to create a special $35 million electoral war chest that put business and Republican candidates on the defensive.[87] Although corporate financial contributions to campaigns increasingly dwarf labor contributions, unions, unlike other organizations with PACs, provide important "in-kind" contributions to political campaigns, such as union-run phone banks and nonpartisan get-out-the-vote drives.[88] These critical in-kind contributions explain why Vice President Al Gore aggressively sought an early endorsement by the AFL-CIO in the fall of 1999 as former Senator Bill Bradley's campaign for the Democratic presidential nomination surged.

In short, labor's growing financial and institutional ties to the Democratic Party do not fit neatly into a story of inexorable political decline in the face of a hemorrhaging membership. Their political significance is more ambiguous. They represent a potential area of strength or weakness, dependent in part on how labor leaders interpret the political and economic environment, and how they choose to respond to it; i.e., on labor's political strategies.

Labor's political strategies are not a central concern of scholars of social policy and American politics more broadly. The handful of contemporary scholars interested in questions related to the ability of organized labor in the United States to articulate and realize its political and legislative goals tend to concentrate on earlier time periods, in particular the 1920s, the

New Deal, World War II, and the immediate postwar era.[89] From about the 1970s onward, interest in labor's capacity for political action was much more limited. The "new" labor historians downplay politics and policy-making in their work, emphasizing instead the subcultures of working people.[90] Social scientists, if they take up the topic of labor and politics at all, tend to focus on electoral behavior, in particular labor's pattern of campaign contributions and the voting behavior of union members and workers.[91] They usually ignore the role of unions in the lobbying process, their impact on public policy, differences between unions over tactics and ideology, the significance of coalition building between labor and other groups, and the causes of labor's major legislative triumphs and defeats.[92]

Labor and the Reagan Democrats

The emergence of the Reagan Democrats in the 1980s reinforced this tendency to treat the politics of organized labor in a one-dimensional way that singles out labor's shrinking membership as the primary explanation for its political defeats and political vulnerabilities. The debates among scholars and popular commentators about the political significance of the Reagan Democrats helped fuel disinterest in the actual political behavior of organized labor. The term "Reagan Democrat" became a shorthand way of connoting the fundamental conservatism of working-class whites broadly and union members in particular in the United States. The political sentiments of the Reagan Democrats and union members were treated as largely synonymous and interchangeable. In the scholarly and popular imagination, the Reagan Democrats replaced the hard hats who stoned antiwar protesters in New York City in an infamous incident in May 1970 that landed on the front pages of newspapers across the country. That incident seared in the popular and scholarly mind an image of labor's bedrock support for the Vietnam War and its deep-seated antagonism toward students and the New Left that went largely unchallenged until recently.[93] Just as those New York construction workers symbolized labor in the late 1960s and 1970s, the Reagan Democrats became a stand-in for card-carrying union members in the 1980s and 1990s. This is a highly misleading view because the average Reagan Democrat—or blue-collar voter—is a different breed politically than the average union member.

Despite the stronger propensity of union members to vote Democratic compared to the working class in general, the view persisted that the Democratic Party was hemorrhaging union members as the Reagan Democrats settled into the Republican camp. Commentators regularly made little distinction between the working-class vote and the union vote, interchanging one for the other. For example, to bolster his point about the waning electoral and political power of organized labor in *Working-Class Hero: A New Strategy for Labor*, Stanley Aronowitz noted that in 1980 "more then forty percent of traditional Democratic voters, especially 'blue-collar' workers, had defected to the Republicans despite the fact that Reagan was the most ideologically conservative Presidential candidate of any major party since Goldwater in 1964." In his review of Aronowitz's book, Seymour Martin Lipset singled out this quote to underscore his own view about rising conservatism among union members.[94] An examination of the broader electoral trends among union members over the past 25 years does not substantiate the claim that union members are fleeing the Democrats en masse to embrace a more conservative agenda, however.

In analyzing the labor vote, it is important to remember that it fluctuates greatly from one election to the next, so using a single election, like the 1980 match up between Jimmy Carter and Ronald Reagan, as a reference point is highly misleading. The white union member vote for major party presidential candidates varies greatly, from a high of about 80 percent in the 1948 and 1964 contests, to a low of about 40 percent in 1972, to 69 percent in the 1996 presidential race.[95] Despite great variation between one election and the next, certain electoral trends are discernable over the past few decades. Between 1972 and 1996, the Republican presidential candidate garnered the majority of union household votes only once—in 1972, when Nixon held a 3 percent edge over George McGovern (see Table 2.1, row 5). The union vote for Democrats dipped during the 1980 and 1984 presidential contests, then rebounded in 1988, 1992, and 1996. In those three contests, the Democratic candidate averaged a 25 percent edge over the Republican nominee, an average that exceeds the Democratic average performance among union households between 1952 and 1976 (calculated from Table 2.1, row 5).[96] In 1992, the spread between the labor vote for the Democratic and Republican presidential candidates was a whopping 31 percent in favor of Clinton; it dipped slightly to 29 percent in 1996. Second only to African-American and Jewish voters, union members remain the most reliable Democratic voters in presidential contests.[97] Union households disproportionately favor the Democratic candidate in presidential contests and Congressional elections. Furthermore, they are much less likely to split the ticket by voting for the Democratic nominee in the Congressional contest and the Republican candidate in the presidential race. A closer look at the electoral data also suggests that unions are particularly adept at keeping their white middle-income members from defecting to the Republicans.[98]

The voting behavior of union members is markedly different than that of blue-collar workers. While union members vote consistently Democratic (except for the 1972 race), the working class by varied margins swung

Table 2.1. Union and Working-Class Electoral Behavior: Presidential Elections, 1952–96*

Election Party	1952		1956		1960		1964		1968		1972		1976		1980		1984		1988		1992		1996	
	D	R	D	R	D	R	D	R	D	R	D	R	D	R	D	R	D	R	D	R	D	R	D	R
Union	61	39	57	43	65	35	73	27	56	29	47	50	59	39	49	44	53	46	57	42	55	24	59	30
W/C	55	45	50	50	60	40	71	29	50	35	43	57	55	43	39	53	42	57	50	49	45	35	53	36
National	44	55	42	57	50	50	61	38	43	43	36	61	50	48	41	51	40	59	45	53	43	38	49	41
Difference Between Union and W/C Vote for Democrats	6		7		5		2		6		4		4		10		11		7		10		6	
Democratic Lead Among Union Households	22		14		30		46		27		-3		20		5		7		15		31		29	
Democratic Lead Among W/C Households	10		0		20		42		15		-14		12		-14		-15		1		10		17	

Sources: Andrew J. Taylor, *Trade Unions and Politics: A Comparative Introduction* (Houndmills, England: Macmillan, 1989), Table 4.7a, p 89; and "Portrait of the Electorate," *The New York Times*, November 10, 1996: 28.

* Excludes minor party candidates. Working class (W/C) is defined as households earning the equivalent of $15,000 to $29,000 in 1996. If you include the next highest income bracket ($30,000–49,000), union votes are skewed even more in favor of Democratic candidates.

Table 2.2. Percentage of whites who voted
Democratic for president by union
membership and class, 1944–96*

	Union Members	Working Class
1944	67	64
1948	79	76
1952	53	52
1956	50	44
1960	64	55
1964	80	75
1968	50	50
1972	40	32
1976	60	58
1980	48	44
1984	49	42
1988	53	43
1992	48	42
1996	69	55

Sources: Frances Fox Piven, "Structural Constraints and Political Development: The Case of the American Democratic Party," in Frances Fox Piven, ed., *Labor Parties in Postindustrial Societies* (New York: Oxford University Press, 1992), Table 11.1, p. 236; Paul R. Abramson, John H. Aldrich, and David W. Rohde, *Change and Continuity in the 1988 Elections* (Washington, D.C.: Congressional Quarterly Press, 1990), Figure 5.1, pp. 124–125; *Change and Continuity in the 1992 Elections* (Washington, D.C.: Congressional Quarterly Press, 1995), Figure 5.1, pp. 134–35; and *Change and Continuity in the 1996 Elections* (Washington, D.C.: Congressional Quarterly Press, 1998), Figure 5.1, p. 102.
* Includes only whites who voted for major party candidates.

wildly back and forth between the Republican and Democratic columns in recent presidential elections (see Table 2.1, row 6). Between 1952 and 1996, the union vote for the Democrats on average exceeded the working-class vote by 6.5 percent in each election (Table 2.1, row 4). The lead of the Democratic presidential candidate over the Republican candidate averaged 20 percent among union households between 1952 and 1996 (calculated from Table 2.1, row 5), and just 7 percent among working-class households during this same period (calculated from Table 2.1, row 6).[99]

Even after controlling for race, union members demonstrate a greater propensity to vote Democratic than the working class as a whole in presidential contests (see Table 2.2). The difference between the white union vote and the white working-class vote for the Democratic presidential candidate averaged 5 percent for the 13 presidential contests between 1944 and 1992, a figure almost identical to the spread in the 1980 election when

48 percent of white union members voted for Carter compared to just 44 percent of the white working class overall.[100] Thus, while the 1980 contest was exceptional in many other respects, it was typical with respect to the distribution of the white union and white working-class vote.

Although union members remain an important part of the Democratic coalition, the view persists that the number of defections among labor's rank and file to the Republicans are significant and mounting. A *Wall Street Journal* article in the spring of 1996 about the AFL-CIO's stepped-up electoral efforts on behalf of select Democratic candidates had the headline: "Labor's Bid to Aid Democrats Faces One Hurdle: Many of Its Members Often Vote for Republicans." Instead of examining overall trends in the voting patterns of union members across several election cycles and comparing them with other major blocs of voters, the article took a snapshot view of recent elections to substantiate its claim. It merely noted that, according to exit polls "about 40 percent of union members voted Republican in 1994. That's up from 32 percent in 1992 and 30 percent in 1990."[101] If the voting behavior of union members is put in a broader historical perspective, as outlined above, it is hard to sustain the claim that more and more union members are embracing the Republicans and a more conservative agenda. Indeed, in the 1998 midterm elections, union members voted 71 percent to 29 percent in favor of Democrats over Republicans and provided the margin of victory for Democratic candidates in a number of tight races.[102]

The widespread use of the term Reagan Democrat to refer to the political behavior of the typical worker and typical union member, i.e., a white, working-class male, is misleading in one final respect. It belies the enormous transformations that labor's membership base has undergone since the 1960s as women, minorities, and public-sector employees, many of whom are middle-class professionals, became a larger proportion of labor's rank and file.[103] Furthermore, while opinions may differ over how much members of public-sector unions like AFSCME are committed to such issues as national health insurance and a more progressive tax system, the new public-sector unionism can hardly be characterized as a collection of Reagan Democrats committed to rolling back government involvement in social policy across the board.[104]

Union members do not behave as Reagan Democrats. Democrats do quite well with union households, both white and non-white, and comparatively poorly among white non-unionists. This is not to say that the labor vote remains largely unchanged in the postwar decades. The important electoral phenomenon is not so much the shift of union members to the Republican camp, but rather the shrinking proportion of white unionists who comprise the electorate, period. Whereas members of white union households made up 25 percent of the electorate in 1952, by 1996 they comprised just 16 percent.[105]

The portion of white union members who voted for the Democratic presidential candidate averaged 65 percent in the first two decades after World War II, with the figure dropping to about 52 percent from 1968 to 1996 (see Table 2.2). This is admittedly a dramatic decline. Deep political changes occurred among workers—both union and nonunion—in the late 1960s and early 1970s. Since then, the labor vote for the Democrats stabilized somewhat, and we do not see a comparable shift on the part of union members away from the Democratic Party.

In short, careless or imprecise use of the term Reagan Democrat compounded the misunderstandings and misperceptions about the political behavior and political significance of organized labor. Many analysts tagged union members as Reagan Democrats, even though the electoral data are at odds with that categorization. The political preferences and behavior of the working class in general, and union members in specific, remain quite distinct, with the latter far more likely to pull the lever for the Democratic candidate despite some erosion of support for the Democratic Party among union members.

Bringing Business and the State Back In

Two additional factors fueled scholarly disinterest in and misunderstandings about the political behavior of organized labor. As scholars sought to bring business and the state back into their analyses of political phenomena, they further marginalized organized labor. The publication of *Politics and Markets* in 1977 by Charles E. Lindblom, who was so closely identified with pluralism, served to legitimize the study of the power of business in the United States, bringing it from the Marxist and neo-Marxist fringes to the perimeter of the mainstream.[106] In arguing that business's "privileged position" in the U.S. political economy is overwhelming and nearly constant, *Politics and Markets* foreclosed for a time the need to consider those variables that might mitigate its influence, such as the institutional setting for business or the role of other interest groups, such as labor unions.[107] The next wave of scholarship to grapple with the place of business in American politics went in two directions, neither of which fostered much interest in the politics of organized labor. One concerned itself with whether the political fortunes of business are constant or variable. The other took up whether the state itself enjoys a privileged position and thus autonomy from the influence of capital and other societal groups.

The former was a direct challenge to Lindblom's contention that the power of business is constant. Instead, David Vogel and others portrayed the political strength of business as highly dependent on how the national and global economy are organized, the ways in which the business sector and individual firms are structured, and the public's perception of the health of the economy.[108] Some scholars also singled out the activities of other interest groups, notably public-interest groups, as important independent variables that helped to explain the rise and fall of business's political fortunes. This focus on other interest groups did not translate into a greater interest in labor per se. Vogel, Michael W. McCann, and others presented the rise of public-interest liberalism as primarily a phenomenon of middle-class, elite professionals with few ties to labor and little interest in the broader socioeconomic issues that were the bread and butter of labor's political activism over the years.[109] In their accounts, business and public-interest groups engage in an intricate minuet, each jockeying for position while labor looks on from the sidelines.

Vogel's work indirectly contributed to the scholarly slight of labor in a second way. In his account of the 1980s, Vogel argues that business's influence on public policy waned during the Reagan years in every area except one—with respect to labor-management relations.[110] In his view, the business community with the help of a sympathetic administration maintained a highly united and increasingly effective front against labor throughout the decade, even as it splintered on the shoals of tax and regulatory policy. He presents business domination of labor as so complete during this period that inquiries about what labor was doing and why were almost irrelevant.

Other analysts, many of them critical of business and the Reagan administration in the 1980s, perhaps unwittingly reinforced this tendency. Kevin Phillips, William Greider, Thomas Edsall, Benjamin Ginsberg, Thomas Ferguson, and Joel Rogers all in some way challenge Vogel's contention that business's influence on public policy peaked in 1981 and fell below expectations during the rest of the Reagan years in every area except labor relations.[111] By bolstering the view that business was all-powerful in the 1980s, not just with respect to labor but in nearly all aspects of social and economic policy, they fed scholarly and popular disinterest in labor's specific role in social policy. In short, why study a gnat harassing an elephant?

A related analytical development at this time was emerging scholarly interest in examining the autonomy of the state in policy-making.[112] This analytical shift away from economic interests and toward political institutions is useful in many respects, but contributes to a tendency to "valorize states" as a counterbalance to the concentration of private economic power,[113] which leaves labor out in the cold. Many state-centered scholars refuse to concede any meaningful part to labor, even in the shaping of the New Deal. Recent debates about the origins of the New Deal hinge on state versus capital, i.e., on the apex of the political institutions versus the most powerful economic interest groups, with labor left largely out of the picture.[114] Given that many scholars will not concede that labor was politically significant in shaping the New Deal, is it any wonder that there is little interest in examining the specific political behavior and strategies of organized labor in subsequent periods, when workers were far more politically quiescent relative to the 1930s?[115]

To recapitulate, labor's eroding membership base represents a potential political liability. Certainly the size and density of the labor movement are relevant in assessing labor's political fortunes. Indeed, labor's hemorrhaging membership is a cause of deep concern, even alarm. That said, labor's membership base should not be used as the sole or even preeminent yardstick to assess its capacity for political action. Organized labor's vulnerabilities on this front must be understood in the context of the potentially more favorable developments discussed here. Unions in the United States face an increasingly hostile political environment. However, in certain respects, labor's technical and strategic capacities improved even as its weight in the economy decreased. Labor's ineffectiveness in the health policy arena is not simply a consequence of its dwindling membership. Rather, it is related to labor's political strategies, and labor's entanglements in the institutions of the private welfare state influenced these strategies, in turn.

The private welfare state remains largely invisible in discussions of social policy. It is, at most, a shadow. In the 1980s, scholars and policy-makers paid more attention to the role of business in the provision of social welfare in the United States as corporations complained loudly about escalating employee health-care costs hurting their bottom line and joined health-care coalitions to tackle the issue of rising costs. This flurry of activity by the business sector, coupled with the general intellectual and ideological climate of the Reagan years that stressed the virtues of the private sector, helped reinforce the view that the corporate sector would lead the way toward a comprehensive health-care solution that would satisfy the needs of the business sector and the broader society.

As more analysts and policy-makers inserted business into the picture, their focus remained circumscribed. When they brought business in, they treated it as a stand-in or substitute for the state in the area of social welfare provision. As shown in greater detail in the next chapter, private-sector benefits emerged out of a particular institutional context, the result of ongoing struggles between employees, employers, unions, and the state about who should shoulder the costs. To focus only on business's immediate bottom-line concerns ignores the complex institutional and political underpinnings of the private-sector safety net, and, in particular, how organized labor is enmeshed in that net. Likewise, it slights how labor-management strife and cooperation at the firm level and in the wider political arena over the decades shaped the development of employee benefits like paid health insurance and, more broadly, the political prospects for universal health care.

CHAPTER 3

The Institutional Straightjacket of the
Private Welfare State

Taft-Hartley, ERISA, and Experience-Rated Health Insurance

Tying Americans' health-insurance protection to "a particular job in a particular company" aptly is described as "an idea as odd as square wheels or solar-powered flashlights."[1] During the formative years of the health-insurance market in the 1940s and 1950s, few anticipated that the United States five decades later would end up with a health-care system that resembles a surreal mosaic. The current system is splintered into countless large and small group plans and individual insurance policies. Rates vary from one group to the next and from one individual to the next based on occupation, gender, ZIP code, sexual preference, family history, medical history, marital status, and personal habits, to name just a few. This mosaic is framed by a growing number of Americans who belong to a health-insurance underclass that is unable to secure good, affordable health care.

For all the irrationalities and inequities of the current health-insurance system, it has a certain institutional logic. This chapter examines the histor ical development of three institutions in particular that organized labor, together with large employers and insurers, helped create and perpetuate. These institutions, in turn, molded the incentives and political behavior of labor and other groups and posed formidable obstacles to achieving universal health care. The first institution is the system of Taft-Hartley health, welfare, and pension plans. Established under the Labor-Management Relations Act of 1947, better known as the Taft-Hartley Act, these plans are a major source of health, pension, and other benefits for tens of millions of Americans. The second is the Employee Retirement Income Security Act

39

of 1974, which set up federal standards for pensions. The act included a little noted and seemingly minor provision—the so-called ERISA preemption—that allows many employers and unions which provide health benefits through self-insurance (rather than by paying premiums to health-insurance companies) to operate group health-insurance plans free of most state-level insurance regulations. The third and final institutional pillar is the practice of "experience rating," whereby the health experience of a particular group determines health-insurance rates. The alternative approach is "community rating," whereby insurance rates do not vary much from one group to the next, or from one individual to the next, in a given community.

This chapter examines the historical development of these three institutions. In doing so, it demonstrates the deep and enduring mark left by these institutions on the U.S. welfare state. They profoundly shaped the contours of the health-care system and the politics of health policy, often in unintended and unanticipated ways. They helped cement the commitment of large employers and unions to a private welfare state in which employment status determines who qualifies for which social benefits. As a consequence, organized labor's commitment to the public welfare state and to national health insurance is not steadfast. In several instances, unions sided with large employers or sat quietly on the sidelines during important struggles over health policy that foreshadowed the 1993–94 war over Clinton's Health Security Act.

A couple of qualifications to this general line of argument are in order at the outset. First, the focus in this chapter on organized labor's culpability must be within the broader political context. Unions gravitated during the postwar years toward a system of private health insurance in a political environment increasingly hostile to the expansion of the public welfare state through measures like national health insurance. In doing so, organized labor made what turned out to be a pact with the devil. Some labor leaders and union staff members were uneasy about the practice of experience rating, about the use of Taft-Hartley plans to provide health and other welfare benefits through the private sector, and about the ERISA preemption. But it does not appear that anyone—labor leaders, insurers, or employers—fully comprehended the far-reaching effects that these institutions would have on the delivery of health care or the politics of health policy over the long run.

The three institutions bound the interests of organized labor more closely to those of large employers and the commercial health insurers, foreclosing the possibility of national health insurance. That said, it is important to keep in mind the significant contributions made by unions in the postwar years to the expansion of health-insurance coverage in the

United States. Unions pushed employers to include dependent coverage and widen the range of medical services covered by any basic insurance policy. They also nudged doctors to commit to explicit fee schedules and monitored cost and quality through their own health plans.[2] Furthermore, unions were instrumental in creating the Kaiser plan in California, which became a national model for prepaid, comprehensive health care, and Blue Cross / Blue Shield, a nonprofit insurer premised on full reimbursement of medical services and community-rated health-insurance policies.[3]

This chapter begins with a brief discussion of organized labor and the early history of the development of health benefits. It shows how the system of job-based social welfare in the United States sprouted in the interwar years primarily at the behest of employers. After World War II, the initiative shifted toward organized labor as many unions sought to secure health and other benefits through collective bargaining rather than by expanding the public welfare state. As will be shown, divisions persisted within organized labor over whether it was better for unions to concentrate efforts on securing health insurance through private means or whether public-sector solutions were preferable.

The second section examines the institutional origins of the Taft-Hartley funds and how they helped solidify organized labor's commitment to a private welfare state, thus shaping the politics of health policy. Organized labor remained committed to these funds in the 1980s and 1990s even though escalating health-care costs and deep structural changes in the U.S. economy threatened the long-term viability of the Taft-Hartley health-care funds and forced unions that administered such funds to cut back or restrict benefits. The third section analyzes how the ERISA preemption further bolstered labor's commitment to the private welfare state. This landmark pension legislation, which the U.S. Congress passed despite loud objections from business, was hailed as a great victory for workers. Ironically, ERISA turned out to be a major impediment to expanding health-care coverage and helped ally business and labor firmly on the side of the private welfare state. The fourth and final section looks at the postwar development of the health-insurance market. It examines why unions ultimately supported a health-insurance system based on experience rating and how that choice affected the subsequent alliances they forged and positions they took on major health policy issues.

ORGANIZED LABOR AND THE EARLY HISTORY OF SOCIAL WELFARE PROVISION

Whether to seek social welfare benefits through the public or private sector has long divided organized labor. The first unions and local worker associations in the United States urged employers to provide certain social welfare benefits. During the building of national unions, labor officials de-emphasized social welfare benefits. In the early part of this century, the American Federation of Labor (AFL) held fast to the belief that workers' organizations could better meet the social welfare needs of union members than government or employer-sponsored programs. It viewed union-run plans as an important selling point to recruit new members and a way to tie the rank and file more closely to the union.[4] In the 1930s, organized labor threw its support solidly behind government programs like Social Security and national health insurance only after union-run social welfare plans, ethnic mutual benefit associations, and employers' social welfare schemes proved wholly inadequate in the face of the economic devastation wrought by the Depression.[5]

In the years immediately prior to World War II, however, unions were ambivalent about whether to pressure employers to provide non-wage benefits like paid vacations, health insurance, and pensions.[6] Labor unionists waged bitter ideological battles among themselves over whether private welfare programs were "a legitimate trade union activity or a form of collaboration with welfare capitalism."[7] In instances where benefits became part of the employment package in the United States, prior to World War II, it was primarily at the initiative of employers, not employees. This was in contrast to Europe, where non-wage benefits proliferated from the 1920s on as trade unions successfully convinced legislators that employers had certain social obligations beyond just providing a wage.[8] In Europe "paid vacations were being won in legislation as a direct result of union pressure."[9]

During World War II, benefit packages multiplied in the United States. Once again, the initiative came from employers, this time in response to new federal policies. Corporations had a strong incentive to begin remunerating their employees through non-wage means because of tax code changes that rendered benefits exempt from taxes and because of the wartime excess profits tax. The freeze on wages imposed by the National War Labor Board (NWLB) also prompted employers to improve their benefit packages to attract and keep good workers in a tight labor market where the government regulated wages.[10]

After the war, labor's stance on the issue of employee benefits shifted. In the mid-1940s, labor leaders for the first time designated collective bargaining over social welfare benefits a top priority.[11] Walter Reuther of the UAW and other labor leaders mistakenly assumed that if collective bargaining agreements burdened employers with high pension and health-insurance costs, then firms would "join 'shoulder to shoulder' with labor-liberal forces to demand higher federal payments to relieve them of this burden."[12] Strident conservative opposition to any expansion of the public welfare state only partially explains why unions abandoned their earlier commitment to a European-style welfare state and turned toward the private welfare state. Reuther and other labor leaders pushed for collectively bargained benefits for a fundamental reason. They viewed these benefits as a way to shore up member loyalty and protect union security, both of which were seriously jeopardized by the Taft-Hartley Act. This milestone labor legislation (more on this below) made it much harder for unions to retain and expand their membership because, among other things, the act restricted the "closed shop," a provision in union contracts stipulating that union membership be required as a condition of employment. In the aftermath of the Taft-Hartley Act, labor leaders looked more favorably on collectively bargained benefits "obtained on union terms," viewing them as the "virtual equivalent of a closed shop."[13]

Faced with an adverse political climate, many labor officials redirected their energies toward the bargaining table and away from lobbying for universal government programs such as national health insurance.[14] This is not the same as saying that unions became apolitical or less political on the social welfare issue. Employee benefits remained a volatile political issue as unions battled employers in the courts and Congress to establish a solid legal basis for collective bargaining over benefits and mobilized their members to counter fierce employer resistance. Unions pushed hard at the bargaining table for old age, medical, and other benefits. In just a few years, the number of union members covered by a health or pension plan through collective bargaining skyrocketed. By 1954, three-quarters of all union members, 11 million workers, were covered by a health plan or pension, up from just one in eight union members six years earlier.[15] The number of workers covered by health insurance under collectively bargained contracts increased, from well below 1 million in 1946 to 12 million in 1957, plus an additional 20 million dependents.[16]

Organized labor was not of a single mind in the late 1940s and 1950s on whether to put most of its energies into collective bargaining for private-sector benefits or continue pushing for public-sector solutions like national health insurance. A 20th Century Foundation survey concluded that as late as 1948 labor officials representing more than 8 million workers—or more than half of the organized workforce—opposed collectively bargained pension and welfare schemes. They favored a state-supported system of health insurance and old-age security. Surveys revealed that workers had deep misgivings about the complex funding schemes necessary for private plans and worried that, if and when the economy sputtered, employers' promises of health and pension benefits would evaporate.[17] In 1949, William Green, president of the AFL, broke ranks with Congress of Industrial Organizations (CIO) president Philip Murray and Reuther of the UAW to publicly oppose collective bargaining for pensions.[18]

In a surprising twist, the AFL craft unions continued to push hard for national health insurance while the industrial unions associated with the CIO quickly accepted the privatization of social welfare provision.[19] The AFL traditionally favored only a limited state role in economic and social matters, believing that greater government intervention worked against the interests of organized labor over the long run. From the mid-1940s onward, the AFL swam against the tide of its voluntaristic tradition, becoming more involved in public social welfare issues than its rival, the CIO. The CIO's industrial unions, whose members tended to work for oligopolistic firms largely insulated from local competitive pressures, were better positioned than the AFL craft unions to establish viable private-sector welfare plans in the immediate postwar years. By 1950, an estimated 95 percent of workers represented by CIO unions were covered by health and welfare plans under collective bargaining agreements compared to just 20 percent of AFL-affiliated workers.[20]

In short, the AFL unions represented a potential wellspring of support for national health insurance. By the early 1990s, however, the craft unions, notably the building trades, were some of the fiercest opponents within organized labor to a single-payer system of health-care reform modeled loosely on the Canadian system. This turnabout on the part of craft unions was in part the result of an institutional artifact that can only be understood by looking more closely at the intervening history of private-sector welfare provision. It is essential to look at the far-reaching and often unintended consequences that the Taft-Hartley Act had on the development of private-sector benefits in the United States.

THE POLITICAL DEVELOPMENT OF THE
TAFT-HARTLEY FUNDS

Over time, the Taft-Hartley Act helped cement the commitment of the building trades and other unions to private-sector benefits. In particular, it fostered an unusual and unexpected political alliance between some unions and large employers around the question of job-based health and pension benefits. That alliance persists to this day and is a major obstacle to establishing either national health insurance or single-payer medical systems at the state level.

Most discussions of the Taft-Hartley Act focus on the ways in which the measure politically muzzled and demobilized organized labor by, for example, placing limits on the right to strike and permitting states to ban the closed shop. Less noted is how the act stimulated privatization of employee benefits and hastened labor's eventual acceptance of and strong attachment to the provision of social welfare through the private sector. The Taft-Hartley Act established the institutional framework for what are now multibillion dollar health, pension, and welfare trust funds largely controlled by unions, not employers.

Commonly known as Taft-Hartley plans, these funds are an important source of private-sector benefits for tens of millions of Americans and their dependents. These plans provide a mechanism for employers to contribute to benefit packages without assuming the administrative burden and expenses entailed in single-handedly running their own benefit programs. The typical Taft-Hartley plan established under collective bargaining agreements requires employers to contribute some negotiated amount to a pension, health and / or welfare fund for each hour worked by the eligible employee. The plans provide health benefits by directly paying for certain covered medical services or through purchasing health insurance for eligible workers and their dependents. In most instances, the union runs the fund. Participating employers are obligated to do little more than pay the contributions on time and submit minimal information to verify employment status of workers. Many employers are not actively involved in administering the plan or designing the benefits, although employers technically are responsible for jointly administering the fund.[21] Taft-Hartley plans are concentrated in industries where union members work for several employers in a given year, such as the construction sector (58 percent of all plans), which is characterized by seasonal, intermittent employment patterns. They are less widespread in the service (14 percent), manufacturing (11 percent), and transportation (8 percent) sectors.[22]

Today about 10 million American workers and 20 million dependents receive pension, health, and/or other benefits from joint labor-management plans established in accordance with the Taft-Hartley Act.[23] More than half of all union members covered by health plans receive their medical benefits through Taft-Hartley funds.[24] As of 1992, about 4,000 of an estimated 7,000 multiemployer plans across the United States were health and welfare funds with the rest pension funds. These plans collectively held more than $230 billion in assets.[25]

The Taft-Hartley Act, which laid the institutional basis for the funds, was the product of several well-known political developments. For years the National Association of Manufacturers (NAM) and U.S. Chamber of Commerce campaigned to scrap or radically revise the National Labor Relations Act of 1935, better known as the Wagner Act. That campaign gathered momentum as public alarm over the political clout of organized labor escalated in 1946 after unions no longer felt bound by the no-strike pledge of the war years and a wave of strikes gripped the nation. Movements for more restrictive labor legislation emerged in dozens of states, and in 1946 the political balance shifted decisively at the national level as the Republicans gained control of both houses of Congress for the first time since 1930. Divisions within organized labor between the AFL and CIO further bolstered the efforts of those seeking to undo the Wagner Act.[26]

Concerns about the proliferation of collectively bargained benefits in the 1940s also fueled the political stampede to revise the Wagner Act, which left unsettled the question of whether management was legally obligated to engage in collective bargaining on social welfare matters.[27] During the 1946–47 fight over the Taft-Hartley Act, there was a push in Congress to clarify the legislative ambiguity of the Wagner Act on the question of employee benefits. One early analyst of the Taft-Hartley Act claimed that "it was welfare bargaining as much as any other subject which produced the public fear and outrage that brought about the Taft-Hartley Act."[28] The 1946 Mine Workers strike riveted national attention on the benefits issue and revealed its political volatility after John L. Lewis, the United Mine Workers (UMW) president, alarmed employers with a demand for a welfare plan paid for by mine operators and administered by the union.[29] The miners' demand that mine owners contribute 10 cents per ton of coal "to the Mine Workers Union for indiscriminate use for so-called welfare purposes" disquieted Sen. Robert Taft (R-Ohio) and other conservative legislators and business executives.[30]

Union health and welfare funds set up through agreements between labor and management were an increasingly important avenue for social welfare provision for more Americans. But there was great variation in how the funds were financed and administered. Estimates of how many employees the union welfare funds covered in the 1940s vary widely. According to one estimate by the Department of Labor, the agreements covered only about 600,000 employees in 1945. By early 1947, the number had more than doubled,[31] and by mid-1949 the coverage had more than doubled again to over 3 million workers.[32]

In the battle over the Taft-Hartley Act, many legislators sought to exclude social welfare benefits from the items over which management must bargain. They also attempted to outlaw any payment by employers to union pension or welfare funds. In making their case for banning labor welfare and pension funds, they charged that employers should not be permitted "to conspire with unions to mulct employees, without their consent, of huge amounts that ought to go into the workers' wages." Conservatives also expressed alarm that unions controlled "these great, unregulated, untaxed funds" at great risk to the "national interest."[33]

Taft and Rep. Fred A. Hartley (R-N.J.) admitted they had little solid information at the time about how existing funds operated. Nonetheless, they argued that immediate legislative action was warranted to assure these funds did not become "a mere tool to increase the power of the union leaders over their men, and even be open to racketeering practices."[34] Not wanting to risk defeat of his contentious legislation by including an explicit prohibition, Taft retained the Wagner Act's vague language regarding collective bargaining over employee benefits. He also agreed to greatly restrict, but not ban outright, union welfare trust funds in the final version of the bill submitted to the Senate.[35] The funds became known as the Taft-Hartley funds.

Concern was growing about the wider significance the funds and other forms of collectively bargained employee benefits might have for providing social welfare in the United States. Taft viewed the restrictions on union trust funds included in the final version of the Taft-Hartley Act as a necessary stopgap measure. He and other conservative legislators made a prescient observation when they warned that the funds would ultimately need to be "integrated with social security" to assure that "the national assistance should not be broken up into a series of industry agreements."[36] Other contemporary observers raised similar concerns about relying too heavily on job-based schemes for the provision of social welfare because such plans "will necessarily vary and result in inequities."[37] In an ironic twist, conservatives suggested that the funds ultimately must be folded into a government program while many liberals endorsed private-sector initiatives in the area of social welfare. Liberal legislators contended that the government should encourage rather than restrict development of such funds because voluntary plans "decrease the responsibility and burdens of the State."[38] Restrictions or prohibitions on the funds, they warned, would "increase the public burden and responsibility and the dependence of the wage earner upon the State."[39]

Some labor officials also viewed the Taft-Hartley funds as a stopgap measure and remained uneasy about relying too heavily on them for providing social welfare. As late as 1953, George Meany lamented the gross inadequacies of the funds and noted that unions were encountering many difficulties as they attempted to establish Taft-Hartley funds and venture "on a large scale into a relatively new and unexplored field." Because prospects for enacting national health-insurance legislation appeared "remote," Meany conceded that organized labor would have to make the most of collectively bargained health and welfare funds.[40]

After passage of the Taft-Hartley Act, welfare funds and the broader issue of collective bargaining over benefits remained a contentious subject.[41] Lewis Schwellenbach, Truman's Secretary of Labor, tried unsuccessfully to persuade the president to include in his 1948 State of the Union Address a call to liberalize the restrictions on union health and welfare funds imposed by the Taft-Hartley Act.[42] Although Truman did not accede to Schwellenbach's request, he remained uneasy about expanding the private welfare state. In advocating a comprehensive public welfare state, the president expressed concern at one point about the proliferation of "a multiplicity of unrelated private plans, which would inevitably omit large numbers of the working population and treat others unequally."[43]

By 1948, ten unions had negotiated health and welfare plans even though the legal issue of whether management must bargain over these matters was unresolved.[44] That issue was settled in 1948 when the National Labor Relations Board (NLRB), ruling in favor of the United Steelworkers, decided in the *Inland Steel* case that pensions qualified under the "conditions of employment" clause in the Wagner Act and were subject to collective bargaining. In 1949, the U.S. Supreme Court upheld the NLRB decision. Although the *Inland Steel* decision established the legal obligation of employers in unionized firms to negotiate over health and welfare benefits, it did not resolve whether employers had a social obligation to provide such benefits. Labor and management waged bitter battles over how much money employers should contribute to employee benefit plans, the items to include in these plans, and whether dependents should be covered.[45] In the wake of the *Inland* decision, business executives stridently mobilized on behalf of proposed amendments to the Taft-Hartley Act to relieve employers of the legal obligation to collectively bargain over employee benefit programs and ban all union welfare funds.[46] No amendment was enacted.

The myth of the consensus years of labor-management relations in the 1950s obscures how contested an issue benefits remained at the bargaining table. In 1949, health and welfare issues were central in 55 percent of all strikes; in the first half of 1950, 70 percent of all strikes were over these issues.[47] The 1949 steel strike finally established the basis for a health program in the steel industry and set a precedent for providing hospital and surgical benefits for employees and their dependents. But it took another major strike in 1959 for the steelworkers to achieve full employer financing of insurance programs.[48] In the automobile industry, it took a decade of squabbling before auto companies agreed to pay the full cost of health-insurance programs in 1961.[49]

To compete with unionized firms for the best workers and keep unions at bay, some nonunion firms provided benefit plans comparable to those in major unionized firms.[50] Over time, some business executives viewed private-sector benefits in a more favorable light for other reasons as well. Some saw employee benefits as a way to thwart expanding the public-sector welfare state. This was particularly apparent during the debate over health care for the aged in the 1950s. At the time, the NAM and other leading business organizations vehemently opposed creating Medicare, a government-sponsored health-insurance program for senior citizens. The NAM implored its members to make health insurance widely available to retiring employees to thwart the push for Medicare. It warned business executives in the early 1960s: "Unless employers accept more of the responsibility for making reasonably adequate protection available at acceptable costs through voluntary means, compulsory governmental coverage may very likely be adopted."[51]

Despite deep-seated concerns about the long-term effect the Taft-Hartley health and pension funds and other private-sector arrangements would have on social welfare provision, the institutional framework laid down in the Taft-Hartley Act in the 1940s was not the expected stopgap measure. Until the passage almost three decades later of ERISA, the funds were not subject to significant changes. Congress periodically held high-profile hearings that focused on corruption and malfeasance allegedly associated with union pension and welfare funds. Although public hearings on the mishandling of select Taft-Hartley plans were a convenient way to malign the reputation of organized labor and put labor leaders on the defensive, they did not result in legislation that placed greater restrictions on the funds or abolished them.[52]

The Taft-Hartley plans gradually took root, as did labor's attachment to them. When organized labor made its last major push for national health insurance in the 1970s, the fate of the Taft-Hartley funds did not appear to be a major concern. At the time, proposals for national health insurance that would put the Taft-Hartley funds largely out of the health-insurance business did not unduly alarm labor officials. In short, unions mustered the political will to defy the institutional logic. In backing Congressional proposals for national health insurance, labor officials stressed to trustees of Taft-Hartley plans that the funds could provide coverage for supplementary health benefits, such as dental care, that were unlikely to be included in a comprehensive health-care reform bill. They also suggested that employer contributions previously earmarked for health benefits could pay for alternative fringe benefits like day care and scholarships.[53]

The Taft-Hartley system of trust funds served unionized workers well, but only for a period. In the late 1970s and 1980s, many Taft-Hartley plans were under severe financial pressures due to escalating health-care costs and enormous structural changes in the economy. As medical expenses skyrocketed, funds were forced to reduce benefits, tighten eligibility requirements, and increase the out-of-pocket expenses for covered workers. Many Taft-Hartley plans depleted their reserves as health-insurance premiums jumped and a severe recession in the construction industry reduced employer contributions to the health and welfare funds. Union officials, who often serve as key administrators of the funds, were in the unenviable position of telling members that they must make do with less. Taft-Hartley plans came under additional financial pressure in the mid-1980s because of cost-shifting by health-care providers.[54] Many union officials redirected money allocated for pensions and wage increases into health plans to maintain existing medical benefits and keep the plans solvent.[55] Workers covered by Taft-Hartley plans began to "no longer feel so secure about their coverage."[56]

The building and construction sector recession in the late 1980s and early 1990s exacerbated the problem of providing affordable and adequate health-care coverage for construction workers through the Taft-Hartley plans. Leo J. Purcell, president of the Massachusetts Building Trades Council, said escalating costs and decreasing revenues "hammered" the health and welfare funds of construction workers in Massachusetts.[57] With fewer jobs available for unionized construction workers, less income was generated for the health and welfare funds.[58] Many health and welfare plans also depend on generating sufficient income from current workers to subsidize the costs of providing health benefits to retired workers. The proliferation of nonunion firms in sectors of the economy that once were strongholds of organized labor, notably construction, further imperiled the funds.[59] As the proportion of nonunionized construction workers grew, employers' financial obligations to contribute to Taft-Hartley plans dwindled. By the mid-1980s, construction workers as a whole were less likely to receive health benefits on the job than workers in most other sectors of the economy.[60]

Some building trades officials at the state level were disenchanted with providing health care through private-sector means like the Taft-Hartley funds. In 1990 the Massachusetts Building Trades Council unanimously passed a measure calling upon the state's Congressional delegation to consider supporting proposals for comprehensive health-care reform based on the Canadian model of national health insurance. The president of the Massachusetts Building Trades Council indicated that members of the building trades, in an important shift, were open to the idea of national health insurance in light of the precarious financial state of their health and welfare funds.[61] In a similar vein, a 1989 report commissioned by the Laborers' National Health and Safety Fund spoke favorably of the idea of a single-payer system.[62] Many national labor leaders, especially those associated with the building trades, fought tooth and nail to preserve the Taft-Hartley arrangements. Even though many of the funds were under acute financial stress by the late 1980s, they were cool to single-payer health-care reform proposals. Instead, labor leaders preferred private-sector solutions based on an employer-mandate formula that required employers to pay a portion of employee health-insurance costs, allowing the Taft-Hartley funds to remain in the health-care business.

It is too easy to attribute their lack of support to the bedrock conservatism long associated with the craft unions. After all, as discussed earlier, craft unions stuck by national health insurance in the 1950s long after supposedly more progressive industrial unions like the UAW turned their attention to the privatization of benefits through collective bargaining. By the late 1980s, some of the rank and file of the building trades appeared more receptive to a single-payer system at the state or national level and the idea of being more politically active on broader political and economic questions.[63]

A deeper explanation lies in the manner in which the Taft-Hartley funds pulled some unions, large employers, and commercial insurers into similar orbits on health-care issues. In at least three important ways, the Taft-Hartley plans realigned the interests of some labor leaders more closely with those of large employers and insurers. First, the Taft-Hartley plans created a potential conflict of interest for organized labor because they catapulted some union officials into the insurance business. Second, some labor leaders viewed the funds as an indispensable device to maintain important institutional ties and preserve a sense of cohesiveness and identity for union locals whose members are scattered across numerous work sites and locales. Both these issues are discussed in greater detail in this section. The third and most important factor, covered in the next section, is that the funds helped spawn an important coincidence of interests between unions and large employers that run self-insured group health plans and have multi-state operations. The passage of ERISA in 1974 helped cement this unlikely coincidence of interests.

By the early 1990s, the Taft-Hartley plans were a major bone of contention within organized labor. Embittered advocates of Canadian-style reform charged that some labor leaders opposed any single-payer plan because of a conflict of interest rooted in the Taft-Hartley system. They singled out Robert Georgine, the president of the building trades department of the AFL-CIO. In 1991, Georgine donned a second hat as chairman and chief executive officer of Union Labor Life Insurance Co. (ULLICO). Established more than 50 years ago, ULLICO is a private company that provides insurance, investments, and benefits management for the Taft-Hartley plans of hundreds of union locals, many belonging to the building trades. During the 1980s, the company hit hard economic times and attempted to reposition itself by exploring alliances with health maintenance organizations and investing in new ventures. By the 1990s, ULLICO appeared to rebound economically. In 1993, it reported $438 million in revenues on assets of $2.1 billion.[64]

Some union officials grumbled that Georgine's position with ULLICO explained why he refused to throw the weight of the building trades behind any health-care reform proposal to eliminate or greatly reduce the role of insurance companies in providing health care.[65] Georgine staunchly opposed the single-payer option at the highest reaches of the labor federation. In early 1991 he cast a decisive vote against endorsing a

Canadian-style system during a contentious meeting of the federation's health-care committee that deadlocked 8–8, which is discussed in greater detail in chapter 7. Robert McGarrah of the American Federation of State, County and Municipal Employees (AFSCME) called Georgine's dual hats as union leader and insurance executive "deeply disturbing."[66] Charging Georgine with a conflict of interest, UMW President Richard Trumka reportedly tried, but failed, to have Georgine disqualified from voting on the critical issue of whether the AFL-CIO should endorse a single-payer plan when the federation's health-care committee considered the issue in the early 1990s.[67] James S. Ray, the legislative representative to the principal lobbying organization for the Taft-Hartley funds, dismissed the conflict of interest charges. He was adamant that Georgine's opposition to the single-payer plan was based on an assessment that a health-care reform proposal modeled on the Canadian system was unrealistic given the political climate in the United States.[68] As for AFSCME's support in 1990–91 for a single-payer plan and its attacks on Georgine, Ray characterized them as a desperate attempt by the public service union to save the jobs of its membership.[69]

Ray and other union officials conceded that their assessment of the poor political prospects for any single-payer plan did not entirely explain why some labor leaders were reluctant to endorse Canadian-style reform proposals that would eliminate or greatly reduce the role of the Taft-Hartley plans in health care. They contended that many local union officials viewed the Taft-Hartley funds as an important organizational device, and that members have a strong attachment to the particular fund providing benefits. Union officials, as fund trustees, derive goodwill from their members. Members are said to prefer the Taft-Hartley arrangements to public programs because the trustees of the plans are free to tailor the benefits packages to meet the specific needs and wishes of the membership. Many local and national labor leaders contend that the Taft-Hartley funds provide an important sense of identity and cohesion for union members who may have few other real attachments to their union or fellow union members.[70]

This is not a simple case of material interests dictating political behavior. In contrast to the building trades, the International Ladies Garment Workers Union (ILGWU) remained an ardent supporter of national health insurance even though its membership was heavily dependent on Taft-Hartley arrangements for medical coverage.[71] The garment workers' strong and consistent support of national health insurance, despite their extensive Taft-Hartley commitments, is not necessarily at odds with the more general argument here about how these funds helped solidify organized labor's attachment to the private welfare state and dampen its enthusiasm for national health insurance. Unlike the craft unions, the ILGWU has a long history of political activism on social welfare issues that stretches back to the turn of the century. The ILGWU also was a pioneer in developing several key features of the private welfare state. It established some of the first union-sponsored benefit programs, union-run medical centers, and multiemployer welfare funds. However, in experimenting with these private-sector schemes over the years, the charismatic leaders of the ILGWU did not abandon their commitment to broader social objectives. They lauded the union's individual accomplishments in the area of social welfare, yet were careful to remind their members that "more important fundamental legislative and political solutions," such as national health insurance, were necessary to meet workers' security needs. They stressed that private solutions arrived at by unions and employers "necessarily are quite limited in their scope."[72] In this respect, the ILGWU was an exception.

To sum up, the institutionalization of union health, welfare, and pension funds through the Taft-Hartley Act furnished craft and other unions with an important mechanism to provide their members with health and other benefits through the private sector. Despite initial uneasiness on the part of legislators and labor officials, these funds proliferated in the 1950s as the movement for national health insurance sputtered. Over the next two decades, the system took root. By the late 1980s, these funds suffered acute financial stress due to the escalating costs of health care, the rolling recessions in the construction industry, the expansion of the nonunionized sector of the workforce, and increased cost-shifting by health-care providers. The system that had become institutionalized was rather rigid, incapable of adjusting to changing conditions.

Although many Taft-Hartley plans were in a perilous financial state, much of the national leadership of organized labor remained committed to the old system. Prisoners of ideas and institutions they helped to create, they opposed any proposal for comprehensive health-care reform predicated on establishing a single-payer system or a greatly reduced role for the Taft-Hartley funds in delivering health benefits. For the most part, the national officers of other unions with sizable Taft-Hartley contingents fought hard to preserve the funds and keep them beyond the reach of state and federal regulators. In doing so unions had an unlikely ally—big employers. ERISA, which established federal standards to protect employees' pensions, was the glue that helped cement this unlikely coincidence of interests.

ERISA, SELF-INSURANCE, AND THE RECONFIGURATION OF INTERESTS

ERISA was enacted in 1974, the year organized labor made its last big push for national health insurance. Viewed as a big setback for business, this major piece of legislation had unintended consequences for health care.[73] It helped perpetuate many health-care system inequities and thwarted labor's quest for universal health care.

The act included a clause that attracted little public attention at the time but had a profound effect on both the development of private-sector benefits in the United States and the political alliances formed subsequently around health-care issues. Section 514 of ERISA preempts state laws that "relate to any employee benefit plan."[74] The courts have interpreted this clause to mean that self-insured employers and Taft-Hartley funds, which essentially execute the same underwriting functions as the commercial insurers, are preempted from state-level insurance regulations regarding such items as benefits, coverage, and quality standards for medical care. States also are not permitted to tax self-insured plans or subject them to state insurance regulations regarding, for example, licensing or the posting of reserves to ensure the financial integrity of such plans.[75] Not surprisingly, large employers and Taft-Hartley funds increasingly switched to self-insurance, whereby they use their own assets to fund health-insurance plans and typically hire outside companies to administer the plans. ERISA created a regulatory vacuum, leaving self-insured group health plans largely unregulated.[76]

National-level labor representatives worked side-by-side with large employers to slip the preemption language into ERISA. Unions pushed hard for the ERISA preemption out of a concern about possible taxation of Taft-Hartley funds; a fear that state-level mandates regarding health benefits would hamstring labor's efforts to negotiate national contracts; and a desire to avoid what labor saw as state interference in the private affairs of collective bargaining.[77] Over the years, a powerful coalition of large employers and unions, joined intermittently by the insurance companies, worked to ensure that the ERISA preemption was not watered down or eliminated.[78] As such, the ERISA preemption helped realign the interests of labor and business. Organized labor stuck by the preemption even though employers used it to perpetuate highly discriminatory practices, such as eliminating promised health benefits for employees who contract AIDS. As a consequence, organized labor found itself on the opposite side of the barricades from groups fighting the preemption and other discriminatory practices in the courts. ERISA helped reconfigure the constellation of interest groups and their preferences in unanticipated ways and bolstered organized labor's attachment to private-sector solutions for health-care reform.

The preemption clause significantly affected the health policy debate at the state level. During the Reagan years pressure mounted on the states to solve the twin problems of escalating health-care costs and an expanding pool of uninsured people. The ERISA preemption clause posed a major obstacle to state-level reform efforts.[79] It helped short-circuit the state-level political experimentation and initiatives that paved the way for nationalization or quasi-nationalization of social welfare schemes like old-age security and workers' compensation in the United States, and universal health care in Canada. For states that desired to experiment with a single-payer plan of their own, for example, or sought to tax self-insured plans to fund indigent care by creating insurance pools, the self-insured Taft-Hartley and employer plans lay tantalizingly beyond their legislative and regulatory reach.

Large employers were increasingly committed to retaining the ERISA preemption as more switched to self-insurance for various reasons, among them a desire not to be subject to state-level insurance regulations.[80] By the early 1990s, most Taft-Hartley funds also switched to self-insurance.[81] Large employers are better positioned to embrace self-insurance than small businesses because they have sufficient asset bases to cover claims and do not risk going bankrupt should any single employee contract an expensive catastrophic illness.[82]

Large employers and unions with Taft-Hartley concerns worked closely to preserve the preemption clause and were joined intermittently by the insurance companies and, later, health maintenance organizations (HMOs). ERISA's exemption of employers who self-insure from state-level benefit mandates unexpectedly was a blessing, not a bane, for the insurance companies. The courts interpreted the preemption provision liberally, exempting more and more categories of employers' health-insurance plans, many of which, critics charge, "bear no resemblance to self-insured plans."[83] The term "self-insured" is a convenient fiction that allows self-insured employers to avoid state mandates while insurance companies provide these self-insured firms the necessary services to run their health benefits programs. The companies agree to cover employee health claims that exceed a specified dollar amount. The courts have interpreted ERISA in other ways favorable to insurers.[84]

The HMO industry is also an ardent defender of ERISA. For years, courts interpreted the federal pension law in ways that made it extremely difficult for patients to sue HMOs and win liability claims for denial of benefits. Over the past couple years, in an important shift, judges on federal district and appeals courts have been more receptive to lawsuits attacking the quality of care provided by HMOs and issued a series of rulings that for the first time dented the protective shield from lawsuits provided by ERISA.[85]

Organized labor remained committed to an expansive interpretation of the preemption clause even as HMOs, insurers, and large employers, with the help of the courts, wielded ERISA in more and more creative ways that disadvantaged workers.[86] National organized labor did not support efforts by individual states to get federal exemptions from the ERISA preemption to overhaul their health-care delivery systems. In the late 1970s and early

1980s, Hawaii's congressional delegation fought in Washington to win a federal exemption from ERISA for the state as it sought to develop a universal health-care program. The delegation encountered strong opposition from business organizations and the national AFL-CIO, even though the Hawaii State Federation of Labor solidly supported the proposed exemption.[87] After years of squabbling, Congress finally agreed in 1983 to exempt Hawaii's statute, but as it stood in 1974 when it mandated fewer benefits. To date, no other state has received a similar exemption.

Unions remained loyal to the ERISA preemption as employers used it to perpetuate highly discriminatory practices involving medical care. Organized labor did not join a number of public-interest groups that mobilized on behalf of John McGann, whose health benefits for the treatment of AIDS fell from $1 million to $5,000 after his employer switched to a self-insured plan. In this landmark case, the courts upheld an expansive interpretation of the ERISA preemption, deciding against McGann.[88] A number of public-interest groups mobilized in 1991–92 on behalf of McGann, including the Lambda Legal Defense Fund (a legal advocacy organization for gays and lesbians), the American Association of Retired Persons, and the Alzheimer's Association. The AARP and the Alzheimer's Association were concerned about the far-reaching consequences the decision would have not just for people with AIDS, but for people suffering a wide range of expensive illnesses. Organized labor was conspicuously silent, even though the McGann case appeared to present an important opportunity to lay bear the inequities of the health-care and health-insurance system as constructed. Some of labor's silence can be attributed to long-standing uneasiness about associating too closely with any issues perceived as "gay" issues.[89] It was also due to how labor's interests were entangled with the two institutions discussed so far—the Taft-Hartley funds and the ERISA preemption.

Coming out forcibly and visibly in support of McGann would entail making it an issue about more than just gay rights. It would mean challenging and exposing the basic inequities of the health-insurance market. In doing so, organized labor would have to touch the third rail of health politics—the ERISA preemption that allows employers and Taft-Hartley funds that self-insure to engage in the very practices that stripped McGann of his health-insurance coverage because he was seriously ill. Instead, organized labor chose to lie low. Union officials continued to fight hard on other fronts to protect the ERISA preemption. For example, organized labor found itself on a collision course with advocates for the handicapped and AIDS activists in 1993 when the Equal Employment Opportunity Commission (EEOC), under the Clinton administration, enlisted the Americans With Disabilities Act of 1990 to challenge employers and unions that attempt to use the ERISA preemption to deny health-insurance coverage to people with AIDS and other costly illnesses.[90]

The Taft-Hartley Act with its provisions for health, pension, and welfare funds administered jointly by labor and management had several unintended consequences. It put unions in the insurance business and gave them a vested interest in maintaining the status quo—a system of social welfare provision rooted in the private sector and specifically based on job-related benefits. ERISA, which came along almost three decades later, was the glue that held together a formidable coalition of organized labor and large employers, joined on occasion by the insurance companies. That coalition opposed any measure that would permit states greater leeway to overhaul their health-care delivery systems or would scrap the ERISA preemption.

DEVELOPMENT OF THE EXPERIENCE-RATED HEALTH-INSURANCE MARKET

Taft-Hartley funds and the ERISA preemption did not create the job-based system of health benefits. Rather, they helped lock it in place and solidified the commitment of organized labor to the private welfare state. The funds and preemption served as protective walls around the private welfare state that eventually posed significant barriers to national health insurance and helped reinforce the inequities of the health-care system.[91] These two institutions overlay a third institution, the experience-rated health-insurance market, which further facilitated the turn toward a private welfare state after World War II.

Large corporations, unions, and the Taft-Hartley funds used their formidable purchasing power to shape the health-insurance market to their advantage during its formative years in the 1940s and 1950s.[92] They established institutional precedents that legitimized what became a market ridden with highly discriminatory pricing and coverage practices, and that solidified the connection between employment status and health insurance. They helped create and sustain the institution of "experience rating."

The term "experience rating" was coined around 1913, but the practice itself dates back to the development of workers' compensation insurance in the 1890s.[93] There was a widespread sense that because different industries had different rates of accidents and injuries on the job, they should be subject to varied workers' compensation rates. During the 1930s, an alternate view of insurance took root as unions pushed for establishing Blue Cross/Blue Shield health plans based on community-rated premiums in which insurance rates do not vary much from one group to the next, or from one individual to the next, in a given community.

The popularity of segmenting the medical market based on the health experience of a particular group grew when commercial insurance companies entered the health-insurance field in the 1950s. After World War II the health-insurance market expanded at a dizzying pace.[94] The commercial insurers quickly adopted experience rating to gain a competitive edge over their main rivals, existing Blue Cross/Blue Shield plans that were premised on community rating. For specific groups deemed to represent a lower risk than that of the average for the insured community as a whole, the experience-rated health plans of commercial insurers provided an attractive and lower-cost alternative to community-rated ones.[95]

In the early years of the developing health-insurance market, unions maintained a strong commitment to national health insurance, which by its very nature ran counter to experience rating. Staff members in the national offices of the AFL-CIO and in the headquarters of major unions strongly favored community-rated health insurance, as did national labor leaders, most notably Reuther of the UAW.[96] As large unions and employers became more sophisticated consumers of health insurance, and as national health insurance receded on the political agenda, unions turned to the private sector and increasingly relied on experience rating as a tool to achieve lower insurance rates for members. The building trades locals, in particular, strongly backed the practice of experience rating.[97] Labor staff members and officials negotiated complex health-care plans through collective bargaining, immersing themselves in the intricacies of the health-insurance market. Their mastery of the ins and outs of the health-insurance market came at great cost, diverting resources, political energy, and time away from the fight for national health insurance.[98] One study of the early development of the health-insurance market concluded that proliferating collective bargaining contracts "played a major role in making experience rating almost universal," which dealt a "mortal blow" to the development of universal health care based on community rating.[99] Unions were so protective of the lower insurance premiums in an experience-rated system that they were reluctant to extend health-care coverage to female employees. They were concerned about how the disproportionate rate of medical claims by women relative to men would spark an increase in the group's insurance premiums.[100]

Large employers, unions, and Taft-Hartley plans were generally deemed lower risks and therefore were favored with lower health-insurance premiums. Under an experience-rated system, a certain statistical logic naturally favored large employers and big Taft-Hartley funds. After all, unlike small businesses, they have large population bases over which to spread the risk of a single costly disease. A certain political logic was at work as well. Under the guise of experience rating, large employers and big Taft-Hartley funds secured a better deal for their employees and members than other groups and individuals because they had the market and political power. Experience rating appears wrapped in the cool objectivity of science; professionally trained underwriters assign higher rates to those groups or individuals considered more likely to require costly medical care. Over the years, experience rating was actually a highly subjective affair.[101]

Unions, together with large employers, helped create the vast medical underwriting establishment in the United States. They also sanctioned the ways insurance companies have spliced the insurance market since World War II into a myriad of risk pools to which an army of underwriters assigns vastly different health-insurance premiums. The commitment of large corporations and unions over the years to experience rating helped enshrine the principle of "actuarial fairness," premised on the idea that each person ultimately is responsible for paying for his or her particular medical risk. To that end, medical underwriters group policyholders and price the policies according to some market logic. Those judged to be higher risks by the underwriters are obligated to pay more to protect themselves. Enshrining the concept of "actuarial fairness" through medical underwriting had a profound effect on the way many Americans think about health care. It helped erode a belief that social welfare provision should be organized around "mutual aid," i.e., that all members of society are obligated to share risks.[102]

Experience rating was a slippery slope for unions. On one hand, it allowed them to secure better coverage at lower costs for many members. On the other hand, through tacit or explicit support of this practice unions were accomplices in creating the current insurance market mosaic. By supporting the principle of "actuarial fairness," unions and large employers also helped open the door to unsavory medical underwriting practices, such as genetic screening, and discriminatory personnel policies, such as pre-employment medical screening and penalties for employees who smoke, drink, eat too much, exercise too little, and have defective genes. They also helped fuel the vast medical underwriting establishment that added so much to the administrative costs of the U.S. health system. By the early 1990s, insurance companies spent more than 37 cents on administrative costs for every dollar's worth of benefits they provided to policyholders.[103]

Unions—at least at the national level—are reluctant to launch an all-out frontal assault on experience rating and the discriminatory medical underwriting practices associated with it. For example, the spread of AIDS in the 1980s had the potential to rivet national attention on the striking inequities of experience-rated, job-based health benefits. Unions and disease-based advocacy groups like the American Heart Association and American Cancer Society were not actively involved in efforts to prohibit

Figure 3.1. Administration expenses of health insurance policies by size of firm. Source: *Reforming the System,* ed. Robert J. Blendon and Tracey Stelzer Hyams (New York: Faulkner & Gray, 1992), 11. © Faulkner & Gray, Inc. Redrawn with permission.

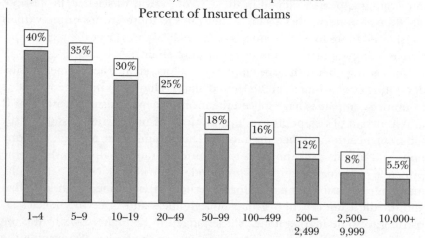

Percent of Insured Claims

40% 35% 30% 25% 18% 16% 12% 8% 5.5%

1–4   5–9   10–19   20–49   50–99   100–499   500–2,499   2,500–9,999   10,000+

Number of Employees Covered

health and life insurance companies from using blood tests and other means to screen applicants for AIDS. Gay rights and AIDS activists battled alone.[104]

In the debates about health-care reform in the early 1990s, unions and Fortune 500 companies stressed how they shouldered a disproportionate share of medical costs, because of cost-shifting, and portrayed small businesses as socially irresponsible for their failure to provide health insurance for employees.[105] However, all this attention on cost-shifting obscured how the experience-rated health-insurance market disproportionately favors large employers and unions to the disadvantage of people without access to health insurance through large group plans. Health-insurance premiums for small businesses average about 30 percent higher than those of big business.[106] Small unincorporated businesses, unlike incorporated firms, cannot deduct the full cost of employee health benefits from their taxes.[107] Furthermore, the administrative costs of group health plans for small businesses are considerably higher. In an experience-rated health-insurance market, commercial insurers invest more time and effort in ferreting out the potential risks in small groups and devising higher rate schedules to insure them. For firms with fewer than 50 employees, administrative costs eat up 25 to 40 cents of every premium dollar (see Figure 3.1). For firms with 500 or more employees, only 5 to 12 cents of every dollar goes to administrative costs, leaving the lion's share for the delivery of medical services.[108]

Experience rating contributes substantially to the expensive red tape ensnaring the U.S. medical system.

During the debate over health-care reform in the early 1990s, unions, Fortune 500 companies, and some analysts attributed the fierce opposition of small businesses against legislative proposals based on an employer mandate to a fundamental conservatism of small business owners. In doing so, they presented the small business sector as one of the primary obstacles to universal health care.[109] The battle lines of social policy appear less distinct with a closer look at the historical development of medical underwriting and the complicity of large unions and employers in establishing a health-insurance system that discriminates against many of the least advantaged members of society. Small employers' failure to provide health insurance is not merely the product of some eternal and largely unchanging Dickensian mentality and primordial conservatism. It is partially the result of a highly discriminatory insurance market that unions and large employers helped create and perpetuate.

Small employers are less likely to offer health insurance to their employees than are large employers.[110] This may indicate a basic and unchanging antipathy by the small business sector to social investment by either the private or public sector. Surveys by the National Federation of Independent Business lend credence to this view. The NFIB found that nearly two out of three small firms polled said they did not believe that employers had a responsibility to provide health insurance for employees.[111] The major trade associations that represent small business, most notably the NFIB, are extremely conservative. In the 1980s and early 1990s, they developed a close working relationship with Rep. Newt Gingrich (R-Ga.) and other leaders of the new Republican vanguard that was based, among other things, on defeating any attempt by the Democrats to enact comprehensive health-care reform legislation.[112] The high-profile battle the NFIB waged against the Clinton proposal helped skew the general understanding of the small business sector's political preferences with respect to health-care reform.[113] That many small firms fail to provide health insurance may reflect something more than bedrock conservative ideology. It may reflect the higher costs small businesses must pay to offer comparable health insurance to their employees.[114]

Many labor leaders and some executives of Fortune 500 firms charged that small businesses were immune to escalating health-care costs because many do not provide health insurance anyway. This is a misleading characterization. Nearly two-thirds of NFIB members—one of the Clinton health plan's fiercest opponents—reported that they provide health insurance for their employees.[115] As far back as 1986, small business owners were citing health insurance as their number one problem.[116] By the early 1990s, nearly two out of three small business owners perceived their health-care costs as out of control.[117] Small business owners were also more likely to report being highly dissatisfied with the U.S. health-care system.[118] Because small business owners are more likely to know their employees personally, they are less able to insulate themselves from the problems associated with having inadequate health-insurance coverage during illnesses.

In one of the most surprising discoveries, small employers, for all their reputed conservatism, looked more favorably on a single-payer system than business executives from large firms. NFIB surveys indicated growing support among its small business constituency in the late 1980s and early 1990s for a single-payer system. Over the years an overwhelming majority of NFIB members, about 90 percent, consistently opposed any government mandate requiring employers to provide health insurance. By the early 1990s, about one in four supported a single-payer system.[119] By comparison, a Roper poll of Fortune 1000 executives found that only 4 percent favored the idea of government-mandated health insurance.[120] At one point during the struggle over the Clinton plan, a top official of the NFIB blurted out during a Congressional appearance:

> I think the cheapest way to deal with the problem of 37 million uninsured people in this country would be for the government to just buy them all a health-insurance policy. . . . The problem is we do not want to tell the people they have to pay for it.[121]

One survey of small business sentiment on health care concluded that "opinions of small business on national health care reform have changed profoundly over the last few years. Small business should not be viewed as a roadblock to reform, but rather as a group that needs to be educated."[122]

Surveys of small business executives also call into question Cathie Jo Martin's contention that firms with greater internal policy capacity in the area of health policy (which tend to be larger corporations) usually have more moderate views on health-care reform and a greater willingness to countenance more government intervention.[123] Greater internal policy capacity does not necessarily make firms more receptive to government intervention in social policy. Precisely because of their enhanced policy capacity, large firms are able to shape the insurance market to their advantage and perpetuate highly discriminatory health-insurance practices. Small firms may be more willing to embrace a comprehensive government solution precisely because they lack the internal capacity to administer affordable health-insurance programs on their own and to shape the insurance market.[124]

Unlike large firms, small firms lack the policy capacity and population base to experiment with firm-based innovations to reduce costs, such as wellness programs, company doctors, elaborate pre-employment health screening, and, of course, self-insurance.[125] Large firms, by contrast, use their in-house policy expertise to engage in crude medical underwriting and redlining insurance practices. They are more likely to use pre-employment medical exams to screen job applicants (83 percent) than are small firms (19 percent).[126] Large employers increasingly require employees and potential recruits to undergo blood, drug, and urine tests, and physical exams. In many cases, workers also must provide information about the incidence of heart disease, cancer, genetic disorders, and health problems in their medical histories.[127] Many efforts at in-house medical underwriting by large employers are highly intrusive.[128] ConAgra Poultry Co. in Colorado required its employees to reveal what prescription and over-the-counter medications they were taking and sign releases that gave the company complete access to their medical records. An employee who refused to do so was fired and subsequently sued the company.[129] Surveys show that employees who regard their health as fair or poor or have a job-related disability are less likely to receive job-based health benefits.[130]

In an effort to control health-care costs internally, large firms established on-site medical facilities and wellness programs reminiscent of the dreaded "company doc" from years ago.[131] These work-site health promotion strategies raise troubling questions about the involvement of corporations in the private lives of employees and about an employee's right to privacy as more Americans receive their medical care, including mental health counseling, at the same place where they work.[132]

Many people castigate the insurance companies for the way the health-insurance market is structured. They see the proliferation of clauses against covering pre-existing medical conditions, the redlining of certain professions, and the great discrepancies in health-insurance premiums for individual and group policies and large and small businesses as the handiwork of profit-savvy insurance companies.[133] Less appreciated is that for many years unions and large employers enjoyed a huge financial advantage in an insurance market that they helped create and that established important institutional precedents for today's underwriting practices.

By sanctioning experience rating, unions and large employers helped usher in a vast array of discriminatory medical practices and construct the underwriting infrastructure that is such a drain on health-care dollars in the U.S. medical system. As large employers became more sophisticated consumers of health care, they used their in-house health policy expertise to engage in medical underwriting practices of their own. They also experimented with a number of personnel innovations that raise fundamental questions about an employee's right to privacy. Because many small employers were priced out of the medical market and do not have the internal resources and policy capacity to innovate and control health-care costs, they were more willing to consider a single-payer solution than were large employers. The health-care cost and coverage crisis affects them more acutely.

Organized labor may not have been aware of all the negative consequences of the health-insurance system it helped create. The consequences only became apparent in recent years as the pool of the health-insurance underclass expanded and escalating health-care costs diverted more and more dollars from wages to benefits. The question raised is why, given all the shortcomings of the system it wittingly or unwittingly helped to construct, has organized labor not extricated itself from the experience-rated, job-based system of health insurance. This closer look at the historical development of three institutions—the Taft-Hartley funds, the ERISA preemption, and the experience-rated health-insurance market—and the interest-group configurations that grew around them over the years offers a partial explanation. The institutions as they developed kept organized labor's gaze fixed on the private welfare state despite a rapidly changing economic and political environment. The private welfare state also provided union members with significant benefits in an uncertain political and economic environment. Such periods of uncertainty may make groups more politically cautious and less willing to seek untested alternatives.

The institutions discussed here did not chain labor to the private welfare state overnight. They gradually pulled it in that direction. A vested interest in preserving these institutions molded labor's political preferences and behavior, predisposing it to private-sector alternatives. As shown in subsequent chapters, the impact of these institutions was uneven.

Institutional factors alone do not explain labor's political strategies and political setbacks in its quest for universal care. We also need to understand how certain ideas that took hold in the late 1970s changed the debate over health care in subtle but important ways. Just as institutions can cause groups to rethink their interests and form new alliances, as shown in this chapter, so can ideas. Chapter 4 focuses on the political trajectory of one policy idea in particular—the employer mandate—that both complemented labor's institutional attachments discussed in this chapter and helped perpetuate its commitment to private-sector solutions for health-care problems.

CHAPTER 4

Labor Embraces a New Idea

The Journey from National Health Insurance to an Employer Mandate

In his State of the Union address in January 1994, President Clinton said his proposed Health Security Act was built upon "what works today in the private sector to expand employer-based coverage." His proposal centered on a requirement that employers pay a portion of the health-insurance premiums for their workers. Clinton underscored that an employer mandate was not a new or radical idea. He hastened to add that mandated employer-based health insurance was proposed two decades earlier by President Nixon, whom he singled out by name in his address. "It was a great idea then, and it's a better idea today," implored Clinton.[1]

This was a remarkable moment in the health-care debate. Two decades earlier organized labor and leading Democrats battled the Nixon plan and resolutely stood by an alternative proposal for national health insurance that eliminated commercial insurers and was to be financed by a payroll tax and a general revenue tax. Labor officials denounced Nixon's proposal, saying that it would not do enough to reduce costs and expand access to quality health care, and that it would ratify a multitiered system of health-care delivery. They also noted that the existing system of employment-based health insurance was ridden with inequities and that tying benefits to jobs gave employers a disincentive to hire full-time workers. The 1973–74 recession, the most severe economic downturn since World War II, heightened their concerns about job-based benefits. By early 1994, many leaders of organized labor were rallying around a health-care reform plan explicitly modeled on the previously despised Nixon plan. Although the Clinton plan added some innovations of its own—notably the complex health-care alliances—at its heart was a requirement that employers pay a portion of their employees' health insurance premiums. Paradoxically, as the attachment between employer and employee became more tenuous, and firms rolled back the private welfare state by slashing health and other benefits, much of organized labor was intent on a job-based system of health insurance. They also were less willing to battle for national health insurance modeled on a single-payer formula.

The analytical issue is why the leadership of organized labor could not or would not extricate itself from the job-based health-insurance system and endorse a national health insurance plan that severed forever the link between employment status and health benefits. The answer is complex and multifaceted. The last chapter showed how several institutions of the private welfare state predisposed labor leaders and other political actors to private-sector solutions for health-care reform and to seek out an alliance with business on the health-care issue. The institutional contours of the private welfare state did not single-handedly determine the particular policy path organized labor set out on and whether it would succeed or fail in its quest for universal health care. Institutions work in tandem with other factors, notably ideas. Ideas, like institutions, can prompt groups to reconsider their interests and forge new alliances.[2]

This and subsequent chapters address why organized labor held fast to an employer mandate despite a drastically changing economic and political environment and what the wider political consequences of that choice were. It is argued that labor's attachment to this particular idea helped refashion its worldview. In the debate over health policy, labor adopted a worldview closer to that of business and at odds with the case organized labor tried to make in other policy realms. To understand the political trajectory of the employer-mandate idea, we need to do more than take a snapshot look at the circumstances that surround its initial adoption and acceptance. Instead, we need to adopt a longer time horizon to consider the nuances of the political and economic context prior to and after its adoption.

A number of health policy analysts portray an employer mandate as a natural, logical response to the political and economic environment. As such, its selection needs little or no explanation. Theda Skocpol contends that the twin legacies of Reaganism—a huge federal deficit and deepening distrust of the government—gave policy-makers little choice but to ensure that new social programs be kept off budget.[3] The employer mandate took on a life of its own long before the Clinton administration embraced the idea, even prior to the spread of anti-government ideas that were the leitmotif of the Reagan era. This policy idea played a critical role in defining the strategies and coalitions around which the health-care debate was waged and may have reduced the likelihood of putting together an alternate winning coalition to promote universal health care in the United States. Organized labor was an important "carrier" of this idea; that is, unions helped create the "fit" between the employer-mandate idea and the political and economic environment in which it emerged.[4]

When the employer mandate was initially adopted, the idea was a "focal point" that served to temporarily reconcile the interests of state, labor, and business leaders so that they could forge a loose coalition on behalf of comprehensive health-care reform.[5] This policy idea became embedded in a compelling causal story that appeared to explain the major shortcomings of the U.S. political economy. This causal story had important consequences for the course of the debate over health policy, in particular labor's political efficacy on health-care reform, and other matters.

This chapter analyzes the early history of the employer mandate, focusing first on its origins in the Nixon years, and then on why labor embraced the policy prescription it once spurned. It begins with the initial introduction of the employer-mandate idea into the national debate over health-care reform, which occurred during the first term of the Nixon administration, and the chilly reception it originally received from the Democrats and organized labor. The next section examines how the failure to pass comprehensive health insurance reform in the 1973–74 period and the lingering recession of the mid-1970s heightened concerns about the plight of the unemployed. As a consequence, the terms of the health-care debate shifted in subtle but important ways that had lasting implications. Economic concerns, as never before, were paramount in discussions of health care. The third and final section examines organized labor's abandonment of national health insurance rooted in the public welfare state during the Carter years, and its endorsement for the first time of the employer-mandate solution. It is suggested that organized labor initially endorsed the employer mandate as the politically expedient solution in the 1977–78 period as key Democrats, notably President Carter and Sen. Edward M. Kennedy (D-Mass.), cooled to the idea of national health insurance and searched for alternatives.

At the time, labor hoped a rightward compromise on its part would make unions part of a broader winning coalition that would not foreclose the possibility of achieving universal health care in the long run. It is important to trace the origins of the employer-mandate idea and of labor's initial endorsement to understand why labor was an important carrier of an idea it previously loathed. By briefly examining what Sheri Berman calls the "back-story," we can better understand how the political space opened to allow this idea to come to the fore.[6]

EMPLOYER MANDATE AND THE GHOST OF RICHARD NIXON

The ghost of the Nixon plan hovered over the health-care reform debate of the early 1990s.[7] Many labor officials privately chastised organized labor for its failure to compromise in the early 1970s on national health insurance and accept a version of the Nixon plan. As a consequence, comprehensive health-care reform slipped through labor's fingers and remained off the national agenda for another 20 years, they contended. The Nixon plan was explicitly on the minds of other would-be reformers as well. Hillary Rodham Clinton courted Sen. Robert Packwood (R-Ore.), fully cognizant of the symbolic importance of getting on her side the legislator who introduced the Nixon plan two decades earlier and extolled its employer mandate.[8]

When the Nixon administration first introduced the idea of an employer mandate in 1971, organized labor and other advocates of universal health care were fierce opponents. By 1978, labor leaders in an abrupt about-face endorsed an employer-mandate solution, essentially abandoning a long-standing commitment to national health insurance. The decisive political variable for organized labor was a shift in the preferences of leading Democrats, notably Senator Kennedy and President Carter. Organized labor viewed adopting the employer-mandate idea as a compromise that could broaden political support over the short run, but that left open the possibility of achieving the ultimate goal of universal coverage.[9] The employer-mandate idea was seen as a "focal point" that could unite important segments of business, labor, and the state on the health-care issue.

In his 1971 State of the Union message, President Nixon identified "improving America's health care and making it available more fairly to more people" as one of his "six great goals."[10] As initially proposed in 1971, the Nixon plan would require employers to pay 65 percent of the cost of insurance premiums for employees working 25 hours or more per week. By 1976, they would be obligated to foot 75 percent of the expense for a basic package of health benefits. A new federal health insurance program would cover poor families.[11] The original proposal also called for federal aid to foster development of prepaid comprehensive care, known today as health maintenance organizations (HMOs).

When he first introduced his proposal, Nixon explicitly defended the employer-mandate feature. He likened the employer requirement to provide health insurance to requiring them to pay the minimum wage or satisfy occupational health and safety standards.[12] Advocates of national health insurance immediately denounced the Nixon plan. Senator Kennedy characterized the employer insurance feature as "wasteful and ineffective" and the proposed family health insurance plan as "poorhouse

medicine" that would perpetuate a multilevel system of health care.[13] He
also charged that the administration's plan would provide the insurance industry with "a windfall of billions of dollars annually." Kennedy was pushing
an alternative bill co-sponsored with Rep. Martha Griffiths (D-Mich.) that
would finance a national health insurance system out of a payroll tax and
general revenues. Their proposed Health Security Act would eliminate the
commercial insurers in health care and provide all Americans with a broad
package of medical benefits without requiring significant cost-sharing by
patients.[14]

The U.S. Congress held extensive hearings on the Nixon plan in 1971.
Organized labor, a strong backer of the Kennedy-Griffiths approach, raised
numerous objections to the White House proposal and, in particular, to the
employer-mandate feature. While UAW president Leonard Woodcock
specifically applauded the provision to nurture the development of HMOs,
overall he had little good to say about the administration's plan. Woodcock
denounced the proposal as too expensive for the average American worker
and reckoned that the plan could cost the typical American family nearly
$1,600 per year, or about 23 percent of its income. He also vociferously ob-
jected to preserving the commercial insurance industry with its high administrative costs.[15] Other labor officials raised similar concerns about the
insurers and what they saw as "half steps" that "would be only another example of government generating an expectation of performance without
delivering it."[16]

Major organizations representing big business were more favorably inclined toward the Nixon approach. Representatives of the NAM and the U.S.
Chamber of Commerce offered their qualified support for the Nixon plan,
but argued for a reduction in the percentage of employee health insurance
costs employers would have to assume.[17] Organizations catering to the small
business community were more reticent about the Nixon plan. The National
Federation of Independent Business went on record opposing the president's
proposal, saying that many small businesses could ill afford the requirement
that they pay for a portion of their workers' health insurance premiums. Under questioning by Representative Griffiths, the legislative director of the
239,000-member NFIB conceded that the administration's plan would be
much worse for small businesses than the Kennedy-Griffiths proposal for national health insurance. In an effort to court the small business sector, Griffiths underscored how her plan, unlike the administration's proposal, was developed with the needs of the small business sector explicitly in mind.[18]

It is hard to identify bedrock conservatism as the driving force behind the
small business sector's opposition to the Nixon plan and its employer mandate. Small business owners appeared more receptive then and later to national health insurance than business organizations like the NAM and the

U.S. Chamber of Commerce that cater more to the concerns of big business.[19] The greater willingness of small business to countenance a larger role for the federal government in social policy was evident in the striking contrast between the stances of big business and small on health policy and in their wide differences over the welfare reform proposal Nixon unveiled in 1970. The centerpiece of that proposal was the family assistance plan that would guarantee a minimum annual income to every American family in which the head of the household was employed. The Chamber led the charge against the plan, and for the first time in its history enlisted the help of paid advertising to defeat a legislative proposal.[20] The Chamber unleashed an "all-out attack" on the family assistance plan, denouncing it as "revolutionary," "radical," and an "outright handout." By contrast, the small business sector appeared to favor Nixon's family assistance plan. Several NFIB polls taken shortly after Nixon presented his welfare proposal revealed solid support among the NFIB membership for the family assistance plan, with about 60 percent in favor, 30 percent opposed, and 10 percent undecided.[21]

With organized labor and leading Democrats solidly committed to national health insurance, the administration implacably opposed, and the business community divided, Congress and the White House remained at an impasse on health policy in 1971 and 1972.[22] In 1973, Congress and the administration again failed to break the legislative stalemate over comprehensive health-care reform. However, that year legislators approved one feature of the Nixon plan as they earmarked $375 million in federal aid to develop HMOs.[23]

The following year, legislators and the White House were more optimistic about resolving the impasse over health policy. On February 6, 1974, Nixon unveiled a revised version of his health plan and the House Ways and Means Committee and the Senate Finance Committee convened their first major hearings on health insurance since 1971. The central pillar of Nixon's new Comprehensive Health Insurance Act was the familiar requirement that employers cover part of the cost of providing their workers with a standard package of health benefits. But in an important shift, employee participation was made voluntary.[24] While Kennedy remained rhetorically committed to national health insurance, in April 1974 he and Rep. Wilbur Mills (D-Ark.), the powerful chairman of the House Ways and Means Committee, introduced the Mills-Kennedy bill, a compromise measure that fell far short of national health insurance.

The Nixon plan and the Mills-Kennedy alternative have a certain aura about them today. Labor officials, Hillary Rodham Clinton, and other latter-day health-care reformers have mused that either measure would have gone a long way toward resolving many of the country's pressing health-care problems in the 1970s, or two decades later in the 1990s. On closer examination, what is striking about these measures is how far they both fell short of universal coverage. They excluded many of the same groups that today constitute the growing ranks of the uninsured. And both required the average U.S. citizen to shoulder much of the expense of his or her basic medical care.

At the start of Ways and Means Committee hearings in 1974 on the revised Nixon proposal, Caspar W. Weinberger, Nixon's new Secretary of Health, Education, and Welfare, defended the employer-mandate formula. Weinberger conceded in his testimony that the White House bill would result in increased costs for employers, but that the added expense did not generally trouble the administration. "We believe that, in the final analysis, when this bill takes effect two years down the road, the increase of employer costs would be only slightly above that which would have been forced by the collective bargaining process," Weinberger testified. He also acknowledged that the Mills-Kennedy bill and the administration's plan had much in common, but that the White House proposal was superior for several reasons, notably that it was not financed by "something as regressive" as a payroll tax.[25]

At several points during her questioning of Weinberger and the administration's plan, Griffiths suggested that employers would have an incentive to discriminate against employees with potentially expensive health problems, and against the old in favor of the young. Other critics noted that the administration's bill would not cover new workers employed for less than 90 days and part-timers who worked less than 25 hours per week. Furthermore, newly unemployed workers would be required after three months to pay for their own health insurance or apply for assisted health insurance through an onerous means-tested program.[26]

The business sector's support for an employer-mandate solution appeared to have cooled by the time the new Nixon plan was introduced. NAM representatives went on record to oppose an employer mandate, saying it amounted to a "hidden tax."[27] A spokesman for the NFIB, the lobbying arm of small business, reaffirmed the organization's opposition to mandates and said that any new health insurance program should be voluntary. If it did become a mandatory program, the NFIB official argued, businesses with less than five employees should be exempted.[28] Representatives of the State Chambers of Commerce urged legislators to pursue a voluntary approach to reform and recommended using tax incentives to encourage employers to provide their workers with minimal health benefits.[29]

Organized labor remained implacably opposed to the new Nixon plan.

In February 1974, the AFL-CIO executive council issued a detailed statement strongly critical of Nixon's latest proposal, charging that it "would leave many Americans unprotected against the high cost of medical care" and would subject the poor and near-poor to "costly and demeaning means tests." The federation denounced the employer mandate, saying that compelling employers to purchase private health insurance policies for their employees "would cost employers at least as much as if they were taxed." The group also objected to the Nixon plan because it would continue the "worse [sic] features of private insurance," notably experience rating.[30] In Congressional testimony, Nelson Cruikshank of the AFL-CIO warned that Nixon's proposal would contribute to the distasteful practice of "skimming," whereby commercial insurers sold health insurance policies to profitable employed groups, leaving the poor, the unemployed, and other high-risk groups to be covered at government expense or not at all.[31]

The labor federation also attacked the Nixon plan because it would hoist a huge portion of medical expenses onto the shoulders of the average American through a high deductible ($450 per family) and a requirement that employees pay 25 percent of covered medical bills up to a maximum of $1,500 per year per family. That was equal to about 13 percent of the median annual household income in 1974.[32] By the administration's own reckoning, three out of four people in any given year would not accrue medical bills that exceeded the hefty deductible and, therefore, would not receive any benefits from the program for that year.[33]

Labor officials explicitly took issue with the employer mandate in their Congressional testimony. Andrew J. Biemiller of the AFL-CIO's department of legislation tweaked anti-labor legislators when he appeared on Capitol Hill. He said that the employer-mandate feature of the administration's bill would further divide unionized and nonunionized workers. Biemiller confidently predicted that, should the administration's bill be enacted, unionized workers would continue to get employers to pay 100 percent of their health-insurance premiums. This would widen the division between the haves of the unionized workforce and the have-nots of the nonunionized sector, thus making it easier for labor unions to organize the unorganized, he warned.[34] Melvin Glasser of the UAW stated in no uncertain terms that the job-based system of benefits in the United States was already ridden with undesirable inequities that any employer mandate would perpetuate. He emphasized that these inequities were compounded during hard economic times, like the 1973–74 recession when the job-based health benefits of millions of workers were threatened as the unemployment rate inched upward.[35] Labor leaders stressed that the Nixon plan provided an incentive for employers either to replace full-time workers with part-timers, for whom they were not obligated to provide health

benefits, or rely more on compulsory overtime rather than hire new workers and provide health insurance.[36]

The bottom line for organized labor was that the new Nixon plan was not
a proposal for universal health care. Labor leaders saw it as an expensive
proposition that would provide many Americans—but certainly not all
Americans—with costly coverage for catastrophic illnesses while the expense of more routine health care would fall squarely on their own shoulders. The bill also did little to remedy concerns about escalating medical
costs and limited access to quality care. At one point, UAW President
Leonard Woodcock warned: "If this health plan is what Mr. Nixon means by
'new federalism,' it should be called the new feudalism, since it would
make all of us serfs of the insurance industry."[37] Labor officials similarly
were disenchanted with the Mills-Kennedy bill, which they dismissed as but
a "modest improvement over the Administration's Comprehensive Health
Insurance Plan."[38] The AFL-CIO contended that "[b]asically, Mills-Kennedy
and the Nixon programs are catastrophic insurance programs designed to
insure against the risk of major illness. Neither provides basic, comprehensive care, because both rely on high deductibles and coinsurance."[39]

Although the Mills-Kennedy plan was not based on the concept of an employer mandate to pay for health insurance, like the Nixon plan it was
premised on retaining the connection between one's employment status
and health benefits. Many groups of U.S. citizens would not qualify for coverage under this bill because of a set of criteria derived from their employment status. Included were new workers and their dependents, people who
worked fewer than 25 hours per week, divorced women who had never
been employed, and new immigrants who were unemployed.[40] In their
1974 testimony on the various health-care reform proposals, labor officials
reaffirmed their support for the Health Security Act, now known as the
Griffiths-Corman bill, which would provide universal health care in the
United States without requiring deductibles or copayments.[41]

Labor's commitment to national health insurance in 1974 was bolstered by
the support it received from consumer advocacy groups, which largely sat out
the earlier debate in 1971 over health policy. In an effort to attract more support from consumer interests, labor officials tailored their Congressional testimony to focus on the "problems of consumers in the health system."[42] Their
efforts seemed to pay off in 1974 because consumer advocate Ralph Nader
and staff members of his Public Citizen Research Group came out solidly in favor of the Health Security Act, as did other leaders of consumer groups.
Nader denounced the Nixon proposal as a "corporate welfare proposal for
the health, drug and medical industries" and attacked Kennedy's compromise
proposal as the product of "congressional fatigue" with health-care issues.[43]

Certain that time was on their side in the summer of 1974, organized labor and other supporters of national health insurance counseled against rushing to pass anything before the midterm elections. They were convinced that any bill Nixon would not veto was a bill not worth passing.[44] Their hopes for securing a veto-proof Congress in the fall elections were bolstered as the Watergate scandal engulfed the White House that summer. After Nixon's resignation in early August, key members of Congress refocused attention on the health-insurance issue and were supported in their efforts by the new president, Gerald Ford.[45] The staff of the Ways and Means Committee drafted a compromise bill that closely resembled the Nixon proposal but incorporated some elements of the other plans. But Chairman Mills refused to take the bill to the House floor that fall because his committee was sharply divided over financing the measure and over some compulsory aspects of the legislation.[46]

No agreement on comprehensive health care emerged after the November elections, even though the Democrats increased their majority to 291 in the House and 61 in the Senate.[47] Although organized labor continued to express its willingness to compromise on a number of issues, it identified the administration's insistence that private insurance carriers run any new program as the primary hurdle for unions. Max Fine, the executive director of the Committee for National Health Insurance (CNHI), founded in 1968 by Walter Reuther of the UAW and serving as organized labor's main vehicle for developing health policy, stated in December 1974 that this was one issue that organized labor could not back down on.[48] "You should be with me when I take a swing around the locals," Fine reportedly said. "They tell me, 'One thing you better not do, Fine, is let those insurance companies in on this!' "[49]

The refusal by labor to endorse the Mills-Kennedy compromise or the subsequent Mills bill caused a rupture with some of its leading Democratic allies, notably Kennedy. At a December 1974 meeting of the CNHI, the senator reportedly acted in "almost a belligerent manner" and stated that he resented the charge made against him that he was "selling out on the health issue." Kennedy said he still believed in the principles of national health insurance as embodied in the Health Security Act. However, he was reluctant to reintroduce the bill in its present form since it would be difficult to get cosponsors "because the bill would be saddled with what he kept referring to as its '$90 billion cost.' "[50]

Labor leaders remained hopeful about the prospects for national health insurance in the weeks immediately after the election. However, their hopes were dashed by early 1975. The first blow came in December 1974, after Mills lost the chairmanship of the Ways and Means Committee following a colorful scandal involving a stripper. The second, and perhaps more significant blow, came in January 1975 when President Ford stated in his

first State of the Union address that he would veto any new spending legislation and instead proposed a tax cut aimed to spur the sullen economy.[51]
The moratorium on new spending applied to health care, and the administration refused to reintroduce the compromise proposal it had unveiled in
August 1974. This resulted in a major shift in how organized labor, legislators, and other government officials viewed health policy, leading to labor's
belated embrace of the employer mandate.

HEALTH INSURANCE FOR THE UNEMPLOYED

Concerns about escalating medical costs and the huge gaps in the
U.S. health-care system dominated debates about health policy in the first
half of the 1970s. Supporters of comprehensive health-care reform argued
that the United States must change its health-care delivery system to expand the medical services available in underserved areas and improve the
nation's standing on such fundamental health indices as life expectancy
and infant mortality.[52] As the recession of 1973 lingered into 1975, economic concerns were paramount in discussions of health policy in a way
they were not before. In particular, legislators and other policy-makers
more explicitly linked their health-care prescriptions with specific analyses
and diagnoses of what ailed the U.S. economy and how to heal its malaise.
As such, the debate over health care changed in subtle but significant ways.

The health-care question increasingly was subsumed in the larger question of what was wrong with the U.S. economy overall. One's view of what
was ailing the economy began to dictate one's view of what ailed the medical system in a way not seen in earlier discussions of health-care reform.
The immediate catalysts for this shift were the expressed determination of
the Ford administration to cap federal spending, and rising public concern
about the plight of the unemployed.

Organized labor continued to support universal health care but redirected its energies toward the plight of the unemployed. As the unemployment rate inched up to a postwar high of nearly 9 percent in the spring of
1975, concern grew because more and more Americans who lost their jobs
also lost the health benefits received through their employers. Although organized labor remained supportive of national health insurance, it devoted
more of its efforts to developing emergency health insurance legislation
targeted at the unemployed.

In doing so, organized labor made two significant but subtle political and
policy shifts in 1975 that facilitated its eventual endorsement of the employer mandate. First, with its newfound focus on how to provide relief for
a specific group of people, recently laid-off workers, labor took an important step toward sanctioning an incremental approach to health-care re-

form based on employment status. There had been an ironclad belief among labor officials that the experience of Medicare had taught them one fundamental lesson—that it was not possible to reform the health-care system in a desirable direction through incremental steps, such as expanding coverage to include certain population groups or specific medical services.[53] Second, labor took a major step away from the principle of universalism. It initially argued for a government-funded program that would provide unemployed workers with the identical package of medical benefits they received from their employers prior to a layoff.

Despite serious concerns about incremental approaches to health-care reform, labor officials backed legislation in 1975 that would require the federal government to pick up the tab for continuing the health insurance plans of laid-off workers. It rejected an alternative proposal that would require employers, not the government, to assume the cost of continuing to provide laid-off workers with health benefits. Leonard Woodcock of the UAW came to the defense of employers on this point. He argued that if a business was in such bad shape to require layoffs, it probably was unable to assume the substantial cost of continuing to provide health insurance for its laid-off employees. Labor officials also initially rejected an alternative bill sponsored by Rep. James C. Corman (D-Calif.) that would make the unemployed eligible for Medicare; thereby creating uniform national standards for health benefits for the unemployed. Woodcock acknowledged that labor's preferred proposal put unions in the difficult position of endorsing an inequity. Laid-off union members presumably stood to benefit disproportionately from any government program based on their on-the-job benefits packages, which were likely to be more comprehensive and generous than those available in any government program based on Medicare, the health benefits program for senior citizens.[54]

The business community remained divided over health insurance for the unemployed. The U.S. Chamber of Commerce supported amending the Social Security Act to provide the unemployed and their dependents with a basic package of health benefits funded out of general revenues. However, a Chamber spokesman warned that the nation needed to resolve several more pressing economic problems before it enacted comprehensive health-insurance reform.[55] The NAM, on the other hand, stood firmly with an administration that implacably opposed legislative proposals to provide health insurance for the unemployed. Like the administration, the NAM derived its views on health care for the unemployed from its larger analysis of the nation's economic woes. The NAM echoed the administration's conviction that any special provision for the unemployed would add to the budget deficit; dry up capital; hurt the overall job picture; and saddle business with higher labor costs, thus slowing the economy's recovery.[56]

Legislative proposals to provide health insurance for the unemployed never made it to either the House or the Senate floor due in large part to jurisdictional disputes. Legislators viewed emergency health-care legislation for the unemployed as a dry run for more comprehensive health-insurance reform and jealously guarded their legislative prerogatives. A struggle erupted in the House between the newly created Subcommittee on Health of the Ways and Means Committee headed by Rep. Dan Rostenkowski (D-Ill.), and the Interstate and Foreign Commerce Committee's Subcommittee on Health and the Environment, chaired by Rep. Paul G. Rogers (D-Fla.). On the Senate side, a milder dispute broke out between the Senate Finance Committee and the Senate Labor and Public Welfare Committee.[57] The turf battle in the House was fueled in part by a committee reform plan adopted in 1974 that put the Commerce Committee in charge of all health-care legislation except that financed through payroll taxes.[58] It was uncertain how that reform would affect any national health insurance legislation. The ambiguous nature of the proposed employer-mandate solutions compounded that uncertainty in that businesses were not required to pay for health benefits through a direct payroll tax in the conventional sense, but would cover a percentage of employee health-insurance costs. The employer mandate was inherently ambiguous. Not wholly a creature of the public or the private welfare state, it was vulnerable to charges that it was, in the final analysis, just a legislative euphemism for a sizable new tax on employers.

Although labor remained cool to an employer mandate, support for this approach appeared to build in surprising quarters in 1975. The American Medical Association (AMA) endorsed a plan that would require employers to offer a standard medical benefits package. The AMA had favored only a voluntary health insurance program. Although the NAM still opposed any mandated solutions, the Chamber of Commerce remained receptive to an employer mandate. However, the Chamber also talked about national health insurance in a larger economic context, as did the NAM and the Ford administration. A leading Chamber spokesman warned that before the nation could enact comprehensive health-insurance reform, it needed to resolve several more pressing economic problems, including slow recovery from the recession, high unemployment, persistent inflation, and the energy crisis.[59]

By the end of 1975, the employer mandate was a viable but uncertain option. Although organized labor inched toward incremental solutions in 1975, it fiercely opposed the idea of an employer mandate. Some segments of business remained open to the concept, but were concerned about what they viewed as more pressing economic questions. As such, the 1975 debate over health insurance for the unemployed helped recast the wider debate over national health insurance and tied it more directly to macroeconomic concerns. When legislators and other policy-makers talked about health care, they were more likely to talk in the same breath about the overall health of the economy.

The following year, Congress held sporadic hearings on health insurance at which labor officials reaffirmed their fierce opposition to the employer mandate. They called it, among other things, a "regressive tax" and a "bureaucratic nightmare" that would be difficult for the government to police and that would fuel job discrimination against handicapped, sick, and older workers. In a written submission to a Congressional committee in 1976, Melvin A. Glasser of the UAW stated: "*We are totally opposed to offering health insurance through employers in any form.* Employment-based health insurance and the private health insurance industry are parts of the problem rather than the solution."[60] Wilbur J. Cohen, the former secretary of the Department of Health, Education, and Welfare and a longtime policy leader on Social Security issues, warned that any mandatory plan for employers was tantamount to federal regulation of the insurance sector. As such it would put the administration in the unenviable position of "fighting and fussing and fuming with the private sector interminably."[61]

The 1976 hearings on health care were significant in one other respect. For the first time, individual corporations focused in a concerted fashion on how rising health-care costs were reportedly hurting the international competitiveness of U.S. products. Victor M. Zink, a General Motors executive, testified that the auto giant would spend $825 million for health care for employees and their dependents in 1976. Zink warned that if GM had to increase the price of its subcompact cars to cover rising employee health costs, "this could be particularly harmful" because these "models compete directly with imports." Several other business executives also appeared before Congress that year as representatives of individual companies—not business organizations—to stress how high medical expenses hurt their economic competitiveness.[62]

LABOR'S INITIAL EMBRACE OF AN EMPLOYER MANDATE

Whereas organized labor inched toward a new position on health-care reform in 1975 and 1976, by 1978 it had taken a giant step in a new direction. For the first time, it publicly embraced the idea of an employer mandate and other proposals based on retaining a major role for the commercial insurers. What explains this important shift? The institutions of the private welfare state predisposed organized labor to endorse the employer mandate. But political, not institutional, factors were the immediate trigger for labor's change of heart. The decisive political variable for organized labor was a shift in the preferences of leading Democrats, notably Senator Kennedy and President Carter. The decision to back an employer mandate appears to have been made without any comprehensive and independent consideration of the wider political and economic context. Labor convinced itself that the employer mandate was a win-win solution that offered a back door to national health insurance and universal health care without burdening the federal tab. Organized labor also convinced itself that an employer mandate was not all that radical an idea. After all, many businesses already were voluntarily providing employee health insurance benefits. Adoption of the employer mandate was viewed as a compromise that could broaden political support over the short run but that left open the possibility to achieve the ultimate goal of universal coverage.

In the 1976 presidential campaign, Carter, after close consultation with the UAW, endorsed a national health insurance system to be funded through employer and payroll taxes and general revenues.[63] Once in office, however, Carter took the position that any national health insurance program would have to wait until medical inflation was brought under control. The centerpiece of his attack on health-care inflation involved various incarnations of hospital cost-containment legislation, none of which Congress enacted.

Frustrated by the impasse over national health insurance, labor and Kennedy stepped up pressure on Carter to send health insurance legislation to Congress in 1978.[64] They also expressed a new willingness to make major compromises to address the administration's two fundamental concerns: retaining a significant role for the insurance companies and ensuring minimal impact on the federal budget. The Committee for National Health Insurance (CNHI), labor's main vehicle for developing health policy, made a major shift in 1978.[65] Working in concert with Kennedy, the CNHI developed a plan based for the first time on the employer-mandate feature. Furthermore, the CNHI proposed that commercial insurers be allowed to stay in the health-insurance business, but under the watchful eye of greater federal regulation.

After making what they viewed as two major and difficult compromises on national health insurance, labor officials and Kennedy were disappointed by what they perceived as a determined effort by the Department of Health, Education, and Welfare to "do in" their new proposal by leaking it to the press in "the most adverse and pejorative way." They charged HEW with stoking the ire of employers by making two misleading claims: first, that the Kennedy-labor plan would require employers to pay the entire cost of employee premiums; and second, that the plan would cost $80 billion, or nearly three times what organized labor had estimated.[66] At a tense meeting at the White House in April 1978, Kennedy, Douglas A.

Fraser of the UAW, and George Meany of the AFL-CIO, told Carter how they had "gone through a major agonizing reappraisal" to devise a compromise proposal for comprehensive health-insurance reform that would satisfy the administration's two stated primary concerns.[67] Fraser underscored for the president how the autoworkers "had come a long way to bite the bullet on private insurers and this had been a very difficult move to make, but we made it." They told the president that given all the compromises they had made, HEW's "unfair and unjust characterization" of their draft proposal was particularly upsetting.

Kennedy then suggested that the president help rectify the situation by appointing a working group on health care that would include experts from labor. However, Carter resisted creating an institutional base for labor's input on health-insurance reform. He rebuffed Kennedy's suggestion and said, "This must be done *within* our Administration."[68] Carter's reluctance to give non-state actors an institutional perch within his administration to develop an acceptable national health insurance plan stood in marked contrast to how Medicare was developed a decade earlier. In that instance, organized labor had worked closely with the Social Security Administration to draft a health-care program for senior citizens, so much so that Martha Derthick describes them as "intimate collaborators."[69]

Instead, Carter was intent on subjecting proposals for health-care reform to a new White House decision-making process. Widely known as PRM, the Presidential Review Memorandum sought to involve all Cabinet officers in major decisions by soliciting their formal comments on important policy proposals. In labor's view, these other departments and agencies, many of which concerned themselves primarily with economic matters and had little expertise in health policy, fueled the administration's already significant fears about the effect any comprehensive health-care reform proposal would have on inflation and the federal budget.[70] Thus, economists, who had established themselves as the "intellectual gatekeepers" for economic policy with the demise of the Keynesian consensus in the 1970s, became important gatekeepers for social policy during the Carter administration.[71] This shows how an institutional artifact, the creation of the PRM process, provided fertile ground for highly economistic views of social policy to take root.

HEW fueled these highly economistic views of social policy rather than neutralizing them, according to labor officials. Organized labor complained that HEW staff members depicted any form of national health insurance in their analyses as inflationary. Those data "then form the basis for less than well-informed attacks by [Charles] Schultze, [W. Michael] Blumenthal and [James] McIntyre," respectively the head of the Council of Economic Advisers, Secretary of the Treasury, and head of the Office of

Management and Budget. Organized labor viewed the PRM process as weakening what had been a "firm commitment" by Carter to national health insurance and of "pulling the plan rightward."[72] Although Carter initially indicated that his two principal considerations in any new health-care program were to ensure a continuing role for the insurers and minimal impact on the federal budget, concerns about inflation dominated all discussions of health-care reform. When the administration insisted on significant cost-sharing by patients, labor officials were firmly opposed. They argued that the administration should back down on the issue because labor had "made a tremendous concession on private health insurance companies' participation." Stuart Eizenstat, Carter's domestic policy chief, shot back that the administration had made an enormous concession of its own by agreeing to introduce any health-care reform proposal in the first place. He said the White House "was under tremendous pressure not to come up with any NHI [national health insurance] plan at all, for the reason that it would be totally contrary to the anti-inflation campaign."[73]

The PRM process was a convenient avenue for economic policy-makers to fan fears about inflation. Those fears were helped along by HEW Secretary Joseph Califano, who in labor's view had a "long record of passive resistance" on national health insurance that predated his tenure with the Carter administration.[74] Disagreement over potential inflationary aspects of a national health insurance program remained central to disputes between the White House and the Kennedy–labor coalition over specific features of the Carter program.

The administration and the Kennedy-labor group eventually agreed on the idea of an employer mandate in 1978, but on little else.[75] Although the administration publicly endorsed an employer mandate, it continued to harbor deep reservations about such a solution. When labor first broached the idea of an employer mandate in early 1978, White House officials expressed fear that it would place "an unusually heavy burden on employers and the Chamber of Commerce and others would be upset."[76] The White House subsequently warmed up somewhat to the idea of an employer mandate, but Califano remained uneasy, even as he acknowledged that this was the only realistic way to finance a version of national health insurance. Califano warned privately in a memo to Carter that, "Any move to employer-related financing, however, brings with it a quantum leap in administrative complexity. *Premium financing engages the Federal government in overseeing health insurance transactions between every employer and employee in the country.*"[77]

White House doubts about the willingness of the business sector to support an employer mandate persisted. While segments of the business community appeared ready to endorse an employer mandate, they apparently were willing to do so only if the system of experienced-rated health insurance was retained. The administration balked when labor pushed the point that any new health insurance scheme should be based on community rating, not experience rating.[78] While labor was instrumental in the developing the experience-rated insurance market, as argued in chapter 3, labor officials still appeared willing to give up the practice in exchange for a comprehensive health-care reform proposal they hoped would result in universal health care.

In July, the Kennedy–labor coalition formally parted ways with the Carter administration over health-care reform. That fall, the CNHI approved a new scheme for national health insurance based on an employer mandate.[79] In May 1979, Kennedy formally submitted to Congress his Health Care for All Americans Act, which became known as the Kennedy-Waxman bill. It would require employers to pay up to 65 percent of employee health insurance premiums in a phased-in program that did not require any deductibles or copayments. In promoting his new legislation, Kennedy stressed the need for any comprehensive health-care proposal to be off-budget and said that this was the primary reason he had done an about-face to endorse an employer mandate.[80] President Carter subsequently introduced a much more modest proposal that basically mandated universal coverage for catastrophic illnesses under an employer-mandate formula.[81]

Kennedy's and organized labor's embrace of the employer mandate and their newfound willingness to retain a large role for the commercial insurers in the medical system antagonized many longtime supporters of national health insurance. In attacking the employer-mandate concept, Representative Corman, champion of the Health Security Act, made prescient observations in warning that "a myriad of unneeded problems and complexities result from gimmicks used to avoid a visible Federal commitment."[82] Corman charged that the new CNHI proposal relied on "two unrealistic assumptions." First, he noted the vexing political ambiguity of any employer mandate, saying that by compelling citizens to purchase a portion of their health insurance through their employers, the federal government essentially was "delegat[ing] to private corporations the power to tax." And second, he contended, it was unrealistic to expect that, in a period of widespread deregulation, Congress would "approve heavy regulation of the insurance industry, presently the sole domain of states."[83]

The AFL-CIO and UAW, who dominated the CNHI, appeared to be solidly behind Kennedy's new legislation. However, there were significant rumblings in the ranks of organized labor over abandoning the Health Security Act. Keith W. Johnson, the president of the International Woodworkers of America, urged the CNHI not to back away from retaining a major role for the government—not the insurers—in the administration of any national health insurance plan. "Health Security was built around a set of broad-based principles. These principles should not be lost in the rush to get a bill passed," he warned.[84] In private many labor leaders conceded that Kennedy's bill did not have a chance given the constraints the federal budget was under. The labor leaders also questioned why CNHI had abandoned national health insurance for legislation that would not go anywhere.[85]

Kennedy and labor purportedly switched to an employer mandate to pick up additional political support, which never materialized. In a testy exchange with Fraser during Congressional hearings in 1979, Corman put the UAW leader and chairman of the CNHI on the spot. The congressman pointedly asked Fraser to tell him what specific support from which specific interest groups did labor acquire by abandoning its longtime commitment to the Health Security Act to endorse Kennedy's new bill. "Basically with the executive branch of this Government," Fraser answered. To which Corman shot back, "It is hard to tell that because you each come here today with great reluctance about the other's proposal."[86]

By the late 1970s, organized labor had abandoned national health insurance and embraced the idea of an employer mandate for the first time. A major reason for the shift was the hope that such a rightward compromise would make labor part of a broader and winning coalition. Despite significant misgivings among longtime supporters of national health insurance, and within the Carter administration, about the feasibility of an employer mandate, organized labor finally took the step in 1978. Its embrace of the employer mandate never had the desired political effect. In the waning months of the Carter administration, Congress remained at an impasse over national health insurance as the Kennedy-Waxman compromise failed to attract new political lifeblood.

Labor's initial endorsement of the employer-mandate idea in 1978 poses an analytical puzzle explored above; at this early stage, the idea of an employer-mandate constitutes the "dependent variable" of the analysis. Over the next decade and a half, labor's commitment to an employer-mandate solution did not waver much despite employers' dogged quest for a more flexible labor market and the most sustained assault on labor by employers and conservative legislators since the 1930s. Later chapters will show how the idea of an employer mandate subsequently functioned as an "independent variable." It took on a life of its own and caused groups to rethink their interests and form new alliances. It helped reconfigure the coalitions around the health-care issue, aligning labor more closely with employers and insurers.

The detailed account in this chapter of the origins of an employer-mandate solution and of organized labor's embrace of the policy prescription it once spurned illuminates several more general analytical points. First, labor's attachment to the Taft-Hartley funds, the ERISA preemption, and the practice of experience rating does not alone explain why labor leaders in the late 1970s became less enamored with national health insurance schemes rooted in the public welfare state and more committed to health-care reform proposals based on retaining the link between employment and benefits. The institutional context described in the previous chapter shaped this outcome, but it did not single-handedly determine it. Although it is important to be sensitive to the complex institutional context described earlier, it is also important to understand how and why key political actors deciphered their political and economic environment as they did.

By the late 1970s organized labor came around to endorsing an employer mandate largely without any serious, independent analysis of the broader economic context beyond consideration of what became a national obsession with inflation and the size of the federal budget deficit. Once leading Democrats re-ordered their preferences, organized labor followed suit. Labor officials largely left state actors to decipher the shifts in the U.S. political economy and thus to define the nation's preeminent social and economic problems. Most labor leaders did not challenge the contention that escalating government spending and inflation were the twin scourges of the United States. In the context of the health-care debate, they generally accepted this view of the U.S. political economy as an uncontested objective fact rather than a potential arena for political debate. State actors, notably leading Democrats, were the major catalysts for new initiatives in health-care reform. Labor leaders eventually endorsed the idea of an employer mandate, understanding their role as passive transmitters of new ideas and political strategies handed down from leading state actors. Given this selective understanding of the political and economic context, embracing the employer mandate was seen as the next logical step.

This is not to suggest that the political constraints of the federal budget deficit and the stagflationary economic environment were just a figment of labor's imagination, or that those factors did not pose significant obstacles to the cause of universal and affordable health care. Rather, these economic problems could have been defined and addressed in various ways. Instead of accepting the conventional wisdom that it was time to just say no to new spending on social programs, labor could have argued more forcefully for military conversion and cuts in defense spending with the end of the Vietnam War and later the end of the Cold War. Instead of giving up on Canadian-style health-care reform due to the burden it allegedly posed for the budget, organized labor could have redoubled its efforts to educate the public and state actors about the enormous cost savings associated with single-payer plans due to lower administrative expenses and other factors. Labor also could have forcefully underscored how Western European countries, with their more extensive public welfare states, spend only half or three-quarters of what the United States spends on health care (as measured as a percentage of GNP) and yet achieve near-universal health care.

Instead, organized labor in the United States pursued what appeared to be the most politically expedient solution at that moment. In contrast to the stance the Canadian labor movement and Canadian advocates of national health insurance took on behalf of universal health care in the 1950s and 1960s, organized labor in the United States did not embed its health-care strategy in a longer-term political strategy derived from a comprehensive and independent analysis of the rapidly changing political and economic context.[87] During the 1980s, organized labor inserted the issue of health-care reform into a wider economic context, but business largely defined that context, not labor. For a second time around, organized labor embraced an employer-mandate solution. Given the enormous economic changes in the United States during the intervening decade, the rationale for an employer mandate rested on even shakier ground in the 1980s than it did in the late 1970s.

CHAPTER 5

Workers and Managers of the World, Unite

Wooing an Elusive Ally

In the summer of 1994, last-ditch efforts to salvage some kind of comprehensive health-care reform consumed labor unions and other supporters of the Clinton administration's Health Security Act.[1] At one point, executives from the major auto and steel companies met with Sen. John D. Rockefeller (D-W.Va.) and his staff to present a check for $300,000 to help the reform effort in the eleventh hour. Dismayed by what he saw as support that was too little, too late, Rockefeller dismissed the six-figure check, as only a multimillionaire could. "I can't take this. It's pathetic," he reportedly declared at the tense meeting, summing up widespread disappointment that big business had not done more on behalf of comprehensive reform earlier.[2]

This was a far cry from the optimism about the potentially constructive role big business would play in health policy that prevailed among labor leaders and others in the late 1980s and early 1990s. The widespread belief was that business, or at least critical elements of big business, was prepared to shift course radically to support a number of health-care reforms that longtime supporters of universal health care in Congress, labor unions, and public-interest groups could live with. In the end, however, the three peak associations for big business in the United States—the U.S. Chamber of Commerce, the National Association of Manufacturers (NAM), and the Business Roundtable—refused to endorse the Clinton proposal, even though the administration, by most accounts, was sensitive to the potential concerns of business in drafting its proposal.[3] Furthermore, Fortune 500 companies did little to counter the all-out assault on the Clinton proposal waged by the small business sector, the Health Insurance Association of America (HIAA), and other stakeholders. "The big guys didn't do shit working on the Clinton plan," said an exasperated Alan Reuther, legislative director of the United Auto Workers (UAW). "The people with the political juice were the small business ones."[4] Reuther and other labor officials based their strategy on the belief that they could cut a deal with business on health care, especially once a friendly Democrat occupied the White House. As it turned out, organized labor fundamentally misread the business community as business support for comprehensive health-care reform proved ephemeral.

From the 1980s onward, organized labor pursued a two-pronged approach to health-care reform. The first was a simultaneous retreat from national health insurance and an embrace of the employer mandate. The second prong was a belief that big business would be a constructive partner in the quest for universal and affordable health care. For a variety of reasons, labor officials staked their health-care strategy on wooing what turned out to be an elusive ally.

When organized labor first embraced the idea of an employer mandate in 1978, it was contemptuous that business could possibly play any positive role in health-care reform.[5] By the end of the 1980s, leading labor officials made the case that business, at least big business, was prepared to be a reliable ally. Labor's optimism about business had political and institutional roots. On the political side, labor leaders made a series of misjudgments. There was a mistaken tendency among labor officials to take the seemingly sympathetic views of executives in the auto, steel, and other heavily unionized sectors of the economy as representing business sentiment overall. Furthermore, the encouraging views of the Chrysler Corporation, in particular, may have blinded organized labor to how tepid support was for comprehensive reform even within the automobile industry.

Organized labor's optimism that business was prepared to be a constructive partner on health-care issues, and the related belief that active business support was necessary for any satisfactory solution, were founded on more than just positive cues coming from Chrysler executives and a handful of other business executives. This was not just a simple case of labor allowing itself to be led down a blind alley by the wishful thinking of a vocal minority within the business community. The misplaced faith that big business would ultimately join with labor and do the right thing on health care has deeper roots. They reach to the heart of how labor officials understood the institutional setting within which organized labor functions, specifically to their understanding of postwar labor and management relations.

Many labor leaders cleaved to a view of labor-management relations that was institutionalized in the 1950s. This view was premised on the belief that if business and labor leaders developed suitable organizational forums that allowed them to meet behind closed doors with one another, they could work out many of their differences through elite-level discussions with little government involvement and public scrutiny. This view, which is closely identified with John Dunlop of Harvard University, ossified into an institution in its own right that constrained labor's autonomy from business and the Democrats.

Chapter 3 examined the impact that three institutions characterized by formal organizations and procedures had on the political behavior of organized labor. This chapter looks at how a different sort of institution, one that constitutes habitual behavior, constrained labor's political free will. This type of institution is characterized by "social patterns" that are "valued in and of themselves" and that "encompass not only explicit rules and expectations but unspoken procedures, routines and assumptions of ways to act socially and politically."[6]

The debate over health-care reform reveals the extent to which faith in the corporatist possibilities for labor-management relations continued to mold the political behavior of organized labor into the 1980s. This faith persisted in the face of a management offensive against labor unparalleled since the interwar years.[7] In the 1980s, the Dunlop view of labor-management relations held enormous sway with AFL-CIO president Lane Kirkland and with John J. Sweeney, president of the Service Employees International Union (SEIU) and the first chairman of the AFL-CIO health-care committee. At the highest reaches of organized labor, Kirkland and Sweeney pushed hard to work with business to solve the country's major health-care problems. They were convinced that the business community would offer significant, perhaps decisive, support if organized labor took a moderate position on health-care reform. The litmus test of moderation was whether labor would push hard for a single-payer system inspired by the Canadian experience with national health insurance or settle for an employer mandate that would leave the job-based system of benefits and the commercial insurers largely untouched.

This chapter analyzes the interaction of labor and business from the late 1970s to the late 1980s on issues related to comprehensive health-care reform. In doing so, it demonstrates how, in spite of vast shifts in the U.S. political economy during that period, institutionalized views about the nature of labor-management relations at the firm level and in the wider political arena persisted.[8] These views contributed to labor officials misreading the interests, policy preferences, and political capacity of business with respect to the health-care issue. They also help to explain why organized labor continued to view the U.S. political economy largely through the eyes of key business leaders and state actors in discussions of health care and was unable to stake out a more independent position on health policy.

This chapter begins by examining the evolution of organized labor's enduring faith in American-style corporatist solutions to social and economic problems. It then discusses the aborted attempts by several labor unions, led by the UAW, to carve out a political position that was more independent of business, the AFL-CIO, and the Democratic Party in the late 1970s and early 1980s. The third section addresses the emerging role of Sweeney and the SEIU on health-care issues in the 1980s, in particular the critical part the union president played in coaxing organized labor to take a more co-operative approach toward business on the health-care question. It shows how the debate over family leave legislation in the 1980s presaged the subsequent battle over health policy in the early 1990s. The fourth section discusses how and why organized labor misread business sentiment on health-care reform and the pivotal role the Chrysler Corporation and Lee Iacocca played in the health-care debate. The final section examines why the UAW and other unions were either unable or unwilling to push the leadership of the AFL-CIO to resoundingly endorse the single-payer route to reform.

THE INSTITUTIONAL LEGACY OF AMERICAN-STYLE CORPORATISM

For a long time now, many labor officials have cleaved to a view of labor-management relations in the United States that first took hold in the 1950s and is closely identified with John Dunlop. In Dunlop's view, labor and management reached a kind of détente in the immediate postwar years that persisted well into the 1980s.[9] This accord was founded on collective bargaining and minimal state intervention in industrial relations, and promised to bring lasting peace to the workplace. Developed during the apparent consensus years of the 1950s, this was a confident vision in which real friction and strife between labor and management would increasingly become a thing of the past as the industrial relations system in the United States matured.

Business and labor were not fundamentally at odds, in Dunlop's opinion. Rather, they lacked suitable organizational structures to work out the differences between them and within their own constituencies. Business groups in particular were thought to lack effective ways to reconcile their internal conflicting interests.[10] In his view, business and labor leaders needed private forums in which to get to know one another better, learn to appreciate the pressures each faced, and see through the haze of rhetorical hot air meant primarily for the consumption of their respective constituencies.[11] Other notable early advocates of this view include Arthur J. Goldberg of the Steelworkers and Walter Reuther of the UAW, who began to take a more accommodating stance toward business in the postwar years.[12] Although Dunlop's view did not go unchallenged, it was never really dethroned.[13] Indeed, Dunlop headed a blue-ribbon commission appointed by the Clinton administration that recommended, among other things, that the United States develop more cooperative labor-management relations through new forums such as works councils modeled on the German experience.[14]

By the 1970s, Dunlop was an enthusiast of American-style corporatism, whereby the state actively seeks to facilitate a more cooperative relationship between labor and management. As chairman of the committee on wage stabilization in the construction industry in the early 1970s and later as Labor Secretary under President Ford, Dunlop experimented with tripartite wage councils and greater regional and national centralization of bargaining.[15] At the instigation of Dunlop, Ford formed the Labor-Management Committee, which was modeled on the advisory committees of prior administrations.[16] The committee, which brought together leading corporate executives and top-ranking labor leaders, sought to find cooperative approaches to substantive issues like rising health-care costs, the energy shortage, inflation, and unemployment. Dunlop's corporatist vision appeared to hit a brick wall in 1975 when business leaders reneged on a previous agreement to drop their opposition to so-called *common situs* picketing in exchange for labor's acceptance of a statutory prohibition against unauthorized strikes.[17] Ford balked at signing the two pieces of legislation after an unprecedented coalition of business groups and right-wing activists pressured him to veto the measures. The president's about-face prompted Dunlop's resignation as Labor Secretary.[18]

Shortly after he resigned, Dunlop severed the formal ties between the administration and the Labor-Management Committee, which he renamed the Labor-Management Group.[19] Health-care costs were a central concern of the new group, which, among other things, developed a number of recommendations for how business and labor could work together to stem medical inflation.[20] Dunlop also was at the forefront of efforts to promote business health-care coalitions through his work with the Robert Wood Johnson Foundation, which committed about $20 million in the early 1980s to promoting such groups around the country.[21]

During this period, some union officials privately raised concerns about how joint labor-management efforts on health care and other issues might hamstring organized labor. UAW staff members, for example, expressed misgivings about the Dunlop group's excessive focus on hospital cost-containment while other big-ticket items like physicians' fees and nursing home costs were ignored. They also were troubled because the group did not consider the possibilities for controlling medical costs through a national health insurance program.[22] These joint labor-business efforts put union staff members in awkward positions and divided their loyalties.[23]

Soon after the Labor-Management Group formed, Dunlop's vision of labor and business elites amicably sitting around a table to privately settle the pressing economic and political questions of the day was put to the test once again. In 1977 another *common situs* bill was introduced in Congress, along with a labor law reform bill that would repeal onerous provisions of the Taft-Hartley Act that constrain union organizing campaigns. President Carter promised to sign the *situs* bill, but would not lobby for it and failed to deliver even a single vote from Georgia's Democratic congressional delegation.[24] Business defeated the *common situs* bill after launching a sustained and massive lobbying campaign that was aimed at both legislators and the general public. As for the labor law reform bill of 1978, some charge that Carter did little to rally public support for the measure in the face of business's spirited attack against it.[25] The Business Roundtable, an exclusive organization of some 200 of the country's leading chief executive officers that included members of Dunlop's Labor-Management Group, helped organize a broad coalition of its own to battle labor law reform. This coalition included representatives of small and big business with important links to the New Right.[26] It waged a "virtual blitzkrieg" against the measure on Capitol Hill, which ended in its death by filibuster in June 1978.[27]

In the immediate aftermath of the defeat of labor law reform and *common situs*, important segments of organized labor appeared ready to bury the Dunlop vision of labor-management relations once and for all. On July 18, 1978, UAW vice president Irving Bluestone proposed that the union examine whether the activities of the Business Roundtable could be challenged under the country's anti-trust statutes. He also suggested that the union do more to educate its membership about "the role which the Business Roundtable is assuming in the right-wing activities within the nation."[28] The following day, Fraser, president of the UAW, resigned from the Labor-Management Group with much fanfare and without pulling any punches.

In his resignation letter, Fraser accused leading business executives of choosing "to wage a one-sided class war" against poor and middle-class Americans and with breaking and discarding "the fragile, unwritten compact previously existing during a past period of growth and progress." He charged that the business community had shifted from a stance of cooperation to one of confrontation. He pointed to its campaign against labor law reform as evidence and characterized the campaign as "the most vicious, unfair attack on the labor movement in more than 30 years." Fraser put the Labor-Management Group's dismal record on health-care reform high up on his long list of examples of the "new class war" waged by business.[29] At the conclusion of his letter, Fraser promised that organized labor would seek new alliances and coalitions in an effort "to help our nation find its way."[30]

Fraser's resignation letter prompted an outpouring of supportive and enthusiastic letters from the well known and the lesser known. Harvard economist John Kenneth Galbraith called it the "best progressive document I've read in years," and a Canadian labor official hailed what sounded like "the beginning of the Democratic Socialist Party." Rank-and-file unionists, retirees, consumers, and environmentalists all wrote to congratulate Fraser and to ask: What next?[31] In his replies, Fraser was vague and noncommittal, seemingly uncertain about how to channel the flood of support he had unleashed. His restrained responses lacked the fervor of his resignation letter. Fraser decidedly nixed the idea of starting a third party, even though he pointedly criticized the Democratic Party in his resignation letter.[32]

The AFL-CIO was measured in its response. When asked about Fraser's departure, George Meany indicated that he, too, might resign from the Dunlop group. But he refrained from directly praising Fraser's decision or seconding the UAW president's criticisms of the business sector. Instead, Meany publicly swiped at Fraser for acting unilaterally and without consulting other labor leaders.[33] The remaining members of the Labor-Management Group also refused to debate the substance of Fraser's criticisms in public. S. D. Bechtel, Jr., chairman of The Bechtel Group, the construction industry behemoth, privately expressed his disappointment with the resignation in a letter to Fraser that was a crisp statement of the Dunlop way. Bechtel reaffirmed his belief that some important disagreements between business and labor "can be resolved through thoughtful, private discussions," and that labor and management "have very definite common interests in selected issues, which can be mutually supported in an effort to correct some of the ills of our country."[34]

Less than three years after his resignation, Fraser and most other labor leaders closed ranks once again to unite around a position strikingly similar to the one articulated by Bechtel in 1978. Fraser had rejoined the Dunlop group, reaffiliated the UAW with the AFL-CIO after a 14-year separation, and repaired his ties with the upper echelons of the Democratic Party. Owen Bieber, who succeeded him as head of the autoworkers in 1983, subsequently joined the Dunlop group, as did SEIU president Sweeney. Organized labor was drawn back into the Dunlop orbit by several factors, all of which had important implications for how the health policy debate played out over the next decade, especially with respect to the question of how closely to work with business on health-care issues. The factors include: the disintegration of the short-lived Progressive Alliance, which Fraser created in the wake of his resignation; the AFL-CIO's largely unshaken belief in corporatist-style solutions and its deepening attachment to the Democratic

Party; the wrenching economic troubles of the automobile industry; and rising discontent among the UAW rank and file.

THE SHORT-LIVED CLASS WAR: THE RISE AND FALL OF THE PROGRESSIVE ALLIANCE

In early 1979, about six months after his resignation from the Dunlop Group, Fraser formed the Progressive Alliance to serve as an umbrella organization for about 100 assorted organizations. Supported primarily by unions, with some help from environmental, civil rights, senior citizen, and consumer groups, the organization was born out of a desire to emulate some of the political strategies of the New Right that were proving so successful. But Fraser and other supporters of the Progressive Alliance did not have a clear idea of how the New Right achieved its political victories and, therefore, what to emulate. The Progressive Alliance never acquired a clear organizational or political identity as a movement or a think tank.

In its founding statement in January 1979, the Alliance criticized the nation's two major political parties for an unwillingness to "serve as vehicles for achieving economic and social justice," but was vague about how it planned to revitalize the parties and participate in electoral politics. The statement indicated that the organization aimed to seed a grass-roots political movement.[35] Four months later, Fraser declared that the Progressive Alliance should eschew direct involvement in electoral politics because it inevitably produced "intense zero-sum conflicts among the constituent organizations of any broad coalition." Instead, the group should pursue what he called "policy politics" and seek to be taken seriously not as a political movement but as "a long-range policy organization."[36]

In his resignation letter from the Dunlop group, Fraser had talked in apocalyptic terms about the need to mobilize against the "new class war" that business was waging in the United States. As head of the Alliance, he recoiled from efforts to mobilize around national issues with a clear class content. Instead, he searched for discrete issues with broad appeal that would address the problem of corporate irresponsibility indirectly.[37] Other Alliance participants argued for more class-based politics that would focus directly on national issues, in particular the role of corporations in the economy. "The question of who profits, of who gets the money will become a political issue and it should become our political issue," one participant advised.[38] Disagreements over what direction to take the Progressive Alliance created a rift between the UAW and AFSCME, two of the most politically active unions. AFSCME president Jerry Wurf and his staff were frustrated by UAW efforts to turn the Alliance into a think tank that would focus on a few specific and immediate issues while putting most of its resources into devising a long-term map to chart the future of progressive politics in the United States.[39]

A month after the rout of the Democrats in the November 1980 election, Fraser met with other union presidents active in the Progressive Alliance to discuss whether the organization should disband, and what role, if any, it should have in rebuilding the party. Several union presidents stressed the need for organized labor to speak in a single voice through the AFL-CIO. They also indicated that the federation, in the wake of Meany's recent retirement, appeared ready to shift direction and become more active in Democratic Party politics.[40] While the union presidents did not reach a definitive decision on the future of the Progressive Alliance at that meeting, by late 1980 its days appeared numbered. The UAW moved closer to the AFL-CIO, the federation moved closer to the Democrats, and the Democrats moved closer to business in the wake of Carter's defeat.[41]

From the creation of the AFL-CIO in 1955 until the UAW's break with the federation in 1967, the key decisions about labor's political activities were made inside the AFL-CIO. The political rift between the AFL-CIO and its more liberal unions widened in the early 1970s when President Meany doggedly refused to endorse George McGovern in his 1972 race against Richard M. Nixon.[42] With Meany's departure in 1979, a rapprochement appeared possible, especially as Lane Kirkland, his successor, sought an influential role for organized labor in the restructuring of the Democratic Party.[43]

The split between the AFL-CIO and the liberal wing of organized labor over the McGovern candidacy obscured important areas of agreement that emerged between them on how to remedy the perceived institutional weaknesses of the Democratic Party. The UAW had endorsed McGovern and provided important financial support to the McGovern-Fraser Commission, which was created after the tumultuous 1968 Democratic convention to reform the party's presidential selection process. McGovern, who initially headed the commission, was succeeded by Rep. Donald Fraser (D-Mich.). Much to the chagrin of the AFL-CIO, dissidents in the Democratic Party established the commission just after the federation had mounted a major effort on behalf of Democratic candidates in the 1968 election.[44] Over time, the UAW came to share the federation's uneasiness about the McGovern-Fraser reforms, which, among other things, increased the number of direct primaries and reduced the number of party caucuses in the presidential selection process. The reforms also ensured greater representation for women, blacks, and other minorities at the nominating convention. The UAW was uneasy about the growing use of the direct primary, believing that it contributed to the decentralization and fragmentation of an already weak party and that it gave an advantage to conservative populists like Governor George Wallace of Alabama. The autoworkers also shared an AFL-CIO concern that the increased influence of women and minorities in the Democratic Party might come at the high cost of putting together a losing ticket that was unappealing to a majority of the electorate.[45]

The McGovern-Fraser reforms clearly strained the relationship between the AFL-CIO and the Democrats. Charles Manatt, who became chairman of the Democratic Party shortly after the 1980 election, sought both to repair the party's relationship with labor and strengthen its bonds with business by establishing, respectively, the Labor Council and the Business Council.[46] In the early 1980s when the Democrats established a second commission to examine the presidential nominating process, Fraser of the UAW supported the effort wholeheartedly, as did Kirkland and the AFL-CIO. They agreed that the party's nominating procedures must be reformed once again to enhance the role of party regulars and roll back some of the other McGovern-Fraser reforms. Fraser envisioned the creation of a more disciplined European-style labor party in which Democratic officeholders would make up a large number of the convention delegates. This would force them to be more accountable to the party platform and the party in general, or so the reasoning went.[47]

In light of the changing of the guard at the AFL-CIO, the federation's newfound interest in restructuring the Democratic Party along the lines envisioned by Fraser, and the UAW's imminent reaffiliation with the federation, the time seemed auspicious for the UAW president to return to the mainstream of organized labor and abandon all talk of class war. In early 1981, Fraser resigned as chairman of the Progressive Alliance, saying his own union members expected him to devote all his attention to the sorry state of the auto industry.[48] By March 1981, the Progressive Alliance disbanded.

In just two years, the UAW and its supporters traveled a great distance ideologically while the AFL-CIO changed surprisingly little despite the departure of Meany. Fraser had launched the Progressive Alliance as a vehicle to challenge the class war he saw corporations waging on middle-class and poor Americans. As he set out to rally the troops, he denounced what he believed was the Democratic Party's complicity in the assault. By 1981, Fraser led the charge to strengthen the hand of labor and political elites within the Democratic Party at the expense of figuring out how to rebuild or reconfigure the party's base at the grass-roots level. As co-chairman of the commission on party reform that year, Fraser embraced a top-down solution for the Democrats at the same time that Charles Manatt, the new party chairman, sought to strengthen ties between the party and business and labor leaders.

When he broke with the Labor-Management Group in 1978, Fraser appeared ready to reject elite-led solutions and the Dunlop way. He indicated his readiness to endorse alternative political strategies, notably grass-roots mobilization and the development of a sharp ideological sword to check the thrusts coming from corporate America. He beat a retreat with the Hunt Commission. The commission agreed to set aside 14 percent of the convention delegates for Democratic officeholders (Kirkland originally wanted a whopping one-third to be selected ex officio).[49] The group believed that the party could best reconnect with its disaffected mass base by granting elected officeholders more clout in the presidential selection process.[50] Fraser endorsed several other potentially top-down solutions for the Democrats: a reduction in the number of required primaries, restoration of the "winner-take-all" rules for congressional district primaries, and "front loading" the shortened primary season to give establishment candidates the electoral edge.[51] These reforms were designed to bind the Democratic officeholders closer to the party, but no additional mechanism was created to bind the officeholders to any coherent ideology or set of policies. In fact, the Hunt Commission did just the reverse. It stripped the midterm Democratic convention of the policy-making authority it exercised briefly in the 1970s. This pulled the rug out from under the party's progressive wing, which was pushing the party to hold a midterm conference in 1982. The progressives viewed such a conference as a way to build party discipline and accountability, and secure an important institutional foothold for the left-leaning forces, including organized labor, in the Democratic Party.[52]

Fraser's enthusiasm for European-style labor politics does not alone explain this about-face. His retreat was prompted in part by changes taking place in the automobile industry as the number of employed unionized U.S. autoworkers was nearly halved in just five years.[53] The UAW responded to these changes by recommitting itself to an updated version of the Dunlop way, called "jointness." This quest for jointness had far-reaching implications. It constrained the UAW's and organized labor's ability to develop an independent political strategy for universal health care based on labor's own comprehensive analysis of the new political economy of the United States in the 1980s.

THE UAW AND THE CONSTRAINTS OF "JOINTNESS"

For a brief moment in the late 1970s, the UAW attempted to stake out a political path for organized labor that was largely independent of business and more focused on mobilizing the grass roots rather than courting leading Democrats. By the early 1980s, it was one of the leading proponents of "jointness," of working together with U.S. corporations to solve the nation's foremost economic troubles. Through its joint efforts with individual automobile companies and its participation in organizations like the Labor-Management Group, the UAW helped redefine the country's economic problems in a way that had important consequences for how the debate over health policy unfolded and for organized labor's broader political strategy. Whereas the battle for national health insurance in the 1970s was waged around issues of social justice and equity, the debate over health care in the 1980s and 1990s revolved around issues of economic "competitiveness." The political fault lines here shifted. For a time, the political fault lines were no longer right versus left, or business versus labor, but rather the U.S. economy versus the world economy.

The Labor-Management Group outlined the new political terrain in a paper Dunlop sent to Fraser in early March 1982 that suggested there were no longer "short-term fixes" or "ideological fixes of the right or left" to alleviate the deep troubles of the nation's economy. The paper contrasted the United States unfavorably with other advanced industrialized countries, including Japan, Germany, and "even Great Britain," which "appear to have workable institutional arrangements" that permit business, labor, and the government to develop policies that advance mutual interests despite ideological differences. It concluded that these countries adapted nimbly to shifting economic circumstances in ways that leave the United States at a disadvantage.[54]

Views like these undergirded the UAW's new commitment to the idea of "jointness." Jointness was a shop floor and collective bargaining strategy that had important implications for the UAW's approach to broader social and economic questions. It was based on the idea that labor and management must cooperate in order to enhance the economic competitiveness of U.S. firms vis-à-vis their foreign counterparts. In the name of cooperation, the UAW leadership in the United States consented to concessionary bargaining, profit sharing, and participation in labor-management productivity discussions.[55] The UAW also sought to persuade the government to relax its regulation of the auto industry.[56] The new emphasis on jointness prompted the UAW to shift course radically on trade issues as well because officials saw jointness as a way to restore the competitiveness of the American auto industry. A new focus on concessionary bargaining, protectionist trade legislation, and other issues related to the perceived challenge of economic competitiveness had important consequences for organized labor's approach to social issues. It brought the UAW closer to the auto industry while distancing it from traditional allies. Those allies included other labor unions, consumer organizations, and advocacy groups that could be counted on to mount a defense of the private- and public-sector safety nets in the face of the deep economic and political restructuring of the 1980s.

This faith in the advantages of a strategy based on jointness when faced with a hostile White House and a deepening recession launched the UAW on the path of concessionary bargaining in the early Reagan years. In December 1981, the union's executive board made a crucial decision to permit an unprecedented reopening of the Ford and General Motors contracts.[57] This decision deeply divided the union and poured salt into wounds already opened by the UAW decision to reaffiliate with the AFL-CIO.[58] In early 1982, an organization called "Locals Opposed to Concessions" formed to resist the $1 billion in concessions proposed in Ford contracts. This action marked the emergence of solid internal opposition to the UAW's leadership. In Region 5, the dissident "New Directions" movement, which advocated more militant resistance, took root. New Directions supporters argued that wage concessions and work-rule changes would not stem the flow of jobs overseas. They also charged that the wide-scale introduction of Japanese-style management techniques into U.S. auto plants was a dangerous step toward enterprise unionism. At the UAW triennial conventions, its leadership found itself beating back motions calling for greater democracy and more rank-and-file participation in union affairs. Even with widespread discontent within its ranks, UAW officials made policy decisions much as they had for three decades. They marginalized critics through control of union funds, staff, and avenues for internal debate. An inner circle of union officials made the major decisions without much input from the rank and file.[59] These heavy-handed tactics further exacerbated divisions within the union.[60]

At the 1989 convention, New Directions movement supporters forcefully challenged concessionary bargaining, sparking a spirited debate about the wisdom of jointness. Dissidents charged that the leadership was insensitive to the rank and file. They introduced a resolution that called for the federal chartering of all large corporations, financial institutions, and foreign-based corporations doing business in the United States. Lew Moye of Local 136 in Region 5 implored the leadership to:

> stop using "competitiveness" as an excuse for caving in to management demands. Competitiveness to maximize profits and to get greater market share from both domestic and foreign competition will always exist in the corporate world. No matter how much we give up competitiveness will only get worse. Instead, we need national policies to restrict lay-offs and plant closings and to force corporations to "compete" without attacking our own job security and living standards.[61]

The internal debates over the headstrong commitment to jointness estranged leading union officials from the most politicized activists within the UAW ranks.[62] Those activists were critical to forging ties with other progressive groups that were essential for waging a successful campaign for universal health care.

The UAW's protectionist stance on trade issues also alienated the union from some of its natural allies. The progressive wing of organized labor, including the UAW, traditionally opposed protectionism because it pitted workers of one country against those of another, and workers in one sector against those in another. Previously, the UAW also had opposed protectionist policies because a sizable number of its members were employed in the agricultural implements and aerospace sectors, both heavy exporters. From about 1980 onward, however, trade issues dominated the UAW's political agenda, in part at the urging of auto executives.[63] In the early 1980s, the union regularly singled out domestic content legislation as the centerpiece of its legislative agenda. In its push for the legislation, the UAW promoted the idea of jointness, saying that the companies backed the bill "in principle," even though the automakers had testified against the measure through their manufacturing associations. After failing repeatedly to get Congress to enact a domestic content bill, the UAW shifted gears and stressed the need for an industrial policy and for "fair trade" legislation designed to restrict imports from countries with unfair trade practices.[64] In the late 1980s, the UAW launched an advertising campaign for U.S. automobiles that stressed "fair trade" and reputed higher quality.

The UAW trade proposals never attracted widespread support from other unions and public-interest groups. The other organizations viewed the UAW proposals as too limited in scope and as largely just an "auto workers special interest bill at a time when companies have successfully created an image of auto workers as overpaid and lazy."[65] Moreover, the UAW focus on trade issues fed the xenophobia of its membership in ways that made working with other progressive groups difficult.[66] The UAW attempted to drum up support for protectionist legislation by directing its anger at the Japanese without making any distinction between Japanese workers and Japanese companies. In lobbying for the domestic content bill, for example, the UAW stressed how the Japanese were the enemy and how U.S. automakers were on the union's side.[67]

Jointness guided the union's approach to trade, other economic issues, and also health care. When he resigned from the Labor-Management Group in 1978, Fraser said he doubted that business could be counted on to play a constructive role in health policy. Yet the UAW continued its joint efforts with the Big Three automakers to control medical costs internally by, for example, requiring second opinions in surgery cases. It also indirectly participated in a private mini-Dunlop group that explored what the private sector could do to stem escalating health-care costs.[68] At the time, some UAW officials and staff members privately raised concerns about entering into joint arrangements with the auto industry to control medical costs. They worried that pressure from Chrysler to agree to cost-containment schemes for health care could cause the union problems with its members, especially in light of the wave of concessionary bargaining and the "current rather sour atmosphere in the plants."[69] UAW staff members also raised doubts about the utility of cost-containment programs, saying most were unsuccessful. Instead of reducing medical costs overall, they merely served "to transfer the costs from the carriers to our members."[70]

Although the UAW privately expressed some misgivings about the joint approach to the problem of escalating health-care costs, for several reasons it was poorly positioned to stake out a path on health-care issues that strayed too far from the Big Three. First, the union's new approach to collective bargaining and trade issues had tied its fate tightly to the idea of working together with the auto industry. This made it more difficult for the union to strike out on its own on some issues while singing the praises of jointness on others. Second, the earnest support of the UAW for protectionist trade policies alienated it from groups that were otherwise natural allies in the fight for a comprehensive health-care solution along the lines of Canada's single-payer system.[71] The battle over trade dominated the UAW legislative agenda, edging out other issues and gobbling up resources. Finally, for an all-out push for universal health care to succeed, the UAW would have had to mobilize its own rank and file.

Ridden with internal divisions and joined at the hip with the Big Three on many trade and collective bargaining issues, the UAW leadership was in no position to lead the charge for universal health care. Despite claims to the contrary, its social unionism was largely a spent force just at the time when health-care reform proposals calling for a single-payer, Canadian-style system were attracting renewed attention and legitimacy.[72] Vocal single-payer contingents emerged in other unions, including AFSCME, the ACTWU, and the OCAW, and advocacy groups, notably the American Association of Retired Persons (AARP), the American Public Health Association (APHA), and even several physicians' organizations. Some members of these groups began to make the case for a single-payer solution in terms of equity, quality, cost savings, and simplicity.[73]

If the UAW leadership encouraged single-payer activists, it would run the risk of encouraging dissidents within its own ranks. Instead, the union straddled the political terrain. It endorsed a vague set of principles on health care at its 1989 convention and mentioned in passing its commitment to "national health insurance," without spelling out what that meant. It also reiterated its support for legislation that would require employers to provide workers and their families with a minimum benefit package.[74] Although UAW leaders advocated for the single-payer approach at the highest reaches of the AFL-CIO, they did little to mobilize their members to put serious pressure on the federation or the Democratic Party to endorse the Canadian-inspired route to reform.

It is important not to overstate or misstate the significance of the burgeoning New Directions movement and other UAW dissidents in the unfolding debate over health care and other social policy questions. The UAW dissidents were not driven by a strong commitment to any specific social and economic policies or to a coherent ideology. They were preoccupied with wresting control of the union away from the current leadership through greater internal democratization and reform, and with ending the UAW commitment to jointness. Beyond that, they supported vague notions of "independent political action" and favored renewing the UAW alliance with the Canadian Auto Workers and the more democratic forces within the Mexican labor movement.[75] This analysis is not intended to equate the dissidents' commitment to rank-and-file militancy with a commitment to greater political activism on a broad range of social and economic issues. The political significance of the dissidents in the debate over health policy is more modest. The dissidents were significant to the extent that they comprised the most politically active members of the UAW and had important ties with activists in other unions and public-interest groups. Thus they potentially served as a critical nucleus to mobilize a broader coalition in support of universal health care.[76]

To recapitulate, even though the UAW advocated on behalf of the single-payer option at the highest levels of the AFL-CIO, its leadership appeared reluctant to mobilize the rank and file to pressure the labor federation to unequivocally endorse national health insurance. Deep economic restructuring in the automobile industry sapped the political energy of the UAW leadership as it waged one unsuccessful battle after another for more protectionist trade legislation. Furthermore, dislocations in the automobile sector spawned rising discontent within the rank and file about the UAW's more conciliatory approach to labor-management relations. Had they attempted to mobilize members in any serious way around the health-care issue, UAW officials might have strengthened the hand of the growing dissident movement within the union, which was calling for greater grass-roots influence in a number of areas.

A MIXED MESSAGE: SWEENEY, THE SEIU, AND
FAMILY LEAVE

When the UAW dropped the social unionism baton, why didn't another union or the AFL-CIO pick it up and lead the charge? The SEIU appeared a likely candidate because Sweeney, its president, actively sought to raise the political profile of his union on social issues. Sweeney, as head of the AFL-CIO health-care committee, pushed instead for a joint labor-management solution rather than a single-payer arrangement. Even though Sweeney could be critical of business at times, he believed that a satisfactory solution on health care would come about because of business participation—not in spite of business participation. Because the business community would never endorse a single-payer plan, this approach was doomed from the start, in his view. Several factors swayed Sweeney, namely the institutions of the private welfare state; his extensive participation in Dunlop-style policy-making over the years, which is examined in this section; and finally, organized labor's fundamental misunderstanding of the shallow roots of the private-sector safety net, discussed in chapter 6.

Health care was a particularly salient issue for the Service Employees for a number of reasons. In its early years, the relatively small union was composed primarily of building-service employees. By the 1970s, however, the SEIU made deep inroads in the hospital industry and the public sector. By the early 1990s, health-care workers comprised nearly a third of its 1 million members, and public-sector employees constituted about half.[77] Much of the rest of the SEIU membership was employed in the service sector, where wages tend to be low, and benefits nonexistent. These service-sector employees increasingly found themselves undercut by employers who subcontracted out janitorial and other services to nonunion firms paying lower wages that did not provide health and other benefits.[78] Sweeney's direct involvement in the union's health-care cost-containment efforts, and experience with stepped-up pressure from employers at the bargaining table to reduce health benefits, prompted him to suggest that the AFL-CIO establish a health-care committee in the mid-1980s.[79]

Another reason health care emerged as an important SEIU issue during the 1980s was because Sweeney sought to raise the political profile of his union. The union president wanted to dispel once and for all the SEIU's image as an organization primarily concerned with protecting the interests of janitors. In a 1986 column that appeared in the union's flagship publication, Sweeney proclaimed that the SEIU was now "proud to be the union both of the janitors and the professionals."[80] During this period, Sweeney moved to position his union under the mantle of social unionism historically associated with the UAW and other unions.[81] One of the union's first high-profile steps in a more activist direction came at the prodding of hospital workers within SEIU ranks who were at the epicenter of the outbreak of the AIDS crisis. In 1983, members of Local 250 in northern California formed an AIDS education committee that put them at the forefront of devising precautionary measures for health-care workers, lobbying the government for more research and education money, and fighting

AIDS-related discrimination. They also pushed the SEIU to sponsor the AFL-CIO's first resolution on AIDS.[82]

The union sought a higher political and policy profile because of dramatic changes in its membership composition. During the 1980s several large state associations of public employees decided to join the SEIU. These public-sector employees wanted good data on public policy issues, such as the impact of state and federal budget cuts on government services. The union responded by expanding its policy staff and, consequently, raising its profile on broader social and economic issues.[83] During this period, as the size of the union's female and minority membership grew, the SEIU, like other service-sector and white-collar unions, focused more of its legislative activities on making redistributive claims on the state. Female and minority union members tend to favor demands for social insurance, public education, job training, welfare, and civil rights legislation because they are more likely to face discrimination on the job and occupy the lower rungs of the socioeconomic ladder.[84]

In the mid-1980s, staff members convinced Sweeney that the family leave bill pending before the U.S. Congress was an ideal vehicle to raise the political profile of the SEIU because half the union's membership were women. Sweeney agreed to a serious commitment to the bill and to conduct a major campaign around it.[85] "It was the first attempt by this union to address the needs of working women as well as working men," explained Kathleen M. Skrabut of the SEIU. She said the "Work and Family" campaign launched in the fall of 1987 signaled the debut of the SEIU as a union with broader social policy concerns. That campaign had three pillars: family leave, universal health care, and an increase in the minimum wage.[86]

The battle over the family leave bill set the stage for later struggles over universal health care in ways that the labor community and other supporters did not understand at the time, but that the business community, especially small business, understood all too well. Big business and small put up a fierce fight against the Family and Medical Leave Act, which would grant several weeks of unpaid leave to new parents and employees caring for elderly parents, sick children, or ailing spouses. That act became a kind of poster child in the larger battle against federal mandates.[87] Even Fortune 500 corporations that already provided family leave benefits to their employees joined in the fray against the measure.[88]

The fiercest resistance came from the small business community, in particular, the National Federation of Independent Business, the feisty and premier lobbying organization for small business. According to John Motley, the NFIB's chief lobbyist at the time, "the whole idea of fighting to the bitter end [on family and medical leave] . . . was to show them that the employer mandate battle was going to be bitter, it was going to be bloody."[89] In 1986, the White House Conference on Small Business singled out the campaign against family leave as one of its top priorities, second only to an overhaul of the nation's liability laws.[90] In the battle over the family leave bill, the 600,000-member NFIB discovered the virtues of just saying no as a legislative strategy. "We had never taken that unbending an attitude" before on legislation, explained Michael O. Roush of the NFIB. "Saying no to something like that" had a "tremendous appeal to our members. It was easy for them to understand." In the subsequent debate over the Clinton health proposal, the NFIB again employed that strategy with great success as it remained implacably opposed to any employer-mandate proposal that would require businesses to provide health insurance to their workers.[91]

The SEIU was at the hub of the fight for family leave, as were a number of women's organizations. The Service Employees helped bring other unions in on the issue and develop a coalition of 250 organizations that included groups ranging from the Women's Legal Defense Fund and the AARP to the Alzheimer's Association.[92] Here there was little talk about joining with business. Rather, the SEIU and other unions rebutted the hysterical claims of the U.S. Chamber of Commerce and other business organizations that the measure would be a financial hardship for business.[93] Advocates of the family leave bill argued that the measure would save businesses money by increasing productivity and helping employers retain a loyal workforce. They also shrewdly positioned the measure so that it would bask in the glow of the calls coming from conservative groups for the defense of "family values."[94] The bill passed both houses of Congress in 1991 and 1992, after an exemption for employers with 50 employees or less was added to the legislation. The House was unable to muster the necessary votes to override a veto by President George Bush.[95] In his first major legislative action as president, Clinton signed the measure into law, despite continued opposition by business.[96]

The ruckus over family leave had important implications for the health-care debate that organized labor did not appreciate at the time. It should have put labor on notice about the deep apprehension within the business sector about employer-mandated benefits of any kind, even among firms already providing a particular benefit. Yet as employers engaged in a pitched battle against family leave, Sweeney and other important labor leaders made the case that business, by and large, was ready to endorse a comprehensive health-care reform proposal that would require employers to pay for a minimum package of employee health benefits.

Sweeney pursued a two-track policy with respect to political action, alternately wearing the radical and conservative cap. From the early to mid-

1980s, he was an outspoken critic of business and the Democrats as Reaganomics took root in the United States. During the tax-cutting frenzy of President Reagan's first six months in office, he expressed disappointment with the Democrats for not doing a better job at protecting the interests of working people.[97] In the wake of Walter Mondale's defeat in the 1984 presidential election and the party's new efforts to woo business, Sweeney charged that the Democratic Party was "trying to become the handmaiden of the big financial interests."[98] He also predicted that a massive debate would soon erupt in the Democratic Party between economic populists and the neo-liberals who say "you must be more Republican on economic issues."[99] Sweeney was strident in his criticism of business in general, and health-care providers in particular, as he denounced the rise of for-profit hospitals and nursing homes and spearheaded aggressive organizing drives to recruit new members.[100] Sweeney's union became known for the comparatively radical approach it took in organizing new members, devoting about one-third of its $30-million national budget to that task. It hired young, fairly radical organizers, which it recruited from community organizations, citizens groups, and the workplace, and tailored its organizing campaigns to the local community.[101]

During his 1995 campaign for the AFL-CIO presidency, Sweeney repeatedly talked about his readiness to call out the janitors and other workers to block the bridges if that's what it took to get justice in the workplace. In his tenure as president of the Service Employees, Sweeney also invested a great deal in more sober, top-down tactics. Shortly after becoming head of the union in 1980, he was invited to join Dunlop's Labor-Management Group as one of organized labor's eight representatives on the body. He also served on the Democratic Party's Hunt Commission and as a member of its Labor Council. In 1989, Health and Human Services Secretary Louis W. Sullivan chose Sweeney as one of labor's two representatives on the Advisory Council on Social Security, which the Bush administration expected would shape its position on health policy.

One of Sweeney's most significant organizational ties was his participation in the National Leadership Commission on Health Care and its successor organization, the National Leadership Coalition for Health Care Reform (NLCHCR). The commission was one of the most prominent private-sector groups created in the 1980s to address the country's health-care problems. Sweeney was the only representative from organized labor to serve on the commission, which drew three dozen people from academia, the health-care field, and business, including insurers and Fortune 500 companies. In 1989, the commission released a report that endorsed a "play-or-pay" model for health-care reform based on an employer mandate.[102] The commission carefully avoided any use of the word "mandate" to describe its proposal, opting instead for what it hoped would be a more politically neutral term— "shared responsibility." The report was endorsed by 30 of the 36 commission members, including Sweeney, and was a precursor to the bipartisan Pepper Commission, a government-appointed panel that endorsed a modified "play-or-pay" solution in September 1990.[103]

As head of the AFL-CIO health-care committee, Sweeney tried to persuade other labor leaders that business would join hands in good faith with labor to find an acceptable solution to the nation's health-care troubles. At the time, companies increasingly were turning to replacement workers to break strikes; holding down wages with threats to relocate production overseas or to low-wage, low-benefit, right-to-work states; shifting more of the costs of health care onto their employees; and vigorously opposing organized labor on issues like plant-closing legislation and family leave. Nonetheless, Sweeney sought to convince other labor leaders that business was sincere in its commitment to work with labor and other groups to find a mutually satisfactory health-care solution. One of Sweeney's "early and consistent views about all this," according to Gerald M. Shea, his longtime assistant, was that "there was potentially common truck to be made between employers and consumers on health-care issues."[104] Labor fundamentally misjudged the business community in several significant respects.

CHRYSLER, IACOCCA, AND HEALTH POLICY

Around 1989, Sweeney and a number of other labor leaders talked more and more about the potential for big business, small business, organized labor, and even parts of the medical establishment to be "singing seductively similar songs on health care solutions" before too long.[105] The immediate catalyst for this optimistic view of business and labor working side-by-side to resolve the health-care issue was a series of remarks that Lee Iacocca, chairman of the board and chief executive officer of the Chrysler Corporation, made in 1989 about health care. On several occasions that year Iacocca said he would support a federal government solution to the nation's pressing health-care problems because rising medical costs were making U.S. products noncompetitive in the global marketplace. UAW president Douglas A. Fraser quipped that Iacocca spent so much time talking about the need for universal health care that he was beginning to sound like an Italian socialist.[106]

When asked why they thought business was willing to work with labor to find an acceptable solution for health-care reform, labor officials invariably brought up Iacocca and the positive signals they believed were emanating from the automobile industry and the business sector more broadly. How-

Jott on health ins ref

ever, in many ways, Iacocca did not represent the views of the automobile sector as a whole on the issue of health care. And the views of the auto industry did not represent wider business sentiment, or even Fortune 500 firms, which by and large provided their employees with comprehensive health insurance.

Labor and many of those who study labor tend to overestimate the degree of progressive sentiment within the business sector. The tendency is to blow out of proportion any sympathetic muttering from a prominent business figure, especially during periods when labor feels under siege on all sides, as in the 1930s and the 1980s. In the 1930s, U.S. Rubber was one of the first to break ranks in the business community as the company staked out a more conciliatory approach to organized labor and suggested that unions were not inherently dangerous and ideologically unacceptable.[107] Major business figures like Owen D. Young and Gerard Swope of General Electric echoed these views, reasoning that unionism was inevitable and that cooperation promised better results than continued resistance.[108] Over the next two decades, this progressive strategy of allowing unions a "positive welcome rather than simply granting them limited legitimacy" gained some supporters within the business sector.[109] But the progressives never came near to gaining the upper hand in the business community in the postwar years.[110] The progressive strategy of labor-management accommodation "attracted more academic attention than it ever won managerial followers."[111] In a similar fashion, Iacocca was a misleading bellwether of wider business sentiment on the health-care issue.

Organized labor's readiness to view Iacocca as somehow representative of wider business sentiment on health policy is surprising in several respects. First, although UAW officials expressed grudging admiration for Iacocca and applauded his attacks on Reaganomics, for years they conceded in private that the Chrysler executive was a loose cannon and an outlier in the business community.[112] They questioned Iacocca's political acumen, cautioned that "Iacocca is given to exaggeration,"[113] and warned that Chrysler executives tend to be overly optimistic in their dealings with legislators.[114] During the delicate discussions surrounding the 1979 government bailout of Chrysler, they admonished Iacocca to devote himself full time to handling the company's problems and to "stop attempting to be the self-appointed spokesperson for the auto industry and corporate America on labor-management relations."[115]

Chrysler's exceptionalism in the business community rested on more than just the force of Iacocca's personality. The Big Three automakers historically have not been joined at the hip with respect to social, economic, and labor policy. For instance, the famous 1937 sit-down strike brought General Motors into a narrow, legalistic acceptance of a unionized workforce on the eve of World War II. By contrast, Chrysler pursued a belligerent approach to labor-management relations until well after the war.[116] During the 1980s, the Big Three divided over trade issues, with Ford and Chrysler adhering to more protectionist policies and General Motors more inclined to sing the praises of free trade.[117] Iacocca was one of the leading business voices raised in support of more corporatist-style policy-making and of an industrial policy to lift the country out of its economic doldrums.[118] In the 1996 contract negotiations between the Big Three and the UAW, the relationship between the autoworkers and Ford was recognized as warm and close; the one with GM as icy; and Chrysler fell somewhere in between. GM was willing to weather expensive strikes over the issue of outsourcing while Ford took a relatively more conciliatory approach.[119]

Just as the 1937 sit-down strike was a defining moment for General Motors, the 1979 government bailout was a defining moment for Chrysler. Chrysler was widely perceived within the automobile sector and the broader business community as far more willing to tolerate a heavier government hand in social and economic policy because of its experience with the bailout.[120] The 1979 bailout opened a rift between Chrysler and the rest of the business community that does not appear to have healed entirely. Chrysler resigned from the Business Roundtable because the elite business organization opposed the bailout.[121] The chasm between the Business Roundtable and Chrysler widened again during the 1993–94 tiff over health policy as the auto company tried unsuccessfully to reduce the influence within the Business Roundtable of insurance industry members, who dominated the organization's key committees forging its stance on health policy.

Chrysler is unique within the business community in another respect. For many years Walter B. Maher, who is widely regarded as a well-informed zealot on health-care issues, headed its public policy department. Maher was director of employee benefits at Chrysler in Detroit before transferring to its Washington office in 1989, principally to focus on health policy. He worked doggedly to make health care a high-profile issue at Chrysler and in the wider business community, beginning with the calculated publication of Iacocca's 1989 column in which the auto executive appeared to endorse a government-led solution.[122] Maher is the rare business executive who draws praise from labor officials and public-interest groups despite the widespread disillusionment with business after the 1993–94 attempt at comprehensive health-care reform failed. Many credit him with needling the business community over the years to do the right thing with respect to health policy. Some of them are even convinced that, given his druthers, Maher would have no problem with a single-payer solution.[123] This may also be the reason why some members of the business community were uneasy about Chrysler's outspokenness on health-care matters.[124]

Labor's readiness to embrace Iacocca and Chrysler as the voice of reason and progressivism on health-care matters was surprising in one final respect. In the mid-1980s, Iacocca was a kind of pop culture hero in the United States, making cameo appearances on popular television shows like "Miami Vice" and appearing in Chrysler's ubiquitous "Pride Is Back" commercials. In the wake of the devastating 1981–82 recession, Iacocca became a national icon of the rebounding U.S. economy and the can-do spirit that Americans so readily identify with.[125] By the late 1980s, his name was also synonymous with the excesses of corporate America. Public officials, citizens, and late-night comedians regularly invoked his name before launching into a tirade or monologue about what was wrong with corporate America.[126] They ridiculed Iacocca for taking home nearly $21 million in salary, stock options, and other compensation in 1986 ($17 million in 1987), the highest of any U.S. executive, while moving to shut down auto plants at home, shift production overseas, and lay off thousands of employees. Iacocca, once extolled as an ideal Democratic presidential candidate, by 1988 found himself the target of Democratic commercials that railed against corporate greed.[127]

Labor's depiction of Iacocca as an ally and the voice of reason on health policy put unions in a paradoxical spot. Labor officials would approvingly cite Iacocca's remarks on health care at length. At the same time they were engaged in a rancorous campaign against the corporate excesses of the 1980s, as represented by Iacocca and other handsomely-paid executives, and lobbied hard for tightening government restrictions on such items as corporate leveraged buyouts (LBOs).[128] What resulted were a number of striking instances of political cognitive dissonance on the part of organized labor. In 1989, the *UAW Washington Report* approvingly republished the infamous column by Iacocca in which the Chrysler executive contended that business executives were more receptive than they once were to making the government responsible for financing health care.[129] Yet in the same issue, on the page immediately following Iacocca's column, UAW officials singled out Chrysler, Ford, and GM for their "astronomical" executive salaries in what they described as "Detroit's annual executive pig out."[130]

For several reasons Chrysler proved an unreliable bellwether of sentiment in the business community on health policy and broader social and economic questions. This is not to say, however, that Iacocca's views on the need for a government-based solution for health-care reform were not echoed anywhere else. Other business leaders drew attention to the problem of escalating costs and indicated their willingness to countenance more government intervention in health care.[131]

Support for a comprehensive solution that would entail greater government involvement in health care was concentrated among executives who hailed from the unionized sectors of the economy, notably autos, steel, and foodstuffs. These sectors generally were more receptive to a government-led solution for a variety of reasons. First, it was harder for them to shift the burden of escalating health-care costs onto their employees because collective bargaining agreements and unionization provided workers with protections that nonunion employees did not have.[132] Second, the contractual obligation to provide their retirees with good health benefits was becoming a more expensive proposition because these companies had older work-forces and more retirees.[133] Finally, unionized firms felt they shouldered an unfair share of the nation's health-care tab in at least two ways. They provided medical benefits to both employees and their dependents, many of whom were employed by companies that provide no or only minimal health benefits.[134] And hospitals and other health-care providers were increasing their rates to offset the expense of providing uncompensated care to the growing population of the uninsured and underinsured and to make up for federal cutbacks in Medicare and other public programs.[135]

For all of these reasons, unionized firms appeared more likely to endorse a government-led solution for comprehensive reform. However, a number of union and nonunion firms balked at the government route to reform long before the Clinton plan was unveiled—indeed, long before Clinton was but a glint in the eye of many Democrats. The most notorious instance was the schism that developed in the NLCHCR, which was launched in March 1990 and counted among its membership about 60 large companies, unions, and advocacy groups. About one-third of its members refused to sign the agreement when it became apparent in late 1991 that the NLCHCR would endorse a health-care solution predicated on a tax increase, government price controls, and, most significantly, a mandate requiring employers to provide health insurance for their employees or pay a penalty tax (the so-called "play-or-pay" option). Several key corporations quit the NLCHCR altogether. The proposal's core group of supporters came primarily from a single sector—steel.[136]

Several major corporations refused to back the agreement because, as major suppliers to the health-care system, they believed government price controls would cut into their revenues. The renegade firms included Kodak, Grace, DuPont, and General Electric, which has a large unionized workforce. Some of the disenchanted firms were opposed to any further government regulation. "Maybe someday we can look at prices and mandates, but we have not exhausted all of the less radical solutions yet," remarked David B. Helms, DuPont's senior benefits consultant.[137] In explaining the surprisingly fierce opposition to the idea of an employer mandate among some members of the NLCHCR, William F. Little of Ford indicated that some firms were more ideologically driven, especially once a policy issue such as health care assumed a high public profile. "If you are opposed to a mandate, you are opposed to a mandate," he said.[138]

The biggest surprise, perhaps, was the refusal of AT&T and the "Baby Bells" (the regional phone companies) to endorse the proposal. Most of the phone companies had joined the NLCHCR as a consequence of contracts negotiated in the 1989 Baby Bell strike, which obligated them to be jointly involved with the Communications Workers of America in seeking national solutions to the health-care problem.[139] The phone companies were loath to sign on to the NLCHCR proposal because they did not want to appear to endorse greater government regulation of the health-care sector at the same time that an unprecedented deregulation of the telecommunications industry was being negotiated in Washington.[140] All the phone companies quickly abandoned the NLCHCR and, except for Bell South, formed the core of a new business-only group of about 25 firms called the Corporate Health Care Coalition.

The criteria for membership in the new business group revealed subtle distinctions that leading corporations made among themselves on the health-care issue. Even though AT&T and the "Baby Bells" contended with heavily unionized workforces, they were welcomed into the new business group. The automobile and steel companies were not welcome. The organization "did not want any companies that were driven by their labor unions," explained G. Lawrence Atkins, the organization's coordinator. The group also excluded any firms that were major health-care providers. Companies with huge retiree health-care costs were also not invited to join because of fears that this single concern would determine the stance they took on health-care reform issues. (Bethlehem Steel Corporation, for example, has two retirees for each employee on its payroll.)[141] Finally, companies widely seen as amenable to the idea of having the "government take this off our hands" were excluded, and here again Atkins singled out the automobile companies.[142]

To sum up, compared to business, organized labor took a less nuanced view of sentiment within the business sector on health-care issues. It overestimated the extent of support for greater government intervention in the medical system. Union leaders were led astray by the views of Chrysler, and Lee Iacocca in particular, on health-care reform and failed to appreciate the automobile company's singular status within the business sector. Furthermore, labor officials did not fully appreciate how the competing interests of corporations in other policy areas might determine what position they ultimately took on the issue of health policy. Companies like GE and DuPont certainly had concerns about escalating employee medical costs. But as major medical suppliers, they were reluctant to endorse any solution that might cut into their revenues. In the case of the phone companies, a deeper concern about the impending deregulation of the telecommunications industry trumped their apprehension about rising health-care costs.[143]

Labor's failure to accurately gauge sentiment within the business sector had enormous political consequences. Kirkland, Sweeney, and other labor leaders premised much of their political strategy on the mistaken belief that business—or at least big business—could be counted on to cooperate with organized labor in resolving the pressing problems of the U.S. medical system. As such they were cool to the growing sentiment in the late 1980s for a single-payer solution. This fueled significant divisions within organized labor that are discussed in greater detail in the next two chapters.

In the decades after World War II, organized labor emerged as a major nationwide electoral organization for the Democratic Party.[144] By the late 1960s and 1970s, that alliance was under severe strain because unions and the Democrats were in disarray over the Vietnam War, race issues, and electoral politics. Nevertheless, once labor made its commitment to an employer mandate in 1978, that commitment remained intact, even as the disarray of the 1970s yielded to a remarkable degree of internal unity for organized labor by the mid-1980s.[145] From the mid-1980s onward, organized labor's faith that business could be a constructive ally in health policy blossomed despite enormous changes in the U.S. political economy that dramatically eroded the bond between employer and employee. Several institutional and political factors explain this outcome. Unions remained captive to the Dunlop approach to labor-management relations, which became institutionalized in the immediate postwar years. The enactment of ERISA in 1974 helped solidify a coalition of employers and organized labor in defense of the private welfare state. Organized labor remained reluctant to break with the Dunlop way despite a string of political defeats, beginning with business's fierce and successful mobilization again *common situs* legislation and labor law reform in 1977–78.

As the corporate onslaught against organized labor gathered steam in the late 1970s and 1980s, some labor leaders argued that unions should take a stance on health care and other issues that was more independent of business and the Democratic Party. UAW president Fraser created the Progressive Alliance in 1979 to challenge the Dunlop-style of labor-management relations, but the new organization quickly closed up shop. Its supporters disagreed on whether it was designed to be a think tank, the catalyst for a new political movement, or the beginnings of a third party. Faced with growing dissension in its ranks, and an unfavorable economic climate in the automobile industry, the UAW recommitted itself to working with business and the Democrats. By committing itself so wholeheartedly to the idea of "jointness," the UAW alienated itself from more natural allies in other labor unions and advocacy organizations that could be counted on to rally for universal health care and national health insurance.

Labor leaders fundamentally misjudged sentiment in the business community. The automobile sector turned out to be an unreliable barometer of wider business sentiment on health policy. Chrysler's Iacocca was a particularly controversial ally for organized labor. Although he talked a good line about the need for universal health care and for a federal government solution, by the end of the decade he was one of the preeminent symbols of the corporate excesses of the go-go 1980s.

Organized labor was prone to take a far less nuanced view of the interests of the business sector than business executives were. Labor mistakenly assumed that the interests of business could be reduced to bottom-line calculations on one particular item—in this case, health-care costs. As this chapter demonstrated, firms, like unions, are a kind of "political coalition."[146] They need to be understood not as unitary actors but rather as complex institutions "whose decisions are the product of the internal political processes as well as external pressures." As such, business decisions in the area of social policy are not merely the product of immediate bottom-line calculations. As Steven Tolliday and Jonathan Zeitlin suggest, noneconomic factors like company history, power struggles, personalities, and ideology deeply affect a firm's political decisions.[147]

Labor leaders made a series of political misjudgments within a very particular institutional context that severely restricted their political free will and impeded organized labor's efforts to develop an independent position on health policy. As a result, unions pursued what was an elusive alliance with business. The AFL-CIO's faith in a corporate-led solution for health care remained solid, even in the wake of the war that big business, and small, waged war against the Family and Medical Leave Act in the late 1980s and early 1990s. Eager to court business, the AFL-CIO leadership, notably Kirkland and Sweeney, maneuvered the federation away from the single-payer position just as Canadian-style solutions were enjoying a new burst of interest and respectability. This strategy was a costly one. As argued in the following chapter, the employer-provided system of benefits in the United States that Sweeney and other labor officials hailed as an essential building block for health-care reform was erected on an extremely weak foundation and was rapidly collapsing nationwide by the 1980s. In going out of its way to show how business and labor saw eye to eye on many health-care questions, organized labor missed an important opportunity to develop a broader critique of the U.S. political economy, one that would resonate with its membership and other potential allies.

CHAPTER 6

Taking Care of Business

The Political Economy of the Health-Care
Cost Burden

The Clinton administration's Health Security Act represented more than the sum of all the health policy prescriptions amassed in its 1,342 pages. The plan was eventually sold to the American public as a prescription not just for what ailed the U.S. medical system, but also for what ailed the U.S. economy and the American worker. In the course of pitching its proposal, the administration made some remarkable claims about the U.S. political economy, claims that organized labor helped legitimize over the years in its eagerness to forge an alliance with business on the health-care issue. In endorsing the Clinton plan and its legislative antecedents, organized labor did not just give its imprimatur to a particular set of health policies. It also endorsed a highly selective understanding of the U.S. political economy, one that contrasted sharply with the case labor tried to make in other policy realms, notably in the 1993 fight over NAFTA.

Much of organized labor treated health policy as if it traveled in its own orbit, subject to the pulls of the need to trim the federal budget and remain economically "competitive," but not to the gravitational pulls of the rest of the U.S. political economy. Paradoxically, at the same time that management was waging a massive and highly effective assault on the very pillars of the postwar compact, including the right to secure full-time and predictable employment with adequate health and pension benefits, organized labor's confidence that business was a constructive partner in health-care reform remained largely unshaken.

The Clinton health plan was developed and sold on the basis of several assumptions about the U.S. political economy and welfare state that emerged during earlier debates over health-care initiatives based on an em-

114

ployer mandate. In its eagerness to forge an alliance with business, labor embraced and promoted these broader assumptions in discussions of health policy over the years. This chapter focuses on three of these assumptions. These three are significant because they molded organized labor's stance on health-care reform and its political strategies, notably the allies it sought and the way it pitched the issue to its rank and file and the wider public. Taken together, these assumptions helped give shape to an alternative worldview, one that was quite favorable to business and that impaired organized labor's political efficacy in health policy.

The first assumption was that the employer-mandate formula was not all that radical, or even new, a solution but merely was built upon the well-established institution of employment-based benefits in the United States. The second and related assumption was that business bore most of the brunt of the private welfare state and thus the increasingly heavy burden of escalating medical costs. The third was that health-care costs imperiled the competitiveness of U.S. firms in the international marketplace. As such, these costs represented perhaps the prime threat to the U.S. economy and were the root cause for most of the economic woes of the U.S. worker.

These assumptions were just that—assumptions. Organized labor treated them as a set of inevitable facts that were not debatable. However, a sustained and independent questioning of these assumptions might have revealed their contingency and highlighted that they were "propositions" rather than uncontestable truths. Instead, organized labor generally accepted them as "hegemonic truths." These assumptions, with labor's help, were embedded in a compelling causal story that appeared to explain some of the major shortcomings of the U.S. political economy. "Appearances" are the bread and butter of politics. Political actors—be they labor leaders, business executives, public-interest groups, or government officials—all compete to create convincing narratives that define the cause of a particular problem in such a way that certain policy proposals appear as natural and obvious solutions. The most skillful political actors are the ones most adept at manipulating the characteristics of issues "while making it seem as though they are simply describing facts."[1] Policy and political outcomes depend in part on how one particular definition and explanation of a problem wins out.[2] New ideas often take flight on the wings of compelling causal stories that come to be accepted as fact, not interpretations.

This chapter scrutinizes each of these assumptions in turn and the causal story in which they are lodged. In doing so, it underlines the "ideological" rather than "truth" nature of these assumptions. Such questioning bolsters the analytical claim that adopting a different set of assumptions—equally plausible—would lead to a different political strategy with possibly different political consequences.

THE WEAK FOUNDATIONS OF THE PRIVATE-SECTOR SAFETY NET

In one of her early appearances before Congress in the fall of 1993, Hillary Rodham Clinton stressed in her opening remarks the importance of building on the job-based system of health benefits, or what she referred to as the "employer/employee partnership."[3] In emphasizing how an employer mandate was a fundamentally conservative—not radical—solution, Mrs. Clinton echoed a theme that was popular with much of organized labor beginning in the late 1970s. When labor officials initially agreed to support an employer mandate in 1978 during the Carter administration, they conceded in private the enormity of what they proposed by describing their new plan as a "program of peaceful revolution."[4] Over the next 15 years, labor and other would-be reformers consistently downplayed the wider political significance of the employer-mandate idea. They instead emphasized how the government would merely require businesses to do what most of them—at least the socially responsible ones—already did voluntarily.[5]

The belief among labor leaders, Mrs. Clinton, and other would-be reformers that business would eventually agree to support an employer-mandate solution because it ratified what most employers did voluntarily, and appealed to the bottom-line interests of business, was a big leap of faith in a few important respects. First, as discussed in chapter 5, business support for comprehensive health-care reform based on an employer mandate may have been broad, but it certainly was not deep, as labor officials belatedly discovered. As shown in this section, the employment-based system of benefits in the United States that Sweeney and other labor officials lauded actually rested on an extremely weak and shaky foundation. Organized labor's talk about pursuing a health-care strategy built upon the existing job-based system of benefits obscured that the system was in the midst of a radical transformation. Firms were experimenting widely with cutbacks in health and other benefits and with new ways of organizing the workforce, notably a greater reliance on part-time and other contingent workers.

Since at least the late 1970s, employers talked among themselves about how the time was coming to curtail private-sector benefits. With the retrenchment of the public-sector safety net and the decline of the unionized workforce, employers felt under less pressure to provide good benefits as a way to prevent the expansion of government programs or to compete with unionized firms for the best workers. A major theme of an important conference titled "Rethinking Employee Benefit Assumptions," sponsored more than two decades ago by the Conference Board, a prominent business organization, was that basic assumptions about employee benefits might no longer be true. In his summary of the gathering, David A. Weeks predicted that benefit packages would probably not continue to improve, and that employees would be required to contribute more for items like health insurance and pensions in the near future. Most significantly, he predicted that companies considered leaders in providing liberal benefits would no longer be given credit for "progressiveness and farsightedness."[6]

Labor's talk since the late 1970s about pursuing a health-care reform strategy that built upon the existing job-based system of benefits obscured a radical transformation. From the Second World War until the 1970s, employer-based health plans covered an increasing proportion of Americans.[7] After that, coverage shrank as the initiative in industrial relations shifted radically from the union to nonunion sector and from labor to management in ways that had important consequences for the private-sector safety net, including health benefits. Many nonunion firms initially provided comparable wage and benefit packages to attract the best workers and keep unions at bay. As firms became more adept at slowing and then stopping the expansion of collective bargaining and union membership, the initiative in the private sector shifted. In an important reversal, innovations in labor-management relations originated in nonunion firms and then spread to union ones.[8] Nonunion firms were the first to experiment widely with cutbacks in benefits and with new ways of organizing the workplace and workforce, notably a greater reliance on part-time and other types of contingent workers.[9] These changes together signified in many ways a collapse of the industrial relations regime established by the labor policies of the New Deal and the subsequent spread of collective bargaining.[10]

What emerged is a several-tiered system of industrial relations ridden with inconsistencies and internal contradictions that has important consequences for U.S. health policy and the shrinking of the private-sector safety net. At the highest levels, some leading business executives appear committed to working with labor leaders to promote labor-management cooperation on issues like productivity, organization of the workplace, and health-care cost containment. At the firm level, however, they engage in sophisticated strategies to keep new plants and operations free of unions and shrink their unionized workforce through outsourcing, subcontracting, and the like.[11] They also seek to reduce their wage and benefit bills by hiring more temporary and part-time workers, and even "leasing" back their former employees from the burgeoning crop of new employee leasing firms.[12]

This period of accelerated political and labor-market experimentation began more than two decades ago as firms sought to meet the perceived challenges of escalating inflation, stagnating growth, increased economic competition from abroad, and growing anti-business sentiment at home. In the mid-1970s, a consensus quickly emerged among business executives about the need to increase their involvement in political activities to meet the new challenges. However, a clear consensus about the specific policies and economic model to pursue as the long-standing agreement in support of commercial Keynesianism eroded did not emerge immediately.[13] Business executives groped around for alternatives and pursued a number of seemingly contradictory or inconsistent policies for a while.[14] Eventually a radically new understanding of the employer-employee relationship took shape, one centered on the "flexible" firm willing to shed labor in short order and embrace a contingent workforce.[15] The flexible firm was seen as the nimble economic actor most likely to succeed in a turbulent and fiercely competitive economic environment.[16]

In the formative years of the contingent labor market, organized labor appeared to underestimate the enormous consequences that a growing reliance on temporary, part-time, and self-employed workers would have for the U.S. labor force and for social policy.[17] Unions and public-interest groups were largely silent as the temporary help industry, "through deliberate and concerted action," successfully persuaded the courts, state legislators, and government administrative bodies to define temporary help arrangements in such a way that legitimized and legalized the widespread use of contingent workers.[18]

Minimal resistance from organized labor and state actors, notably the Carter and Reagan administrations, helped spur on this search for greater labor market flexibility. In 1978 the Carter administration reluctantly moved toward endorsing a health-care solution based on an employer mandate. Paradoxically, several months earlier it gave state sanction to greater experimentation with internal labor market structures that would weaken the attachment between employer and employee, and as a consequence, the link between employment and health benefits.[19] In the fall of 1977, Carter issued a memorandum to Cabinet members and agency directors encouraging them to make much greater use of part-time workers. The White House's new policy had an important demonstration effect on big business. By the late 1970s, many big firms were no longer reluctant to hire large numbers of part-timers on a permanent basis and emulated the federal government's wide-scale experimentation with part-time arrangements.[20]

As the Carter administration helped legitimize the widespread use of part-time employment, the Reagan administration helped sanction greater use of temporary workers. The Reagan administration's best known contribution to creating a more flexible workforce was its decision to fire striking air traffic controllers in 1981 and bring in replacement workers. This action is widely credited with popularizing the practice of hiring temporary and permanent replacement workers to break strikes and unions.[21] The Reagan administration helped sanction the creation of a "just-in-time" workforce in other important—but less well known—ways. In 1985, the administration promulgated new regulations that allowed the federal government to employ some people for up to four years without providing them benefits comparable to regular federal employees.[22] Three years later, the federal government's Office of Personnel Management decided that the use of temporary workers supplied by outside agencies or contractors did not obligate the government as an employer. In effect, the decision overturned long-standing civil service regulations understood to prohibit the use of temporary workers. This paved the way for the widespread use of "temps" throughout the federal government.[23] The federal government also subcontracted more work out to the private sector, often to firms whose employee benefit packages paled in comparison to those received by the typical federal worker.[24]

Temporary employment, which had trended upward since the 1970s, shot up in the late 1980s and early 1990s,[25] as did the number of part-time and self-employed workers.[26] Despite the dramatic growth in the flexible workforce, the plight of contingent workers remained marginal to most discussions of health-care reform even though these workers are more likely to be uninsured or underinsured.[27] For example, the Consolidated Omnibus Budget Reconciliation Act (COBRA) of 1985 required that employers continue to offer group health insurance coverage to full-time employees after certain events that would otherwise cause a loss of coverage (such as job loss, retirement, or a change in marital status). However, this landmark legislation did not extend this protection to part-timers or other members of the contingent workforce. During Congressional hearings on the 1987 Minimal Health Benefits for All Workers Act, there was little discussion about what ramifications the proliferation of part-time, temporary, and contingent employment in the U.S. might have for any health-care legislation premised, as this one was, on an employer mandate.[28] When this issue came up briefly, labor leaders remained confident that the 17.5–hour cutoff for benefits would not prompt employers to reduce the weekly hours of their part-timers to avoid paying their health benefits.[29] At minimum, these political developments underline labor's failure to fully comprehend the changing nature of the employment contract within the U.S. political economy and the related failure to insert this understanding into relevant political and policy debates.

Despite the ongoing restructuring of the U.S. economy and expansion of the contingent workforce, the employer mandate remained an attractive option to labor and the Democrats. In its final report in 1990, the bipartisan, blue ribbon Pepper Commission endorsed an employer-mandate solution.[30] Proposal supporters, which included almost all the ranking Democrats, stressed a familiar theme about how the Pepper plan built upon the existing system of job-based benefits and thus was evolutionary, not revolutionary. Republican opponents denounced the mandate as "essentially a head tax on labor."[31] The major dissenter on the left was the only dissenter and Democrat to raise any fundamental questions about the fairness of the employment-based system of benefits, especially in an age when employers were demonstrating a greater willingness and capacity to restructure internal labor markets. In his dissent, Rep. Pete Stark (D-Calif.) underscored the jerry-built nature of the system, its perennially uncertain status within the U.S. welfare state, and the plight of contingent workers.[32]

In subsequent discussions surrounding the various comprehensive health-care reform bills introduced in the 1991–92 period, the health-care issue was seldom tied to broader economic questions associated with the search by employers for greater labor market flexibility nor to issues concerning the future viability of the private welfare state. On a few rare occasions, some policy experts and legislators challenged the whole premise of perpetuating an employment-based system.[33] For the most part, however, few called into question the long-term viability of the employment-based system of benefits at a time when employers sought to create a more flexible labor market.[34]

To sum up briefly to this point, the employer mandate incorporated in the Clinton proposal and its legislative forerunners was pitched as a fundamentally conservative solution to the nation's health-care woes. By making the case for an employer mandate based on the argument that most employers already provided health benefits for their employees, and that the solution as such was a moderate one, labor unwittingly helped draw public attention away from the enormous transformations taking place in the labor market and from employer culpability in these changes. It also downplayed the huge gaps and inequities on which the private welfare state was built. As a result, labor, trapped by ideas it had adopted earlier, helped minimize how vulnerable the institution of job-based benefits was to shifting political and economic winds. In reality, employers in many sectors of the economy retained enormous capacity to engineer a retrenchment of the private welfare state in quick order.

THE DOWNSIZING OF THE PRIVATE WELFARE STATE

In making their pitch for Clinton's Health Security Act and its legislative antecedents, proponents portrayed the job-based system of benefits, and the business sector more broadly, in a highly selective and sympathetic light.[35] Mrs. Clinton and other defenders of the Health Security Act and prior proposals based on an employer mandate bent over backwards to underscore how the weight of escalating health-care costs fell heaviest on the American business sector.[36] In doing so they distorted the reality of the health-care burden in the United States in at least three critical respects. First, it is individual Americans and their families—not the business sector—who shoulder the lion's share of the nation's medical tab. Second, that burden varies greatly between one individual and the next as participation in the employer-sponsored system of health benefits varies by race, gender, ethnicity, income, and locale. And third, the burden of health-care costs on individual Americans and their families has grown steadily in recent years because employers were quite successful at engineering a retrenchment of the private welfare state in short order. As the social and political pressure to maintain the private-sector safety net eased up, employers were poised to shred significant pieces of it. In portraying business as primarily a victim in the face of escalating health-care costs, proponents of reform, including organized labor, drew attention away from how business had already set off on a long march to downsize the private welfare state. Business accomplished that downsizing through shifting more of the expense of health care and other benefits onto employees and by lowering employee expectations about the benefits they are "entitled" to receive by virtue of their employment.

The Unequal Burden of Health-Care Costs

Despite widespread claims to the contrary in the early 1990s, the burden of health-care costs weighs heaviest on the U.S. public, not the business sector. While business spent an estimated $238 billion on medical expenses in 1991, aggregate spending by U.S. families equaled $456 billion.[37] That year the United States spent $6,535 per family on health care; about two-thirds of that paid for by families and the rest by business.[38] It also is not obvious that health-care costs ascribed to corporations are necessarily "corporate" costs. Some economists vigorously contend that employees—not businesses—ultimately absorb the higher health-care costs because workers receive lower cash wages to offset any increase in what employers pay for health insurance and other benefits.[39]

In holding up the system of employment-based benefits as a model to be built upon, proponents of employer-mandate solutions minimized the enormous gaps and gross inequities on which the private welfare state is erected. In certain important respects, it is a misnomer to refer to the health-care system in the United States as an employment-based system. It is really more like a block of Swiss cheese that excludes wide swaths of the population. For all the talk from the 1970s to the early 1990s about the need to build upon the "employer/employee partnership," just over half of the population received medical coverage through employment-based benefits when Clinton took office (see Table 6.1).[40] Most employers *did not* offer health insurance through the workplace, and many who did required employees to assume a large portion of the cost.[41] By one estimate, only 43 percent of the population depended primarily on health insurance paid for by private-sector employers.[42] President Clinton and others often cited Hawaii, the only state with an employer mandate on the books, as a model of health-care reform. Contrary to the conventional wisdom, the results of Hawaii's experience with an employer mandate are mixed. In the early 1990s, Hawaii's uninsured population was rising sharply. By 1993 more than 11 percent of Hawaii's residents did not have health insurance, a proportion that surpassed that of six other states.[43]

In pushing the employer-mandate solution, proponents generally ignored how employee benefits have long operated alongside wages and salaries as an important reward structure that stratifies the workplace.[44] As a consequence, they also slighted how these stratifications intensified in recent years as employers sought to create a more flexible workforce.[45] Historically, labor market variables were strong predictors of who receives benefits like health insurance coverage and pensions in the United States. Critical labor market variables include the racial, gender, and ethnic composition of occupations, how physically demanding a job is, whether the workforce is unionized or not, and the worker's locale. For example, women are less likely to receive health insurance through their employers because they are more likely to work part time, to predominate in low-paying, nonunion jobs, and to experience greater job mobility. (Thus they are more vulnerable to clauses in group health plans that exclude coverage for new employees and that exclude pre-existing medical conditions for a designated period of time.)[46] Hispanics are more than twice as likely to be uninsured as whites (see Figure 6.1). In 1990 a private source of health insurance covered only 48 percent of Hispanics, compared with nearly 77 percent of non-Hispanic whites, and 52 percent of African-Americans.[47] Barely one-third of agricultural workers receive medical benefits through employment, compared with 83 percent of government workers, 81 percent of manufacturing workers, and about half of all construction workers.[48] There are also enormous regional disparities, with people living in the South and West almost 60 percent more likely to be uninsured than individuals in the East and Midwest.[49]

Medical coverage also varies significantly in relation to income. People earning less than $25,000 per year are three times more likely to be uninsured as those earning $75,000 or more annually (see Figure 6.2). Only about one in four low-wage workers (bottom 10 percent of earners) receives health insurance through his or her workplace compared to 90 per-

Table 6.1. Erosion of employer group health insurance coverage, 1979–92: percentage of employees participating in employer- and union-sponsored group health plans

	1979	1981	1983	1985	1987[1]	1989	1990	1991	1992
Civilian Wage and Salary Workers[2]	61.2%	62.0%	61.0%	60.2%	56.6%	56.5%	55.8%	55.5%	54.2%
In poverty	30.5	30.7	27.2	23.6	18.7	16.9	15.3	14.9	14.4
Not in poverty	62.8	64.1	63.5	62.8	58.9	59.0	58.5	58.4	57.0
Working full time, full year	81.9	83.2	82.1	80.8	76.1	75.5	74.5	74.4	72.9
In poverty	56.7	57.0	54.7	46.0	40.4	38.2	33.9	30.9	33.0
Not in poverty	82.3	83.8	82.8	81.6	76.9	76.2	75.4	75.3	73.7

Source: Carolyn Pemberton and Deborah Holmes, eds., *E.B.R.I. Databook on Employee Benefits*, 3rd ed. (Washington, D.C.: E.B.R.I., 1995), Table 8.10, p. 261.
[1] Data for 1987 and later years are not directly comparable with earlier years because of a change in the questionnaire.
[2] Excludes self-employed workers.

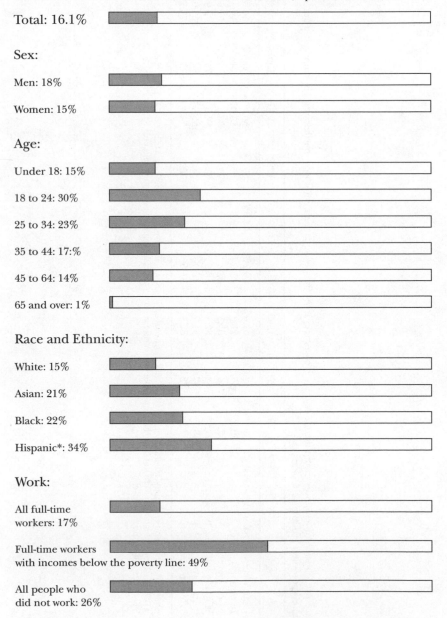

Figure 6.1. The uninsured: percentage of people in the U.S. without health insurance, 1997. Source: U.S. Census Bureau, "The Official Statistics" (September 1, 1998): 2.

Total: 16.1%

Sex:

Men: 18%

Women: 15%

Age:

Under 18: 15%

18 to 24: 30%

25 to 34: 23%

35 to 44: 17:%

45 to 64: 14%

65 and over: 1%

Race and Ethnicity:

White: 15%

Asian: 21%

Black: 22%

Hispanic*: 34%

Work:

All full-time workers: 17%

Full-time workers with incomes below the poverty line: 49%

All people who did not work: 26%

* May be of any race.

Figure 6.2. Health insurance and income, 1997: percentage of people never covered by health insurance during 1997, by household income. Source: U.S. Census Bureau, "The Official Statistics" (September 1, 1998): 3.

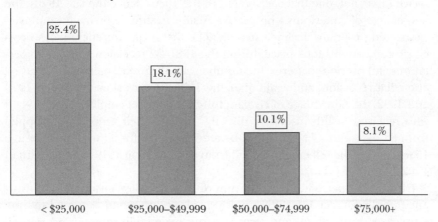

Household Income of Employees Covered

cent of all high-wage workers (top 10 percent of earners).[50] The financial burden of the employment-based system is lopsided, falling more on the less-well-off than on the well-to-do. Whereas Americans belonging to the top income decile pay on average 8.4 percent of their income into the medical system, households near the bottom rung typically pay about 19 percent.[51] Furthermore, the provisions in the federal tax code that permit companies that offer group health plans to deduct the expense of health benefits from their taxes are structured in a highly regressive manner that disproportionately favors employees in the upper-income brackets.[52]

All the public attention on the burden that health-care costs purportedly pose for business helped eclipse not only the inequities of the job-based system, but also that employers in recent years proved willing and capable of shifting more of the medical expense onto employees. Employers imposed higher deductibles and copays, reduced coverage for employees and their dependents, and eliminated coverage for certain ailments and treatments.[53] Beginning in the early 1980s, demands by employers for nonwage concessions escalated dramatically, not just in the area of health benefits, but across the board, including pensions, cost-of-living allowances, and life insurance. The extent of concessions demanded by management was unprecedented.[54] Increasingly, medical benefits were a major arena for labor-management strife despite all the concurrent talk among labor, business, and political leaders about the dawning of a new age of cooperation on the health-care issue.[55]

Employers did not shift the burden of medical care and other benefits onto their employees overnight. Rather, it was a steady erosion of the private-sector safety net, one that accelerated in the 1980s. Since the late 1970s, the percentage of Americans who receive health insurance through employer-sponsored programs declined steadily. The first major retrenchment in coverage and benefits took place during the 1981–82 recession. Defying expectations and previous patterns, the number of uninsured Americans increased after that recession, and again after the 1990–91 recession.[56] Between 1979 and 1992, the percentage of civilian, full-time workers employed year round who received health insurance directly through their employers dropped from 82 percent to 73 percent. Job-based coverage for all workers over age 15, excluding the self-employed, fell from 61 percent in 1979 to 54 percent in 1992 (see Table 6.1).[57]

During that period, the proportion of Americans receiving health insurance wholly financed by their employers also plummeted. Among full-time employees in medium- and large-size private establishments who participated in medical care plans in 1979, nearly three out of every four were enrolled in plans for individual coverage entirely financed by their employers. By 1993, the figure stood at just 37 percent.[58] Many employers required workers to cover a larger portion of their health-care costs through higher payroll deductions. A study by the Kaiser Family Foundation found that "employers who ask workers to pay part of the cost through payroll deductions had raised the workers' share to 22 percent on average by 1996, from 13 percent in 1988."[59] As a result, the proportion of employees offered employer-subsidized health insurance who declined to sign up for coverage de-

Figure 6.3. Percentage of personal consumption expenditures spent on medical care. Source: *Reforming the System*, ed. Robert J. Blendon and Tracey Stelzer Hyams (New York: Faulkner & Gray, 1992), 73. © Faulkner & Gray, Inc. Redrawn with permission.

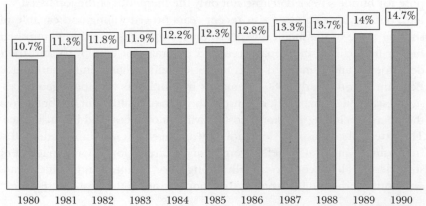

clined sharply. Another significant contraction of the private welfare state is in the area of dependent coverage. Many employers either eliminated coverage for spouses and/or children of employees or required workers to foot more of the bill for family health insurance.[60] Some government studies attribute much of the rise in the uninsured population between 1979 and 1986 to reduced coverage for dependents.[61] Overall, the percentage of personal consumption expenditures spent on medical care rose from about 11 percent in 1980 to nearly 15 percent in 1990 (see Figure 6.3).

Assault on Retiree Benefits

The employer assault on the private welfare state accelerated in other ways in the 1980s, including drastic changes in retiree health benefits that had important implications for the battle over universal health care in the 1990s. ERISA, the federal pension legislation discussed in chapter 3, imposes fairly tough standards on employers to ensure that they honor their commitments to private pension plans. However, retiree health benefits, like other job-based medical coverage, remain an "uncertain promise."[62] Firms experimented with new ways to shed the health-care commitments they made to retirees by, for example, declaring bankruptcy and shutting down operations only to re-open under a new name. Because health-care benefits often only accrue in the final year of employment before retirement, many firms also downsized employees approaching the retirement age and hired fewer older workers overall.

The issue of retiree benefits first drew public attention in mid-1986 when the LTV Corporation abruptly terminated payment on the health and life insurance policies for its 78,000 retirees after filing for bankruptcy under Chapter 11.[63] Following intensive lobbying by labor, Congress eventually passed the Retiree Benefits Bankruptcy Protection Act of 1988, which was supposed to provide greater protection for retiree benefits in bankruptcy proceedings. However, court cases brought under that measure disappointed workers and organized labor and did not bring about the anticipated relief to retirees.[64]

The issue returned again to the limelight in April 1989 when 1,700 members of the United Mine Workers went out on strike after Pittston Coal declared that it would stop contributing to the mining industry's health and welfare funds. The nine-month strike was a rallying point for coal-mining towns across Appalachia and a cause célèbre nationwide for labor and political activists. During the strike, coal miners, with the help of their families and communities, engaged in widespread acts of civil disobedience, including blocking roads and participating in the nation's first sit-down strike since the 1930s.[65] The mineworkers eventually called off the strike in early

1990 after Pittston agreed to restore some of the benefits and pay a portion of what it owed to the trust fund.

The struggle over retiree benefits for miners was in many ways a dress rehearsal for organized labor's contradictory stance on the Clinton plan. During the Pittston strike, the leadership of the AFL-CIO dipped briefly into the waters of civil disobedience and took a more confrontational position toward employers over the issue of retiree benefits for mine workers. Even though the employer assault on retiree health benefits intensified in the late 1980s, the federation was committed to the belief that the crushing expense of the private welfare state would, largely on its own, prompt employers to work with labor and legislators to find a mutually acceptable solution for the woes of the health-care system.

Labor's wishful thinking and contradictory position on the issue of retiree benefits, and health benefits more broadly, are epitomized in an August 1989 article on the subject that appeared in the *AFL-CIO News*, the flagship publication of the labor federation. In the piece, the AFL-CIO was described as hopeful that the "urgent situation" over retiree health benefits "will prompt labor and management to work together in seeking health care reform by containing costs in their own plans and in calling for the enactment of a permanent national health-care solution." These expressed hopes came at the end of a lengthy article that documented how numerous employers, including TRW, Pillsbury, and Quaker Oats, had succeeded in shifting more of the expense of retiree health benefits onto current workers or had reduced or eliminated such benefits altogether.[66] Ironically, the article appeared the same month that leading labor officials were arrested during a sit-in demonstration at the county courthouse in Lebanon, Va., to protest the drastic cuts in retiree benefits by Pittston. This was the first time in recent memory that federation leaders were arrested during a strike.[67]

The battle over retiree benefits in the mining industry was part of a wider trend to roll back retiree benefits in many other sectors of the economy. Employers' determination to curtail retiree benefits intensified in the late 1980s in part as a consequence of a new rule proposed in 1988 by the Federal Accounting Standards Board (FASB), the private organization that sets the rules governing corporate accounting practices.[68] The FASB recommended that companies be required to include on their balance sheets the future cost of providing retiree health care for employees expected to retire at a later date.[69] Organized labor initially viewed the new FASB rule on retiree health-care liabilities as a welcome catalyst to force employers to finally face up to the extent of their obligations to the private welfare state, thus kindling their interest in a comprehensive legislative solution to the health-care dilemma. What labor failed to anticipate was the tenuousness of those obligations. Business was situated to cast off its commitments to retiree benefits in quick order, and without the public outcry anticipated by labor. The employers' rapid response to this rule change reveals the fragility of the private welfare state in the United States, and, in particular, employers' tenuous commitment to health-care benefits.

The FASB rule change, which was promulgated in 1990 and went into effect in late 1992, did galvanize companies around the issue of retiree benefits—but not in the way organized labor expected. It forced many companies to face the long-term cost of promises made to employees for health benefits after they retire. The cost of accounting in the present for retiree benefits promised in the future set off alarms as estimates of the unfunded liability for retiree benefits ranged from $227 billion (General Accounting Office) to $1 trillion (Washington Business Group on Health).[70] Many employers responded to the rule change by shredding retiree health benefit packages promised to workers.[71] In 1988, 62 percent of surveyed firms provided coverage to retirees under age 65, compared with just 52 percent in 1992.[72]

Perhaps more significant than the reduced number of firms that offered retiree benefits after the rule change was a dramatic change in the way companies structured their benefit programs. Many firms stopped basing their programs on the principle of a "defined benefit," choosing instead to offer their employees a "defined contribution."[73] In other words, they no longer committed to providing a fixed benefit package—such as a guarantee of comprehensive health insurance for early retirees before Medicare kicks in.[74] Corporations informed their employees that they would set aside a fixed amount of money in a separate account to go toward a specified service. Employers inoculated themselves from escalating benefit costs through defined contribution plans, agreeing to pay only a fixed amount and not the entire cost of a particular item.[75]

Many labor leaders continued to believe that business, when confronted with the stark reality of the actual costs of retiree health benefits, would be compelled by bottom-line logic to endorse an extensive reform of the health-care system based on an employer mandate that would shore up the private welfare state. Business responded instead by testing the political waters and whittling away at health-care benefits for retirees, along with other pieces of the private-sector safety net. Firms intensified their efforts in the aftermath of the FASB ruling, emboldened in part because of their apparent success in reducing obligations to retirees without much of a focused public outcry.

The effectiveness of this effort to shrink the private welfare state was premised on a conscious strategy by employers to change employee expectations. For all the initial hand-wringing about escalating medical costs, many firms gradually viewed the health-care issue as a welcome opportunity to chip away at the entire benefit package. It was also time to put to rest once and for all the belief that firms have a social obligation to provide health insurance and other benefits to employees. One management publication pointedly noted that although the postwar "deal" between employers and employees regarding benefits lives on, the latest debate over health policy "does raise interesting strategic decisions and gives employers an opportunity to reevaluate the deal."[76] The Conference Board, a prominent business organization, echoed this view. It concluded in one report: "The concept of 'entitlement' may be obsolete in a mature economy that must compete with countries that do not provide entitlements, especially in a globally competitive world."[77] As part of their offensive to reevaluate the "deal," employers began, among other things, to stress the "voluntary" nature of the benefits they did provide and how insurance is meant to cover only catastrophic events, not routine care.[78]

The debate over retiree health benefits during discussions of Clinton's Health Security Act revealed to what extent the public and the politicians now accepted the new downsized "deal" between employers and employees regarding the private welfare state. Retiree health benefits were a central issue in formulating the Clinton plan. Companies with extensive and expensive retiree commitments were initially drawn to the Clinton proposal because it would lower the eligibility age for Medicare and cap a firm's health-care costs at between 3.5 and 7.9 percent of payroll.[79] To the surprise of organized labor and companies with extensive retiree overhangs, these two provisions came under fierce attack.

Instead of heaping praise on companies that had not shredded retiree benefits, legislators and those corporations, both big and small, that provided no or only minimal health coverage for workers took aim at these businesses. Executives from leading corporations like Pepsico and General Mills got into a nasty and uncharacteristic public spat with auto executives when they depicted the comprehensive health benefits the Big Three automakers provide to their employees, dependents, and retirees as socially and economically irresponsible.[80] Union officials and auto executives alike were surprised that those companies made that charge stick in the court of public opinion. Alan Reuther of the UAW described the "intense hostility" that progressive Democrats displayed toward retiree benefits provided by the Big Three as "shocking," again underlining that labor was not in tune with important political shifts.[81] To their astonishment, even liberal Democrats like Rep. Pete Stark (D-Calif.) did not defend the generous safety net of the automobile industry.[82] The automakers responded to the attacks on their relatively generous retiree health packages by warning: "Absent some remedial measure such as that contained in the administration proposal, market forces will eventually force almost all employers to eliminate early retiree coverage."[83]

To recapitulate, organized labor contributed, perhaps unwittingly, to this ongoing and generally successful effort by business to chip away at the "entitlements" of the private welfare state, notably retiree and other health-care benefits. Labor leaders and the White House emphasized how the burden of escalating health-care costs fell heaviest on business, not the public. In taking this approach, they misrepresented the nature of the health-care cost burden and helped draw public attention away from the ways in which business for years had chipped away at the private-sector safety net that had shielded millions of Americans for decades. They helped distort not only business complicity in the assault on the private welfare state, but also its complicity in the restructuring of the U.S. political economy, to which we now turn.

HEALTH CARE AND ECONOMIC "COMPETITIVENESS"

The employer offensive to create a more flexible and lower cost workforce was premised on more than stressing the erosion of "entitlements" in all walks of life and taking a harder line at the bargaining table. Corporations also paid greater attention to the amount and the kind of information employees received about a firm's economic situation. In particular, they emphasized how U.S. corporations faced dire competitive conditions at home and abroad, and, as a result, employees must make do with less.[84] The issue of escalating medical costs provided a fortuitous opportunity for business, with the help of organized labor, to bolster this selective understanding of the U.S. political economy.

In tapping big business as a key ally in the health-care debate, organized labor largely accepted the Fortune 500's definition of what ailed the American economy and hence the U.S. worker. Much of organized labor jumped on the "competitiveness" bandwagon. In public statements, labor and business leaders regularly sang off the same song sheet. Their refrain was a simple one—higher medical costs made American products less competitive in the international marketplace, which severely hurt the U.S. economy and the U.S. worker.

The tight link that labor leaders made between the health-care issue and the competitiveness question boxed organized labor into a remarkable spot, as demonstrated by a report released by the SEIU in 1992 as the debate over health policy heated up. While the report mentions in passing how "[s]low productivity growth and structural changes in the U.S. economy" contributed to falling wages, it identifies health-care costs as the main villain for the woes of the U.S. worker. It blames the country's "out-of-control" medical expenses for a host of sins, including falling wages, the plummeting savings rate, the large federal budget deficit, the precarious financial situation of the states, slowing economic growth, and, notably, the "noncompetitiveness of American businesses." The report portrays the growing health-care cost burden as an important cause of the restructuring of the U.S. economy that wrought so many hardships for so many U.S. workers—rather than as a consequence or symptom of that restructuring.[85] In his appearances before Congress during the struggle over the Clinton plan, Sweeney regularly cited this report. In one appearance, he claimed that if health-care costs had grown only as fast as the economy over the past decade, the United States could have "reversed one of the most damaging economic trends of the last decade, the decline in real wages for most workers."[86]

The close association that organized labor made between rising health-care costs, economic competitiveness, and the livelihood of the average U.S. worker predated the debate over the Health Security Act by a number of years. In discussions of health-care reform from the 1980s onward, much of organized labor started to treat as fact what were highly contested claims about the U.S. political economy. Labor leaders worked side-by-side with corporate leaders and government officials to portray stemming health-care costs as the magic bullet that would critically wound, if not slay, the dragon of intensified economic competition that was reportedly pricing U.S. workers out of the global marketplace and eating away at their standard of living. They portrayed U.S. employers as largely willing—but increasingly unable—to offer health benefits because of this intensified competition.

In taking this stance, organized labor conceded important political and intellectual ground to business in several key areas related to the competitiveness question and broader economic issues. By largely accepting without question the dominant view that the economic troubles of the United States stem largely from a failure to compete effectively in global markets, labor contributed to the general tendency in academic and political circles to "overstress the international side of our domestic problems."[87] Organized labor accepted an image of the U.S. economy and of U.S. firms drowning in imports produced by either low-wage, low-benefit developing countries that were irresistible havens for U.S. direct foreign investment, or by other advanced industrialized countries that enjoyed significant cost advantages over U.S. firms because of lower medical expenses. Instead of challenging or qualifying such premises in discussions of health care, labor joined in the chorus. Labor officials failed to critically evaluate three of the core premises of the economic competitiveness argument as they were applied to the health reform issue: that escalating health-care costs pose a major threat to the profitability of U.S. firms; that the health-care costs for U.S. firms are way above those of competitors in other advanced industrialized countries and thus are pricing American goods out of the market; and that economic competition from lower-cost producers abroad is the prime threat to the economic livelihood of the U.S. worker. All three premises are questionable.

Profits

Beginning in the 1980s, business harped on how health-care costs eat up a huge portion of corporate profits.[88] Business and labor representatives widely publicized the results of a 1989 survey by the NAM that concluded that employers' medical expenses equaled more than one-third of business profits.[89] This finding was used to bolster the argument that business had a compelling dollar-and-cents incentive to support comprehensive health-care reform. Organized labor did not challenge the contention that health-care costs imperil profits; indeed, labor officials regularly made reference to how employer spending on medical plans equaled, by their reckoning, an alarming 61 percent of before-tax profits by the early 1990s.[90]

In its eagerness to make common cause with business on the health-care issue, labor contributed to a widespread misperception about the extent to which medical costs hurt corporate profits. It is true that employer spending on health care, if measured as a percentage of profits, did jump in the first half of the 1980s.[91] A more nuanced look at these figures calls into question the claim that rising health-care costs imperil the profitability of U.S. firms. The jump in the early 1980s was due in part to a drop overall in corporate after-tax profits.[92] Also, spending on health care as measured as a percentage of corporate profits was surprising stable from 1985 to 1991, defying claims about how health-care costs imperil U.S. firms. More significantly, employer spending on wages and salaries, and on total compensation as a percentage of after-tax profits dropped significantly after 1985.[93] Although health-care costs may have been rising, employers had great success at squeezing wages and other forms of compensation.

Health-Care Costs, Relatively Speaking

To underscore the severity of their health-care cost crunch, business executives often stressed what they pay out in direct costs for health care as compared with foreign competitors. This was a central theme of a major conference of economists and business leaders in Little Rock, Ark., shortly after Clinton was elected president. At the conference, Harold "Red" Poling, chairman of the Ford Motor Company (who was acting as the chief spokesperson for business), emphasized how "health care costs give Japanese auto makers an advantage over Ford of $500 per car." Poling also said

that Ford spends as much on health care as it spends on steel.[94] Labor officials repeated these figures, eager to buttress their case about how an ir-
refutable bottom-line logic would force business to seek a satisfactory legislative solution with the state and labor. This was a highly selective
understanding of the burden that health-care costs reportedly place on
U.S. firms. First, comparing what U.S. firms pay directly for health care relative to their foreign competitors ignores the higher indirect costs that
many European and Japanese firms shoulder due to the relatively higher
corporate and personal income taxes they must pay to support more extensive public welfare states. For example, in Germany health care is financed
through a payroll tax that is equal to about 13 percent of a company's total
employment costs. This amount generally exceeds what even the most generous U.S. firms spend on health care for their employees.[95]

In lamenting how higher health-care costs make U.S. firms uncompeti-
tive vis-à-vis multinationals headquartered in other advanced industrialized countries, U.S. labor leaders overlooked that European and Japanese
firms were highly competitive even though their benefit packages were far
more generous, and more costly, than those offered by American firms.[96]
In discussions of health care, organized labor missed an opportunity to
show how health care and other benefits that U.S. workers received were
paltry compared to what workers in other advanced industrialized countries received.

The "Threat" from Abroad

In rising so ardently to the defense of U.S. firms allegedly battered by lower-
cost competitors from abroad, organized labor absented itself from wider
and more penetrating debates about the U.S. political economy. Labor
leaders ended up on the sidelines in discussions about whether American
multinationals were increasingly shedding their national identity for a
global identity, and whether, as a result, their interests were fundamentally
at odds with those of the average U.S. worker.[97] Labor's obsession with the
competitiveness angle of the health-care issue helped buttress the dominant view that structural forces in the international political economy (notably the speed and ease with which capital could seek out lower-cost
havens) were to blame for many of the economic woes of the U.S. worker.
The woes included stagnating wages, growing income inequality, shrinking
benefits, and increased job insecurity despite a robust GNP. Although this
view did not go entirely unchallenged, it fell upon others, namely icono-
clastic economists, to take it on. For instance, economists Paul Krugman
and David M. Gordon forcefully challenged the conventional wisdom that
rising imports from lower-cost producers from abroad were the root cause

of the economic difficulties of U.S. workers.[98] In a similar vein, health-care economists Uwe Reinhardt and Mark Pauly questioned the popular view among business and labor leaders that the overall percentage of GNP devoted to health care in the U.S. economy "is too high for the nation's long-run competitiveness" and that higher health-care costs are to blame for stagnating wages for workers.[99] In discussions of health-care reform, labor rarely raised such issues.

The aim here is not to settle whether the analyses of these economists are more accurate than those offered by other observers. The main point is that in the context of the health-care debate, organized labor did not challenge the dominant interpretation of the changing U.S. political economy. Labor generally accepted and promoted the view that rising health-care costs were to blame for reduced economic competitiveness and stagnating wages. This was an analysis essentially proposed by business.[100] Labor's ability to develop a coherent, compelling, and independent political program to address the economic dislocations of the 1980s and 1990s was impaired, as was its specific strategy on health-care reform, because of its fealty to a business-centered worldview of the economic consequences of escalating medical costs. As Kim Moody observes, "By the 1990s, it was enough to utter the word 'globalization' to obtain the submission of many workers, unions, or even nations to the needs of capital."[101]

Labor leaders viewed their initial embrace of the employer mandate in 1978, and their periodic recommitment to this solution, as the optimum strategic choice. In their quest for universal health care, unions consistently took a circumscribed view of the political and economic environment in which they operated. For labor, concerns about inflation, and later the anti-tax, anti-deficit, pro-competitiveness concerns of business and the Democrats, delimited that environment. As employers sought greater labor market flexibility and whittled away at the private welfare state, labor continued to take a narrow view of its political environment. Labor leaders consistently portrayed the employer mandate as the natural—and optimum—strategic choice even though the option took on a life of its own and became an imprisoning idea.

This is not to suggest that the single-payer option was necessarily labor's only and best alternative. Rather, this suggests that labor forfeited the opportunity to use health care as a building block to construct an alternative interpretation of the woes of the U.S. worker and of the U.S. political economy. Instead of heralding the resilience of the private welfare state, organized labor could have shown how the shadow welfare state, inadequate and inefficient to begin with, was besieged by a complex set of political factors—and not merely the pressures associated with a compulsion to be more competitive in a global market.

In endorsing the Clinton proposal and its legislative antecedents based on an employer-mandate solution, organized labor endorsed a highly selective understanding of the U.S. political economy. It generally accepted that, in this age of widespread economic restructuring and a manic search on the part of employers for greater labor market flexibility, the institution of job-based benefits was a well-established, stable one that had long shielded most Americans and would continue to do so. By holding up the existing system of employment-based benefits as a model of social responsibility, organized labor minimized or whitewashed gross inequities lodged in that system that, during earlier campaigns for national health insurance, it had highlighted and taken issue with. It thus helped promote the misperception that business shouldered most of the burden of the private welfare state and, in particular, the burden of escalating health-care costs. In doing so, organized labor was an accomplice in minimizing the retrenchment of the private welfare state.

Organized labor argued that escalating health-care costs were the scourge of the U.S. economy because they imperiled the competitiveness of U.S. firms, thus hurting the average worker. Labor leaders chose to overlook that U.S. firms were highly profitable despite escalating health-care costs; that the benefits of U.S. workers paled in comparison with those of employees in other advanced industrialized countries; and that the competitive threat from low-wage, low-benefit producers was overstated in ways that had the effect of politically taming the U.S. workforce. This embrace of a worldview that interpreted the causes, consequences, and nature of the health-care cost burden in a manner that was uncritical of business's role led labor to self-defeating political strategies. In pursuing an elusive partnership with business on health policy, organized labor may have forfeited the chance to serve as an engine to generate a powerful social movement or reform coalition mobilized around the health-care question and broader issues associated with the restructuring of the U.S. economy. The next chapter will focus in greater detail on the political consequences of organized labor's decision in the 1993–94 period to pursue that elusive partnership with business and the White House on health-care reform.

CHAPTER 7

Adrift and on the Defensive

Labor and the Defeat of Clinton's Health Security Act

In the 1993–94 struggle over health-care reform, organized labor proved politically ineffective. Unions, which played a critical part in the passage of a number of major pieces of social welfare legislation, notably Medicare, were not only unable to put together a winning coalition, but also found themselves divided and on the defensive as they struggled to prevent further erosion of the private-sector safety net of the U.S. welfare state. By the summer of 1994, organized labor was battling alternative measures supported by business and conservatives that were likely to shrink—not expand—the existing private-sector safety net. Labor officials were alarmed at what they characterized as the rightward drift of the health-care reform debate, in particular the growing support for proposals based on a watered-down employer mandate that would not guarantee universal coverage and that called for greatly limiting the tax deductibility of employment-based health benefits.[1]

Organized labor's capacity for political action depends on many factors, not just the size of its rank and file, as argued in chapter 2. To understand labor's relative ineffectiveness in the 1993–94 debate over health policy, it is important to keep in mind the preceding analysis about how the postwar institutional and ideational context conditioned that debate. Although that context defined the terrain, it did not on its own determine the precise path organized labor took once President Clinton indicated that comprehensive health-care reform was a priority of his administration. Besides issues of institutional continuity, several political factors conspired to reinforce organized labor's tendency to stick to a policy path on health-care issues charted primarily by business and leading Democrats during the preceding years. These factors, which are analyzed in greater detail in this chapter, further help to explain why organized labor failed to play a more meaningful role in the 1993–94 skirmish over health policy.

This chapter begins with a discussion of the divisions within organized labor over health-care reform in the months leading up to the 1992 election. It then looks at how unions quickly distanced themselves from the single-payer option shortly after Clinton's election in November 1992. The third section explores simmering divisions within organized labor over health-care reform despite a stated public commitment to forging a united front with the Clinton administration on health policy and how the struggle over the North American Free-Trade Agreement (NAFTA) exacerbated the divisions. The following section examines why organized labor was unable to use the NAFTA experience as a basis to put together an effective reform coalition that would, at minimum, help stem the rightward drift of the health-care debate. The fifth section discusses how the institutional context, notably several key institutions of the private welfare state, further antagonized these divisions within organized labor and structured the politics of health policy during this period. The final section focuses on organized labor's failed attempts to regain the initiative in health policy. In particular, it examines how two critical pillars on which labor erected its health-care strategy over the preceding 15 years came tumbling down in rapid succession in early 1994. The first was the belief, examined in chapters 5 and 6, that business would be a constructive and reliable ally in the cause of comprehensive health-care reform. The second was an assumption, analyzed in chapters 4 and 6, that the proposed employer-mandate solution would have widespread support because it built upon the job-based system of benefits and would neither burden the federal budget nor ignite a tax increase.

GROWING DIVISIONS WITHIN ORGANIZED LABOR OVER HEALTH-CARE REFORM

Labor's attachment to the institutions of the private welfare state, the employer mandate, and a worldview sympathetic to business spurred unions to pursue self-defeating political strategies. However, organized labor was not of a single mind about health-care reform in the late 1980s and early 1990s.[2] The impact of institutions and ideas was uneven. Just at the moment that single-payer proposals and the Canadian medical system were attracting wider attention and gaining respectability among policy-makers and the general public, some labor unions were bitterly divided over the issue. Several AFL-CIO officials eventually neutralized the remaining support within organized labor for a single-payer system. John J. Sweeney, chairman of the federation's health-care committee and president of the

Service Employees International Union (SEIU), played a pivotal role here, as did Lane Kirkland, AFL-CIO president.

Sweeney and Kirkland cautioned unions to avoid endorsing any specific legislation in order to increase the likelihood of building a consensus with other groups, including business.[3] This was a major theme of a series of hearings on health-care issues that the AFL-CIO conducted around the country in the fall of 1990.[4] Yet the federation's efforts to mobilize its membership on the health-care issue fell flat around this time because it refused to support any specific proposal and due to deep divisions between unions and within unions over the single-payer option. Many local labor organizers reported that members wanted to rally around a specific proposal, but beyond the call for health care for all, there was no specific program.[5]

The showdown for organized labor over national health insurance came in late 1990 and early 1991 as several unions pushed the AFL-CIO to endorse a single-payer solution. Although Kirkland and Sweeney took an open-ended approach in public, in private they strongly opposed any Canadian-style solution. Behind the scenes, and consistent with the analysis presented earlier, Sweeney advocated on behalf of a variant of the employer-mandate model, believing it to be the most acceptable to business because it built upon the existing system of private-sector health benefits.[6] This approach was also attractive to him because it would not force unions that provided health benefits through the Taft-Hartley funds to give them up.[7]

At a critical and contentious meeting of the federation's health-care committee on January 31, 1991, Robert M. McGlotten of the AFL-CIO argued that the single-payer approach was not politically viable because legislators did not want to take on the insurers. He warned that if organized labor insisted on endorsing such a proposal, it would find itself politically marginalized as the debate over health-care reform unfolded. Several union presidents disagreed with McGlotten's assessment. UAW president Owen Bieber countered that it was still too early to assess the political feasibility of a single-payer plan because organized labor had done so little to educate legislators, the public, and its members about this solution. He pointedly noted that John D. Rockefeller (D-W.Va.), the dean of health policy in the Senate, had reported that no one from organized labor had been to see him to discuss the question of a single-payer plan.[8] After much squabbling, the health-care committee deadlocked eight to eight at this meeting over whether to endorse the single-payer option.[9] Faced with such an impasse, the AFL-CIO executive council responded days later by endorsing what appeared to be a "let a hundred flowers bloom" approach to national health-care reform and issued a statement supporting vague "principles" for health care.[10]

Like the original Hundred Flowers campaign four decades ago in China, this one quickly lost its bloom. Kirkland and Sweeney clearly remained committed to the employer-mandate formula and to undercutting the single-payer position. And they brought the full weight of the AFL-CIO bureaucracy and the Democratic Party to bear behind the scenes on supporters of the single-payer path. At the 1991 annual February meeting of the federation's executive council in Bal Harbour, Fla., the council enlisted the help of Majority Leader George Mitchell (D-Maine) and Speaker of the House Tom Foley (D-Wash.). Speaker Foley told union officials not to expect enactment of "any legislation that involved anything but tinkering with the job-based system." The day before the executive council meeting, Kirkland told a gathering of the American Medical Association, the federation's longtime nemesis, "Gone are the old, hardened attitudes and purely political exercises." He proudly announced that organized labor was "in common cause with many of our traditional adversaries in the business community—including the National Association of Manufacturers and some of the nation's biggest corporations."[11] Kirkland and his supporters used official union publications to sideline the single-payer option. Around 1991, discussions of the Canadian model dropped largely out of sight in the *AFL-CIO News*, the official federation publication, and in the SEIU's *Service Employees Union*, which previously ran several favorable and detailed stories about the Canadian system. That summer eight union presidents sent an angry letter to Kirkland complaining about indications he had given Rep. Dan Rostenkowski (D-Ill.) that all the AFL-CIO unions, including the single-payer contingent, would support the employer-mandate measure that the chairman of the House Ways and Means Committee was pushing on Capitol Hill. In their view, the proposed bill did not even conform to the general principles adopted by the federation six months earlier in Bal Harbour.[12]

Three months later at the AFL-CIO biennial convention, Sen. Edward M. Kennedy (D-Mass.) set the tone for the gathering when he stressed the need for political pragmatism on the health-care reform issue and promoted his Health Security bill, which was based on an employer mandate.[13] Speaker after speaker rose to denounce the Canadian model as politically unfeasible. The 11 international unions that favored the Canadian plan were conspicuously silent on the convention floor.[14] At the gathering, delegates passed a vague resolution that reaffirmed the federation's commitment to an unspecified restructuring of the health-care system.[15]

The real drama at the convention took place off the floor. As Sweeney proclaimed labor's unity on health-care reform at a press conference, a member of AFSCME distributed a letter from its president, Gerald McEntee, that took issue with Sweeney and pitched a single-payer system. The drama heightened as Sweeney released a report from the National Leadership Coalition for Health Care Reform that called for an employer-mandate solution and applauded employers' new willingness to make common cause with labor on health issues. The NLCHCR counted among its membership International Paper, which had turned to replacement workers to crush a bitter 16-month strike in Jay, Maine; Dayton-Hudson, which had refused to bargain with the UAW; and Northern Telecom, which had succeeded in virtually eliminating unions from its workforce. Asked at the press conference why labor leaders now trust employers to do the right thing on health care when they cannot be trusted to respect workers' rights generally, Bill Wynn, president of the United Food and Commercial Workers (UFCW), answered: "Our employers came to their senses."[16]

Eager to court business, Sweeney and Kirkland maneuvered the federation away from the single-payer position just as Canadian-style solutions were enjoying a new burst of interest and respectability.[17] Although they kept the AFL-CIO from officially straying down the single-payer path, they could not quell completely the growing sentiment in several unions for a Canadian-style solution. As a result, the AFL-CIO was forced to adopt a "wait-and-see" approach to health-care reform that, not surprisingly, failed to inspire the rank and file.The approach left labor fragmented and tentative just as the health-care issue lurched once again into the national spotlight with the election of Clinton in November 1992.

CLINTON, ORGANIZED LABOR, AND THE MARGINALIZATION OF THE SINGLE-PAYER OPTION

Almost immediately after the election, labor appeared to close ranks quickly and effortlessly around Clinton on the health-care reform question. In fact, divisions simmered between unions, and between the leadership and the rank and file. And the twin battles over NAFTA and health-care reform in the summer and fall of 1993 helped bring some of these divisions to the fore and debilitated organized labor. These divisions had institutional and political roots that reinforced one another. On the institutional side, as suggested in chapter 3, was labor's commitment, especially the commitment of labor leaders, to the Taft-Hartley funds and the ERISA preemption. On the political side, as discussed in chapters 4 and 6, was its commitment to an employer mandate, which meant seeking an alliance with business on health-care reform and distancing itself from the single-payer forces.

Shortly after the 1992 election, a debate broke out within organized labor about the type of relationship to seek with the first Democratic administration in more than a decade. Unions, which had played a vital, but largely unrecognized, role for the Democrats in the 1992 campaign, were divided over whether to prod Clinton to pursue a bolder agenda on health-care reform and other matters than he had promised during the electoral campaign.[18] Much of organized labor eventually chose to blend into the political landscape defined by Clinton and the Democrats rather than attempt to broaden and reshape that landscape.

Days after Clinton was elected, AFSCME and the UAW, two critical anchors of the single-payer coalition, rejected a proposed postcard campaign on behalf of a single-payer plan, as well as the idea of organizing a bus caravan to Little Rock, Ark., to press their views. "We made a conscious decision not to do a grass-roots campaign," explained Alan Reuther, legislative director of the UAW. "We saw it as setting our people all up to be pissed off at Clinton."[19] Officials from the two unions reportedly told other health-care activists that they would only work from "inside" the Clinton team to influence the course of health-care reform.[20] The defection of the UAW and AFSCME was perceived as "deeply wounding" to the single-payer coalition.[21]

The UAW and AFSCME followed in the footsteps of the United Steelworkers of America (USWA), a long-time single-payer supporter that moved to the "play-or-pay" position in the early 1990s. Explaining the steelworkers' shift, former president Lynn Williams said:

> We also believed, with our knowledge of the Congress and its members, and our sense of all the complexities of the general atmosphere surrounding this issue in America, that to win a single payer plan was impossible, that to attempt it would be to lose an historic opportunity to move forward with the result that increasing millions of Americans would continue to be without health-care coverage in the foreseeable future.[22]

Several other unions, including the Communications Workers of America (CWA), the Teamsters, the International Ladies Garment Workers Union (ILGWU), and the Oil, Chemical and Atomic Workers (OCAW), were less reluctant to pressure Clinton in the weeks immediately following the election.[23] However, as the outlines of the Clinton plan took shape in the coming months, most of the single-payer unions attempted to straddle the health-care question. Although they remained ostensibly committed to a single-payer solution, they increasingly found virtue in the plan the White House appeared to be putting together.[24]

AFSCME's McEntee, who was a pivotal voice for a single-payer plan over the years, was again a pivotal figure in swaying organized labor to go easy on the new president. At a meeting of the AFL-CIO health-care committee in early 1993, AFSCME reportedly voted in favor of managed competition, breaking with the single-payer contingent on the committee for the first time. The committee deadlocked eight to eight, with supporters of managed competition on one side and single-payer advocates on the other.[25] A statement issued by the federation's executive council in February 1993 shortly after the deadlocked vote did not mention the single-payer solution. Instead, the federation commended President Clinton for his leadership on health care and issued a two-page list of vague principles that it said should guide the drafting of any health-care reform legislation. It had little to say, however, about what labor was prepared to do politically to make universal health care a reality.[26]

Despite the lack of any major legislative or political victories for labor in the months leading up to the official introduction of the Health Security Act in the fall of 1993, organized labor's commitment to the president did not waver much, at least in public.[27] In the summer of 1993, Ralph Nader's Public Citizen attempted to enlist labor in its efforts to plan a major event to launch a campaign for Canadian-style reform that fall. But the consumer advocacy organization was unable to mobilize much support from organized labor because union officials said they did not want to get involved in any activity that might be construed as opposition to the president.[28] Clearly, the institutional and ideological influences discussed earlier were in full operation by now, especially among labor leaders. Even after Clinton decided to make the passage of NAFTA a top priority, relations between labor leaders and the White House remained cordial. When Clinton appeared as the keynote speaker at the AFL-CIO's 20th convention in October 1993 at the height of the struggle over NAFTA, Kirkland vowed, "By and large, his agenda is our agenda, and we are and will be his most loyal troops."[29]

NAFTA AND HEALTH-CARE REFORM

This close identification with Clinton's agenda vexed labor with a serious case of political cognitive dissonance that undermined its stated quest for universal health care. This is most apparent in the drastically different approaches that organized labor took simultaneously in its campaign against NAFTA and in its fight for Clinton's Health Security Act. At the same time that organized labor was engaged in a pitched battle with business and the White House over the free-trade agreement, it attempted to make the case that both the administration and business could be counted on as constructive partners on health-care reform. The political message was decidedly mixed and inconsistent. Notably, Lee Iacocca, who was the leading business spokesman on behalf of comprehensive health-care reform, was a leading figure in the campaign for NAFTA and reportedly a key figure in enlisting Clinton in the battle for the free-trade agreement.[30]

In the struggle over NAFTA, labor leaders faulted U.S. multinationals for what they characterized as a ruthless and unwarranted effort to shift production to low-wage countries with more lax environmental and labor standards.[31] Unions sought to make the treaty a referendum on how corporate America was failing the average U.S. worker and his or her family.[32] In discussions of health care, however, labor officials conceded, as they had for years, that U.S. corporations were under mounting and dire competitive pressures from low-wage, lower-benefit producers at home and abroad, and that escalating health-care costs compounded those pressures.[33] For example, *Steelabor*, the flagship publication of the United Steelworkers of America, reported in fall 1993 that Lynn Williams, president of the union, put his full support behind the Clinton plan "primarily because it is the right thing to do" and because "universal health care will also make the economy more competitive."[34]

As an analytical aside, it should be noted that labor's contrasting approaches to NAFTA and the health-care debate dramatically underline the inadequacy of any explanation of labor politics that emphasizes labor's shrinking membership and related political weakness. In the case of NAFTA, labor chose to confront business and a Democratic president in seeking to defeat the free-trade agreement. By contrast, labor leaders eagerly sought the cooperation of business on the health-care issue, even though the strategy was fraught with contradictions. The latter strategy only makes sense when keeping in mind labor's imperfect but longstanding attachment to the private welfare state's institutions for health-care provision and to the idea of an employer mandate.

In the case of NAFTA, unions sought to energize their grass-roots supporters for what they hoped would be a highly partisan fight that, simply put, would pit labor against capital. In doing so, organized labor forged unprecedented alliances with consumer, environmental, farm, labor, and civil rights groups at home and abroad.[35] In the case of health-care reform, however, organized labor threw its lot in with an avowedly nonpartisan group composed of a loose-knit coalition of consumer, provider, business, and public-interest groups called the Health Care Reform Project, which was slow to get off the ground.[36] The members of this coalition were united by their shared commitment to the general idea of comprehensive reform of the U.S. medical system and by an expressed willingness to work with Congress, the administration, and the two main political parties to find an acceptable solution.[37]

In the late summer of 1993, more than 100 Democratic House members called upon the president to focus on health-care reform legislation rather than NAFTA.[38] Clinton refused to retreat on NAFTA because, among other things, the free-trade agreement had taken on enormous symbolic significance for his young administration.[39] In the weeks that followed, Clinton embarked on what was subsequently described as an "almost obsessive campaign" to secure passage of the treaty, brooking opposition from two of the three Democratic leaders in the House, organized labor, and important consumer, environmental, and other public-interest groups.[40] By the time Clinton unveiled the broad outlines of the Health Security Act in an address to Congress and the nation on September 22, 1993, organized labor and many Democrats were already distracted by the growing demands of the anti-NAFTA campaign they were waging.[41]

As the smoke cleared from the NAFTA battle following Congressional approval of the treaty in November 1993, it appeared for a moment that organized labor might finally stake out a political path that was more independent of the Clinton White House. Labor leaders, embittered over the way the administration had conducted its campaign for ratification of the trade agreement in the eleventh hour,[42] used uncharacteristically harsh language to denounce the White House.[43] Teamsters president Ron Carey warned: "We need to develop political alternatives so that we can't be taken for granted."[44] Several union leaders vowed to punish at the polls those senators and representatives who had supported the treaty, a promise that went largely unfulfilled.[45] The AFL-CIO did, however, cut off funding to the Democratic National Committee for a period of almost six months, leaving the DNC's campaign for health-care reform, which was already strapped for money, in a real pinch.[46]

Labor leaders acknowledged that their membership was alienated by the great lengths the administration went to pass a measure that they perceived as deeply detrimental to their interests. They also warned that the business-Republican alliance Clinton had forged for NAFTA would not hold in the health-care debate. Kirkland and other labor leaders conceded that the NAFTA setback had deflated the rank and file's enthusiasm for Clinton, thus jeopardizing the prospects for his Health Security Act.[47] In early December 1993, the AFL-CIO introduced a plan to train union activists on how to educate the rank and file about the Clinton plan.[48] However, federation officials postponed sending their staff members into the field for several weeks because of the rank and file's continued hostility to Clinton over NAFTA.[49] Over the next few weeks, the Clinton administration intensified its efforts to smooth the ruffled feathers of organized labor as senior labor officials appeared to distance themselves from the glowing endorsement they had given to Clinton's Health Security Act in early October.[50]

Despite Kirkland's personal reaffirmation of labor's commitment to the Clinton framework for health-care reform in early 1994, debilitating divisions simmered within organized labor.[51] The complex nature of the Clinton proposal compounded the divisions over health-care reform. Training sessions for union activists tended to concentrate on providing detailed explanations of how the Clinton plan would work in practice and reassuring union members that the Health Security Act would not make them worse off. Little time was devoted to explaining the political rationale behind labor's support of the Health Security Act and to discussing how to rev up the rank and file for a fight for comprehensive health-care reform.[52] It appears that rank-and-file union members were not the only ones who felt uneasy about the complexities of the Clinton plan and who needed to be convinced that the Health Security Act would not leave them worse off. Asked what he thought of the Clinton plan, Robert M. McGlotten, legislative director of the AFL-CIO at that time, bluntly said after the fact, "It scared me to death."[53]

The single-payer activists among organized labor's rank and file remained reluctant to heed the leadership's call for a united front with the Clinton administration on health-care reform. For many years, the rank and file of those unions who were the most active on health-care issues, including the UAW, AFSCME, and the ILGWU, had heard from their leadership about how a single-payer plan was the only way to go in terms of access, affordability, simplicity, savings on administrative costs, and preservation of freedom of choice for patients. Then they were told to mobilize in support of a complicated, untried plan that was rooted in the existing job-based system of benefits and that retained a sizable role for the major commercial health insurers. Moreover, the plan was hatched by a president who had just kicked sand in labor's face during the NAFTA struggle.

THE GROWING RIFT: ORGANIZED LABOR AND THE PUBLIC-INTEREST COMMUNITY

Two related developments emboldened these rank-and-file activists to stay on the single-payer course in defiance of their national leadership. First, public-interest groups with whom organized labor had established closer ties during the NAFTA fight were making direct appeals to labor's rank and file on behalf of Canadian-style solutions. Second, a new movement to establish a labor party as an alternative to the Democrats and Republicans emerged in the early 1990s and singled out national health insurance as one of its top priorities. This movement represented no immediate threat to the Democratic Party or a serious challenge to the pro-Democratic Party line of the AFL-CIO leadership. However, it provided a new venue for disgruntled labor activists to pursue an alternative political agenda and link the single-payer issue to other broader social and economic concerns. It also provided an opportunity for political activists to focus not just on the legislative battle of the moment but on the development of long-range strategies to engineer a major and enduring political shift.

In the 1993–94 period, single-payer activists from Nader's Public Citizen consciously courted labor's rank and file through visits to union locals in which they explained why, in their view, the single-payer approach was superior to the Clinton plan. Single-payer activists revved up labor's rank and file with facetious slogans that poked fun at the alleged lack of political imagination that went into developing and selling the Clinton plan. Two of the slogans that sparked chuckles from union members were: "Hey, hey, ho, ho, arguably better than the status quo"; and "What do we want? Universal health coverage. When do we want it? As soon as the savings are available."[54]

These efforts to appeal directly to the locals over the heads of their national leadership jeopardized the new climate of détente between the leaders of organized labor and liberal-leaning public-interest groups that had emerged in the struggle over NAFTA. From the early to mid-1970s, there were promising efforts to build bridges between labor and the blossoming community of liberal public-interest groups. For example, labor made a concerted effort to enlist consumer advocates like Nader and Sidney Wolfe in its 1973–74 campaign for national health insurance.[55] From about the mid-1970s onward, however, relations between the mainstream of organized labor and public-interest groups soured somewhat due to a variety of reasons.[56] But in the struggle over NAFTA, liberal public-interest groups and the mainstream of organized labor overcame some of their historic antagonisms to work together with a degree of cooperation that perhaps was unprecedented. Efforts by liberal-leaning public-interest groups to appeal directly to the rank and file on behalf of Canadian-style health-care reform created a new source of tension.

In the late 1980s a handful of public-interest groups and labor activists began working together to lay the foundation for a third political party and in early 1991 formally launched the Labor Party Advocates. Their efforts further heightened tensions within organized labor and between the national leadership of organized labor and certain public-interest groups. The 100,000-member Oil, Chemical and Atomic Workers union was the main catalyst behind efforts to organize a third party.[57] Third-party activists in the OCAW and other unions placed national health insurance at the center of a new social agenda around which they hoped to organize a viable labor party. In contrast to many other labor leaders, OCAW officials regularly expressed doubts in public about the degree to which business could be counted on to cooperate with labor to find an acceptable health-care solution. They viewed the issue of universal health care as a pillar on which to build a wider critique of the role of corporations in the United States.[58]

OCAW officials did not shy away from drawing a connection between the health-care issue and broader questions about the role of corporations in the United States.[59] In its coverage of health-care matters, the OCAW's leading publication documented the problems of the U.S. medical system and explained why Canadian-style reform could ameliorate many of these difficulties. Unlike most other unions, the OCAW published detailed articles about the political context out of which national health insurance in Canada was born.[60] Over the years the OCAW also pointedly challenged what it viewed as the AFL-CIO's wait-and-see approach to health-care reform and any employer-mandate solution.[61] The OCAW and other third-party activists viewed the health-care reform cause as an important bridge to link labor with political activists from other organizations. A critical tie was forged, for example, between the OCAW, whose leaders endorsed a single-payer plan in 1989, and the Physicians for a National Health Program (PNHP), an organization of doctors established in 1986 that was committed to Canadian-inspired health-care reform.

The OCAW was one of the few single-payer unions that did not attempt to straddle the health-care issue in the 1993–94 period. Instead, it unequivocally rejected the Clinton plan.[62] A number of other unions tried to have it both ways. They said nice things about the Clinton plan, yet attempted to keep one foot, or at least one toe, in the single-payer waters. For example, Willie L. Baker of the UFCW said, "We thought single-payer was a great way to go. We just didn't think the votes were there. We had a Democratic majority but not a philosophical majority."[63] In justifying their retreat on the single-payer question, many representatives of organized labor dismissed Canadian-style reform proposals as not politically feasible or politically viable. They stuck to this position even though single-payer proposals attracted the greatest number of cosponsors, and even though the Congressional Budget Office, which was required to "cost out" all health-care reform proposals, had deemed single-payer plans very cost effective.[64]

Single-payer advocates had few illusions at the time that they could muster the votes necessary to pass a Canadian-style reform proposal in the 103rd Congress, even though the single-payer option was enjoying a renaissance of respectability.[65] Indeed, months before Clinton unveiled his Health Security Act, Rep. Jim McDermott (D-Wash.), the leading single-payer advocate on Capitol Hill, predicted in private that no comprehensive health-care reform measure would be enacted by the 103rd Congress.[66] In pushing the single-payer approach, these advocates aimed to accomplish several other things. First, they hoped to keep the Clinton plan from slipping more to the right. Second, they aimed to prevent any "incremental nonsolution" from passing and then being hailed as a comprehensive solution. Finally, they wanted to spark a real and ongoing national debate on the single-payer approach and ensure that the approach would emerge from the health-care debate in 1994 as a credible option.[67]

These divisions within organized labor over health policy were mirrored elsewhere as other public-interest groups attempted to straddle the Health Security Act and Canadian-style reform.[68] In the spring of 1993, Citizen Action, a strident single-payer advocate, aligned itself more closely with the White House and took it upon itself to neutralize opposition among single-payer activists to the Clinton plan.[69] By early summer of 1993 a serious schism developed between Citizen Action and Public Citizen over health policy.[70] Like organized labor, Citizen Action and other major public-interest groups, including the AARP, the American Public Health Association, Consumers' Union, Families USA, and the National Council of Senior Citizens, were contending with significant rumblings in their ranks because they refused to endorse the single-payer path above all others.[71] Similarly, leading officials and staff members of these organizations conceded that their most politically active members favored Canadian-style reform.[72]

In the 1993–94 period, labor divided over whether to assume a more confrontational stance vis-à-vis the Democrats. Differences over the single-payer approach further divided labor and opened up schisms within the public-interest community. Lingering hostility to President Clinton because of his zealous support of NAFTA made it difficult to mobilize the rank and file on behalf of his proposal, as did the mixed, inconsistent, and, at times, contradictory messages that organized labor employed simultaneously in the NAFTA and health-care debates. Furthermore, the mainstream of organized labor, which erected important bridges with liberal-leaning public-interest groups during the struggle over NAFTA, was unable, for various reasons, to use these connections to forge a winning coalition for health-care reform. "Labor was fractured. It couldn't really decide what it wanted," explained longtime congressional staffer David Abernethy.[73] Another key Capitol Hill staffer on health matters described labor unions as "being at war with each other" over health policy.[74]

THE HEALTH SECURITY ACT AND THE INSTITUTIONS OF THE PRIVATE WELFARE STATE

The inherited institutional context compounded divisions over health-care reform. Unions that depend heavily on Taft-Hartley funds for their health benefits were generally reluctant to give them up, which had far-reaching consequences for the debate over the Health Security Act and other comprehensive reform proposals. These unions fought long and hard to get a provision included in the Health Security Act that would permit Taft-Hartley funds with 5,000 or more members to opt out of the proposed health-care alliances if they so wished.[75] The main lobbying group for the Taft-Hartley plans, the National Coordinating Committee for Multi-employer Plans (NCCMP), hailed the Clinton plan with its 5,000-member cutoff. The cutoff would serve as a welcome prod to force smaller, less efficient Taft-Hartley funds, which had resisted efforts over the years to merge, to finally do so to remain independent of the alliances.[76] In giving his endorsement to the Health Security Act, NCCMP chairman Robert Georgine stressed that, under the Clinton plan, many Taft-Hartley funds could do business as usual.[77]

This opt-out provision for the Taft-Hartley funds ended up strengthening the hand of large employers, many of whom had lobbied hard for such a provision for themselves.[78] Once organized labor successfully made the case that large Taft-Hartley funds should be free to choose whether or not to join a health-care alliance, it became that much more difficult for unions to argue that all large employers be required to participate in the alliances. Kirkland of the AFL-CIO testified on Capitol Hill that while organized labor did not like the provision in the Health Security Act that would permit large employers to remain outside the alliances, "if it's necessary to broaden support for the plan, we're prepared to live with it."[79]

Some union officials went ballistic over organized labor's efforts to preserve the independence of large Taft-Hartley funds and to keep them out of the alliances. They contended that by doing so labor was sanctioning the deleterious practice of carving up the health-care market in a way that essentially perpetuated the practice of experience rating.[80] The health-care alliances would be dumping grounds for less healthy people in need of greater—and more costly—medical care. Furthermore, by securing an opt-out provision for organized labor, they charged, unions helped open the door to a lengthy debate over just how low to set the cut-off point for requiring private-sector employers to join the alliances.[81] In discussions of the Health Security Act, a cut-off point as low as 100 employees was seriously considered (which in effect would have allowed more than half the workforce to remain outside the alliances).[82]

The institutional context antagonized the divisions within organized labor over health-care reform in a second respect. Not wanting to appear as if they had totally sold out on the issue of Canadian-style reform, unions with strong single-payer contingents pushed the Clinton administration to incorporate single-payer language into the Health Security Act, reportedly against the wishes of AFL-CIO president Lane Kirkland. They were joined by a number of public-interest groups, notably Consumers Union, which called upon the White House to provide federal financing to help individual states establish single-payer programs if they wished.[83] In the end, the White House included a measure in the Health Security Act that would allow individual states to create single-payer systems. This neither fish-nor-fowl legislative compromise proved to be highly controversial. "All hell broke loose at that point," said congressional staffer David Abernethy.[84] Business leaders denounced the state-level single-payer provision as a stalking horse for national health insurance a la Canada. Corporations that self-insure were particularly upset. They contended that the proposed single-payer provisions of the Health Security Act flew in the face of the ERISA preemption.[85]

Not surprisingly, unions that rely heavily on Taft-Hartley funds to provide benefits to their members sided with corporations on this point. These unions feared that the single-payer provision in the Health Security Act would permit states either to force unions to give up their Taft-Hartley funds or to dictate to labor how to run the funds.[86] In short, the single-payer provision appeared to put the ERISA preemption, so cherished by employers that self-insure and unions with Taft-Hartley funds, on a collision course with the Health Security Act.[87] Labor's extreme sensitivity to the ERISA issue reportedly prompted the AFL-CIO to pull its support from eleventh-hour compromise legislation proposed by Sen. George Mitchell (D-Maine) in the summer of 1994 because it appeared to threaten the sanctity of the preemption by permitting government surcharges on Taft-Hartley funds.[88]

Even some unions without sizable Taft-Hartley commitments, notably the UAW, did not favor allowing individual states to create single-payer plans. The UAW and other unions with multistate contracts feared that the emergence of a hodgepodge of single-payer plans at the state level would impede efforts to negotiate and implement uniform contracts that span several states.[89] This fear of jeopardizing multistate contracts and weakening the ERISA preemption through state-level initiatives reinforced a long-standing tendency within organized labor to look askance at state-level social reform.

Historically, the AFL-CIO and its antecedents have been ambivalent or downright hostile toward attempts to extend the safety net on a state-by-state basis. Among other things, federation officials feared giving up control of the social welfare agenda to the states. They feared that the most socially backward and poorest states would set the national standard for social welfare. They also doubted the capacity of individual states to develop and implement adequate social welfare programs on their own.[90] Gerald M. Shea, who headed the federation's health-care reform campaign in 1993–94, dismissed state-level initiatives, calling them a "drain on political energy for national action." Furthermore, he said he doubted that labor and other activists could prevail by pursuing universal care on a state-by-state basis.[91] In the 1993–94 period, the national leadership of some unions that had once been ardent single-payer supporters pressured single-payer advocates at the state level to change their tune. AFSCME pushed hard to get the Coalition for Universal Health Insurance for Ohio (UHIO), which first introduced a state-level single-payer bill in 1990, to support the managed-competition approach favored by the White House.[92] The national leadership of the AFL-CIO did not mount any high-profile efforts on behalf of California's Proposition 186, which would create a statewide single-payer system. The initiative was placed on the November 1994 ballot thanks to a state-level labor-community coalition that gathered over 1 million signatures in record time.

Despite all the time and energy that union officials and some public-interest groups devoted to getting single-payer language incorporated into the Health Security Act, organized labor won few kudos for its efforts from the diehard members of the single-payer coalition.[93] "This was their badge of loyalty to the cause," said Barbara Markham Smith, a former legislative aide to single-payer advocate Rep. Jim McDermott (D-Wash.). She dismissed labor's efforts as a "meaningless trophy."[94]

ORGANIZED LABOR ON THE DEFENSIVE

These divisions within and between organized labor and public-interest groups, together with the distractions of the NAFTA fight, made it difficult for organized labor to take the offensive on health-care reform. Preoccupied with NAFTA until November 1993, organized labor left the field clear for opponents of comprehensive health-care reform—most notably the Health Insurance Association of America—to define the terms of the public debate. The HIAA saturated the airwaves in select television markets that fall with the devastating series of "Harry and Louise" commercials.[95] At least as early as October 1993, key union staff members indicated in private that Clinton's Health Security Act was in trouble.[96] After the NAFTA vote in November 1993, labor was unable to recapture the initiative on health care. Valuable time was spent attempting to repair rifts between its grass roots and the treetops, as well as between the White House and labor. As such, organized labor's campaign for health-care reform did not get into full swing until about February 1994, just as the Clinton plan was in its death throes. By that point the Clinton administration appeared much weaker than it had a year earlier because of several major political setbacks. Those setbacks included an indelicate handling of the issue of gays in the military, embarrassing delays and mistakes in making appointments to the executive branch, the bruising battle over the budget, and the growing scandal surrounding the Whitewater land deal.

In early February, the two central assumptions on which organized labor had staked its health-care strategy for more than a decade finally came crashing down in quick succession. The first was the belief that business could be counted on as a constructive partner in health-care reform if organized labor distanced itself from any Canadian-style solution. The second was the conviction that an employer-mandate solution would ultimately triumph because it built on the existing system of job-based benefits and placed no additional burden on the federal tab.

Despite an intense lobbying effort by the White House, the Business Roundtable, an elite business organization comprised of 200 or so leading CEOs, refused to endorse the Health Security Act. Instead it voted on February 2 to back the rival plan sponsored by Rep. Jim Cooper (D-Tenn.), which did not require employers to pay the costs of employee health insurance.[97] The following day, the Chamber of Commerce, in an important retreat, unequivocally disavowed the Clinton plan.[98] The National Association of Manufacturers (NAM) likewise distanced itself from the Clinton plan in no uncertain terms.[99] Labor officials tried to counter the Chamber of Commerce, NAM, and Business Roundtable setbacks in early 1994 by imploring business leaders, notably executives of the Big Three automakers, to reaffirm publicly their commitment to comprehensive health-care reform. Their attempts to encourage leading automobile industry CEOs to author a high-profile op-ed on behalf of the Clinton administration's efforts were unsuccessful. "There was this deafening silence when we needed business to take a stand," said Mary Kay Henry of the SEIU.[100]

The second major blow to labor's strategy came at about the same time. The appeal of the employer-mandate solution rested on what turned out to be two questionable assumptions—that it would not be considered a tax increase, and thus would not affect the federal budget in any significant way.[101] In early February, Robert Reischauer, head of the Congressional Budget Office (CBO), swept away the "tortured fiction" that had sustained labor's deep faith in an employer-mandate solution.[102] He told legislators that the federal government must treat the health insurance premiums that firms would be required to pay for their employees under the Health Security Act as a tax increase for business. Kirkland subsequently conceded that this decision by the CBO was a major blow for labor.[103]

In light of a string of political setbacks on health-care reform and other issues in late 1993 and early 1994, labor leaders debated whether organized labor should recommit itself to the single-payer path.[104] Teamsters president Ron Carey called on President Clinton to alter his strategy on health-care reform after the business community resoundingly deserted the Health Security Act in February 1994.[105] Several unions, including AFSCME, the UAW, and the ILGWU, were reportedly ready to put up substantial sums of money on behalf of the single-payer solution and entered into discussions with one another and legislators about conducting a major publicity campaign for it.[106] This effort sputtered due to continued disarray and disagreement within and between unions, liberal public-interest groups, and legislators.[107] AFSCME attempted to persuade sympathetic legislators and other labor officials that a successful publicity campaign could be waged around a theme that the public was entitled to "health care as good as Congress gets." Congressional Democrats, fearful of inciting another round of Congress-bashing, initially quashed the idea. Advertisements belatedly appeared after a delay of several months, by which time the moment for comprehensive health-care reform had passed.[108]

In short, organized labor's efforts to mold the health-care debate in early 1994 were sporadic at best. For the most part, the debate over health-care reform was conducted in a vacuum in which labor seldom raised broader issues about economic restructuring, the responsibilities of employers to their employees, and the role of insurance companies in the U.S. medical system. The harshest criticism of the job-based system of benefits and the commercial health insurers came from maverick legislators in the U.S. House, not leading figures in organized labor.[109] Representative McDermott was one of the few to call the insurers directly to task and challenge the business community's new united front against an employer mandate.[110] In early 1994, he remarked:

> What is fascinating to me is the retailers, and now the Chamber of Commerce, are getting up here and begin by saying that America cannot do what they can do in every other industrialized country in the world. That is a terrible admission, and I would like to hear these people talk about why it is America is so weak and so uncreative that the business community cannot find any way to participate in a mandatory way as they do in every other country in the world.[111]

Rep. Pete Stark (D-Calif.) forcefully challenged the whole premise of an employer-mandate solution. "It seems to me we jump through a whole lot of hoops to mandate an employer who will then jump through a lot of hoops to not make you or me an employee," he declared.[112]

For the most part, the leaders of organized labor raised few of these deeper structural issues in their public discussions of health-care reform in the 1993–94 period. In their appearances before Congress, they tended to give a qualified "yes, but" endorsement to the Health Security Act and, in some cases, to follow this up with some pleasantries about the single-payer approach.[113] Few dared to raise the third-rail questions associated with health care and economic restructuring and the role of corporations in the new work order in the United States. One notable exception was Tom Gilmartin of the Teamsters, who directly tied the health-care question to broader issues of economic restructuring in his testimony. When asked why, given the concerns he had just raised, organized labor did not speak out more loudly and forcefully on behalf of a single-payer system, Gilmartin told legislators: "That is certainly a question our general executive board and president ask quite often."[114]

There are defeats, and then there are defeats. Washington's failure to pass comprehensive health-care reform legislation in the 1993–94 period represented more than just one more missed legislative opportunity for universal health care and one more legislative defeat for organized labor. The failure to agree upon a solution in the face of heightened expectations fueled cynicism within the general public and within labor's rank and file about what, if anything, government is capable of accomplishing. It fed into the anti-government, anti-tax sentiments that organized labor had tried to quell since the tax revolt of the 1970s and the Reagan revolution of the 1980s.[115] Whereas Canadian advocates of universal health care endured numerous political setbacks in the 1950s and early 1960s but came out emboldened to fight another day, organized labor in the United States did not emerge from the 1993–94 struggle with its political base fortified. It also lacked a viable long-term political strategy to achieve universal health care and shift the political debate in a more desirable direction.[116]

It is not the contention here that the private welfare state institutions and the idea of an employer mandate mortally wounded the Health Security Act. Rather, this analysis shows how the institutions of the private welfare state represented a severe impediment to forging a winning political strategy and coalition that could secure universal and affordable health care over the long haul. In this sense, they contributed to the defeat of comprehensive health-care reform in 1994. These institutions helped realign the interests of labor more closely with those of business and the insurers. They also contributed to tensions within and among unions and liberal-leaning public-interest groups that impeded efforts to form a durable coalition. These divisions made it that much more difficult for labor to lead rather than follow in the health-care reform debate. They also reinforced organized labor's long-standing tendency to defer to the leadership of the Democratic Party on social policy questions. In short, the institutions of the private welfare state and the employer-mandate idea were mutually reinforcing; both, in turn, molded but did not determine labor's political choices and behavior.

These institutions are not entirely to blame, however, for why organized labor was not more effective in furthering the cause of universal health care in the 1993–94 period. Labor leaders made a number of political missteps as well, including the failure to develop a coherent political strategy and message that resonated with the rank and file. They pursued a strategy premised on two unfounded assumptions: First, that some inexorable bottom-line logic would compel business, or at least the Fortune 500, to strike a mutually acceptable deal on universal health care; and second, that the employer mandate was a way to avoid many of the controversial fiscal questions raised by a proposed expansion of social welfare provision in the United States. As such, they did not embed their approach to comprehensive health-care reform in a deeper, coherent, and independent understanding of the U.S. political economy during a time of widespread economic restructuring.

In the battle over the Health Security Act, the Clinton administration echoed the view that escalating health-care costs were the root cause of the woes of the U.S. firm, and hence the American worker. For President Clinton, this was an important shift away from the picture of the U.S. economy that he had painted on the campaign trail. As the Democratic Party's presidential candidate in 1992, Clinton certainly did not launch any stinging broadsides against corporate America. However, he did gingerly suggest in his stump speeches that a complex mixture of factors was to blame for the fact that more Americans were working harder than ever just to maintain an economic foothold. In short, "It's the economy, stupid." These factors included an inequitable tax system, inadequate government and corporate investment in infrastructure, education, economic development, and environmental protection, and the "biggest imbalance in wealth in America since the 1920's."[117] Following his bruising battle over the budget, which dominated his first seven months in office, Clinton emerged with a reduced vision of what was ailing the U.S. worker. In short, "It's the health-care costs, stupid."[118] After Clinton unveiled his Health Security Act, administration officials ran with the theme of how escalating medical expenses lay at the heart of the nation's economic woes.[119] Although labor attempted to develop a more comprehensive and multifaceted understanding of the nation's economic woes in its campaign to defeat NAFTA, in discussions of health care it reinforced this more one-dimensional view of what ailed the U.S. economy and the average worker.

If labor had pursued the single-payer option in a more forceful and united fashion, there might have been short-term political costs to pay with the administration. However, in the case of NAFTA, labor was quite willing to defy the administration and suffer those costs, which turned out to be minimal. Moreover, Clinton's record on labor issues already fell well below expectations and was, frankly, disappointing. In terms of access and appointments, his record was better than that of his two Republican predecessors. But from the get go, the administration was unwilling to spend real political capital on behalf of organized labor and issues important to the average worker, be it an increase in the minimum wage or a ban on hiring permanent replacement workers during strikes.

This focus on organized labor's missteps in the health-care debate should in no way minimize the fact that labor was up against formidable institutional obstacles and formidable political obstacles. It faced a conservative and polarized political environment in which its opponents were intent on killing any comprehensive health-care reform measure.[120] Its opponents could muster enormous resources, financial and otherwise, to that end.[121] Furthermore, the media and opponents of the Health Security Act generally distorted the public debate on health-care reform and increased anxiety among middle-class Americans who had good health-care coverage that the Clinton plan or other untried alternatives would jeopardize that coverage.[122] Leading media outlets, in particular *The New York Times*, helped marginalize and delegitimize single-payer solutions while banging the drum loudly for managed care, and often gave disproportionate attention to non-labor groups.[123] However, these obstacles, while not insignificant, cannot fully explain the defeat of the Health Security Act and why organized labor was not more effective in shaping the public debate and furthering the cause of universal, affordable health care in the United States.

In her explanation of the defeat of the Health Security Act, Theda Skocpol faults the administration for not doing more to shape the public debate over health-care reform by educating the public about the details of the Clinton proposal. The details she had in mind included the rationale for an employer mandate, the health-care alliances, and the heavy regulatory hand underpinning the Health Security Act. Yet the right message will not, on its own, assure passage of major social policy legislation, especially in the face of decided ambivalence by big business and the absence of a crisis on the order of, say, the Depression.[124] Ultimately, advocates of universal health care need to figure out how to create and nurture durable political alliances glued together by something more than just the right message for a specific policy. This is especially so today in an age when budgetary concerns drive social policy.[125] Major social policies ultimately raise fundamental questions not just about which is better—more government or less—but about what constitutes a fair and just society and who should bear what burden to that end. That question is inherently controversial. And during periods when the winds of retrenchment blow hard, that question is inescapable.

To enter into a broader public debate about how the employer mandate would work and the reasons for it would mean opening up a broader discussion about why the United States has such a jerry-built system of employer-sponsored benefits in the first place. It would mean confronting not just the question of whether employers should provide benefits like health insurance, but what social obligations, if any, employers have in exchange for the right to do business in the United States. In doing so, the Clinton administration would have had to confront many of the volatile issues raised by the wrenching restructuring of the U.S. economy that has been under way for more than two decades.

In presenting the idea of an employer mandate to the public, Clinton and organized labor together might have raised some of these deeper questions about the U.S. economy and triumphed in the court of public opinion. But to do so would have required building more than just a fair-weather coalition, with elements of business, that entered into a marriage of convenience over health-care reform after a messy public spat over NAFTA. Given Clinton's conservative Democratic Leadership Council credentials, his deep ties to the financial sector, and his lack of any solid political or ideological grounding, it is unlikely that he would have begun this public debate on his own accord. However, organized labor together with public-interest groups might have been able to drag him in that direction. This certainly would not have brought about the passage of any single-payer legislation in the short- or medium-term, nor have assured enactment of the Health Security Act. However, it might have altered the debate over health care such that the quest for universal health care and the plight of the uninsured remained viable, credible issues on which to build a coherent reform coalition over the long haul. As shown here several issues precluded this option: the institutional constraints of the private welfare state; internal divisions within and between organized labor and public-interest groups over health-care reform; labor's dogged commitment to working with business to solve the nation's health-care dilemmas; and its general lack of political imagination.

CHAPTER 8

Conclusion

The Peculiar Politics of U.S. Health Policy

> Successful politics is always the art of the possible. It is no less true, how-
> ever, that the possible is often achieved only by reaching out towards
> the impossible which lies beyond it.
>
> MAX WEBER

More than 25 years ago, organized labor and the Democrats battled President Richard M. Nixon's health-care plan. They stuck by an alternative proposal for national health insurance loosely modeled on the Canadian system and premised on eliminating the commercial health insurers and the link between employment and health benefits. By 1993, much of organized labor, together with leading Democrats and a number of public-interest groups, was rallying around a reform plan explicitly modeled on the previously despised Nixon plan. President Clinton's Health Security Act incorporated a key feature of the Nixon proposal—the so-called employer mandate, which would obligate employers to pay for a portion of their employees' health-insurance premiums. Despite enormous changes in the labor market since the 1970s, namely efforts to create a more flexible workforce by expanding the number of part-time, temporary, and other contingent workers, the commitment of organized labor and the Democrats to an employment-based system of health benefits rooted in the private sector became more intense.

The institutional context of the private welfare state goes a considerable distance in explaining why organized labor and the Democrats largely abandoned a grander vision of national health insurance. It also helps explain why Clinton's Health Security Act crashed and burned. The institutional context was an impediment to forging the durable, broad-based coalitions necessary to overcome the formidable obstacles to achieving universal and affordable health care in the United States. Even with such coalitions in place, it is unlikely that the 103rd Congress would have passed a major health-care reform bill. However, organized labor and its allies might have come out of the 1993–94 battle in a better position to continue the long march for universal health care. As such, the quest for universal health care would have been more than just the battle of the moment. It would have been, as in the Canadian case, the rallying cry for a long-term strategy to realign the political center of social policy and the agenda of the major political parties.

This analysis walks a fine line between showing the importance of institutions and falling into the trap of institutional determinism. While institutions are important, they are seldom the "sole 'cause' of outcomes."[1] In explaining political outcomes in social policy, notably health policy, a textured understanding of the institutional context will get you far, but only so far. It is also important to have a good grasp of the larger political economy in which these institutions operate, the ways in which political actors interpret their environment, and the political consequences that flow from how they decipher that environment.[2]

This brief final chapter first addresses some of the broader analytical implications of this study. It concludes with a few observations about the future direction of organized labor and health policy in the United States.

INSTITUTIONS OF THE PRIVATE WELFARE STATE

The debate within political science over the significance of institutions has gone through several waves—some that overlap and others that crash against one another.[3] The analysis here fits most comfortably within the historical-institutional framework. Namely, it uses postwar health policy as a window through which to view how specific institutions molded the goals, strategies, and worldviews of political actors, notably labor and business, often in unintended or unanticipated ways.[4] As demonstrated in the preceding chapters, the political terrain is seldom a tabula rasa on which individuals and groups are free to etch and pursue their interests. Institutional landscapes mold group interests and political behavior. Indeed, institutions not only shape the goals and strategies of groups, but also may determine the specific types of groups that emerge in the first place.[5]

In the case of health policy, institutions were highly constricting. Several critical institutions of the private welfare state in the United States grew up ensnared in certain interests. These institutions helped realign the interests of organized labor more closely with those of business and the insurers. They also helped solidify a coalition of labor, business, and insurers in favor of experience-rated health-insurance plans and the so-called ERISA preemption and opposed to enacting national health insurance. Furthermore, they enabled a more business-friendly view of the U.S. political economy to congeal and then ossify. In the process, elements of organized labor became isolated from key potential allies in health-care reform—including gay activist organizations and liberal public-interest groups like Public Citizen. Bitter divisions also arose within organized labor as unions battled among themselves about whether to support the single-payer path and whether to preserve the Taft-Hartley system of health benefits.

This analysis highlights just how sticky institutions can be; in short, why institutions persist and shape behavior. However, institutions are not like mountains, largely fixed, unchanging, and crisscrossed by familiar and well-trod paths. They are more like sand dunes whose contours change over time, often in ways that are confusing to the traveler attempting to cross the political desert and arrive at an oasis of social policy reform. Political actors often retain a fixed view of a particular institution and continue to base their political strategies on that view long after the political and economic winds fundamentally alter its contours. Just as it is hardest to get an accurate view of the lay of the desert as a sandstorm whirls about, during periods of rapid political and economic change the new contours of old institutions may be the hardest to discern.

This disjuncture in perception between what a particular institution was and how it has changed over time has important political implications. For example, over the last two decades many unions abandoned their once dogged commitment to fighting for a universal system of health care that eliminates job-based benefits and commercial health insurers. They shifted course and endorsed an employer-mandate solution. Labor leaders defended this shift on political grounds and contended that they were merely asking the state to mandate what most employers already did voluntarily. But the system of employment-based benefits is an institutional accident with complex economic and political underpinnings. And it was crumbling just at the moment when organized labor sought an employer-mandate solution.

Just as there is no readily apparent logic to how the sand dunes are arrayed after a sandstorm, institutions are not always logical, consistent, or predictable.[6] The landscape is further complicated because shifts in one institution may have far-reaching and unintended consequences for other institutions down the line. Moreover, institutions shape strategies and mold preferences. For example, the Taft-Hartley Act sanctioned the creation of a peculiar set of institutional arrangements for providing medical care and other benefits through the private sector. The AFL-CIO, initially cool to the concept of the Taft-Hartley health and welfare funds, over time warmed up to these private-sector arrangements as the funds proliferated and became an important organizing device and a lucrative financial opportunity for some union officials. The Taft-Hartley funds subsequently became a real impediment to creating a universal health system that eliminates job-based benefits and the commercial health-insurance companies.

The institutional context not only defined the coalitions, but also the worldview and strategies around which the fight for health-care reform was waged. From the early 1980s, organized labor sought to forge an alliance with business on health policy. In doing so, unions acquiesced to a redefinition of the terms of the health-care debate. Whereas earlier struggles for universal health care, notably in the 1940s and early 1970s, were waged around issues of social justice, concerns about the economic competitiveness of U.S. companies predominated in the 1980s and 1990s as organized labor staked its strategy on working closely with business. In the end, labor appears to have misread the business sector. Business support for a comprehensive health-care reform plan that unions could live with, even if they could not love it, was ephemeral. The decision to seek a close alliance with business and support an employer-mandate solution was a costly one for unions. It yielded few political gains, but exacerbated cleavages within and between organized labor and important public-interest groups.

A group's strategic choice can lead it or prime it to accept more encompassing arguments about the "definition of the problem" at a later point. Unions made a strategic choice in 1978 to abandon national health insurance and endorse the employer-mandate idea. This had enormous political consequences. Unions subsequently were locked into a definition of the health-care problem—which then locked them into particular coalition-building strategies that were untenable and ultimately self-defeating. The institutions of the private welfare state coupled with the ruling discourse about the basically cooperative nature of labor-management relations in the United States reinforced these strategies.

HEALTH POLICY AND THE "HEALTH" OF THE ECONOMY

The institutions of the private welfare state sit at the center of this analysis. But the institutional context does not wholly explain why organized labor pursued the health policies that it did and why it was unsuccessful in its quest for universal health care. This account highlights the importance of two additional and related factors, namely the ways in which political actors decipher their environment and the central role that ideas, even a single policy idea, play in the process.

As E.E. Schattschneider reminded us several decades ago: "The definition of the alternatives is the supreme instrument of power."[7] In the case of the most recent skirmishes over universal health care, organized labor, which was so central to earlier battles over health policy, failed to define meaningful alternatives. Instead, labor echoed business's view that escalating health-care costs coupled with intensified economic competition at home and abroad put the U.S. corporation and the U.S. worker in peril. This was a view at odds with many of the economic facts on the ground.

The assumptions about the U.S. political economy and welfare state that political actors hold near and dear turned out to be important variables. Such assumptions facilitate or impede the shift from one policy path to another.[8] In the case of health policy, a single policy idea—the employer mandate—helped legitimize a set of assumptions about the U.S. economy that were highly favorable to business. Over time it reinforced labor's tendency to take a cooperative stance toward business and to pursue the Dunlop way. It also impeded labor's capacity to develop a coherent, alternative understanding of the U.S. political economy and formulate social and economic policies compatible with that alternative interpretation (and consistent with one another).

As demonstrated in chapter 6, the Clinton administration's Health Security Act was developed and sold on the basis of several assumptions about the U.S. political economy and welfare state that emerged during earlier debates over health-care initiatives based on an employer mandate. Labor embraced and promoted these broader assumptions during the 1980s. The employer-mandate idea thus functioned not just as one of the "switchmen" that launched organized labor onto a new policy path with respect to health care, but also served as a convenient hook on which to hang and legitimize a number of new assumptions about the U.S. political economy.[9] Taken together these assumptions helped shape an alternative worldview, one sympathetic to business. These assumptions also drew attention away from the sobering fact that employers were quite successful at whittling away the private welfare state by shifting more of the costs of health care onto employees.

This somewhat narrow focus on the political trajectory of a single idea, the employer mandate, has broader analytical implications for how we think about the role of organized labor in politics, and the significance of ideas more generally in explaining political outcomes. Much of the literature on ideas in political science focuses on a cluster of related ideas and related policies, for example, Keynesianism, Stalinism, monetarism, or decolonization. Those related ideas or policies are the lens that define, if not a new political and economic era, at least a new and compelling political or economic model.[10] Although it is important to consider the role of clusters of ideas—be they "programmatic beliefs," "worldviews," "principled beliefs," "causal beliefs," or "policy paradigms"—in ushering out one era or model and ushering in another, we should not ignore or underestimate the far-reaching consequences of a single idea.[11] Adopted initially out of political expediency and as yet not linked to any grander vision or framework, such ideas can have important unintended consequences. In periods fraught with uncertainty, when the sun sets on one cluster of ideas and policies, such as Keynesianism, and a new day has yet to dawn on another cluster, such as Reaganism and monetarism, single ideas often provide the raw materials out of which a new paradigm, ideology, or worldview is molded or legitimated. In this instance, labor's endorsement over the years of a single idea—the employer mandate—helped legitimize a worldview premised on a strong coincidence of interests between labor and business in the face of the vast restructuring of the U.S. economy. This, in turn, had important consequences for the political efficacy of organized labor and for the fate of universal health care in the United States.

The preceding chapters demonstrate another broader analytical point: that there really is no such thing as a politics of health policy per se.[12] Health-care issues must be analyzed within a larger political and economic context. It is essential to examine not just the actions and preferences of labor, business, and the state with respect to specific health-care policies and proposals, but also the objectives political actors pursue simultaneously in other key areas of the political economy, such as labor-management relations, electoral politics, and tax and regulatory policies. By taking this broader view of health policy, analysts are forced to reconcile the often competing and contradictory views and impulses of business and organized labor in social policy. For example, how do we assess International Paper's active participation in and expressed commitment to labor-management health-care coalitions at the national level in the late 1980s at the same time that it engaged in an acrimonious battle with its workers in which it enlisted replacement workers to break a strike?[13]

Inserting health policy into the larger debate over the U.S. political economy is also a way to wrest the issue of health policy away from the health-care experts. In recent years the debate over health policy increasingly operated "with the language, methodology, and mind-set of bureaucratic actors."[14] Such a politically charged issue as health care is seemingly stripped of politics. Whether they intended to or not, many health-care experts nonetheless succeeded in precluding wider public participation in the debate by treating health policy as if it somehow operates outside of the normal push and pull of the political economy that shapes other realms of social and economic policy.

By contrast, this study demonstrates how health policy is inextricably bound up with larger questions related to the current restructuring of the U.S. economy, the political consequences of which are hazy and largely unexamined by political scientists. That restructuring has had far-reaching consequences, including an explosion of innovations in the organization of work unparalleled since the Depression, a stagnation in real wages for the average American since the early 1970s, and a whittling away of health-care, retirement, and other job-related benefits that comprise the private-sector safety net in the United States. Except for vague and dire calls from business representatives and labor officials about the need to cut medical costs to remain "competitive," the health-care debates of the 1980s and 1990s generally took place outside of a larger debate over the future of the U.S. economy and the future of the public and private welfare states. One consequence of this is that analysts and advocates took a compartmentalized view of the role of business in health care. They concentrated on business's stated concern about how escalating medical costs threaten the competitiveness and profitability of U.S. firms. But seldom did they examine that concern within a larger political and economic context. This helps explain the excessive optimism among analysts, policy-makers, and labor leaders in the late 1980s and early 1990s that business could help lead the way to an acceptable health-care solution.

Organized labor responded as if the political economy of the 1980s and 1990s were a replay of the late 1920s and 1930s. Labor jumped onto the competitiveness bandwagon, confident that cutthroat competition from lower-benefit or lower-cost producers at home and abroad during a period of perceived economic malaise would force U.S. firms to support comprehensive health-care reform. After all, ruinous interstate competition in the 1930s prompted industries to eventually support national social welfare legislation.[15] Firms in the 1980s and 1990s, however, did not face a situation analogous to the interwar years when fierce competition, in the face of scarce demand, and shrinking product markets presented an opportunity to forge cross-class alliances in support of Social Security.[16] Despite the burden of rising health-care costs, the 1980s and 1990s were halcyon days, economically and politically, for much of business in the United States in the wake of the 1981–82 recession. By the mid-1980s, the competitiveness of U.S. manufacturing firms had improved dramatically because of good productivity growth, large appreciations in foreign currency values, and a decline in unit labor costs.[17]

Ruinous competition was not the only reason that a key cadre of employers eventually agreed 65 years ago to support Social Security. Employers came to view this landmark social legislation as a bulwark against more radical solutions proposed by organized labor and other groups. The popular Townsend movement, which demanded that the federal government provide each person aged 60 and older with a monthly pension of $200, served as an important prod. It induced business and the Roosevelt administration

to enact a broad social welfare agenda to neutralize growing public sentiment for more radical proposals.[18] Faced not just with ruinous competition
but also a burgeoning and threatening social movement, employers accepted a legislated solution. As John Commons argued, employers do not
normally accept legislated social reform "until they are faced by an alternative which seems worse to them than the one they 'willingly accept.' "[19] In
the 1990s, no social movement congealed around a more radical alternative, in part because organized labor did not anchor a "radical flank" to realign the political debate over universal health care.

Unions were highly constrained by the institutional contours of the private welfare state and broader shifts in the U.S. political economy. And
certainly other features of the political and institutional environment constrained organized labor: its longstanding "barren marriage" or "abusive
relationship" with the Democratic Party[20]; the formidable institutional barriers to creating a third party in the United States; the rise of a more forceful right flank in American politics; and the disproportionate resources
that its opponents—notably the business sector—could muster. Although
these obstacles are real and significant, they do not entirely explain labor's
political inefficacy on the health-care question and why it abandoned national health insurance and embraced the employer-mandate option. A
central argument here is that its own lack of political imagination constrained labor. On the health-care issue, organized labor chose to accept
the given political environment and concentrate most of its political activities and resources on what appeared to be achievable in the short
term. But much of politics is about developing a vision that supersedes
the given political environment; then using that vision as a tool or
weapon to undermine, chip away at, delegitimize, and ultimately trans-
form the existing political environment. For example, Rep. Newt Gingrich (R-Ga.) did not accept his party's minority status in the U.S. House
as a permanent feature of the political landscape. He developed a long-
term strategy that by the early 1990s succeeded in mainstreaming what
were considered fringe political ideas circa the 1970s, when Gingrich appeared to be howling in the political wilderness. Two decades ago, virtually no analyst expected that his strident rejection of the go-along-to-get-
along stance of the more moderate Republican leadership would yield
the first Republican House of Representatives in 40 years or that it would
catapult him into the speakership.[21]

By comparison, organized labor was singularly unimaginative. It neglected to develop a long-term strategy to secure universal health care embedded in a broader vision of how to restructure a decidedly unfavorable
political environment. It failed to seize the political opportunities that did
present themselves. In the case of health policy, organized labor was unable

to develop its own independent understanding of the U.S. political economy. It accepted at face value many of the questionable claims that business made about the connection between rising health-care costs, economic competitiveness, and the economic livelihood of the average U.S. worker.

THE FUTURE OF ORGANIZED LABOR AND UNIVERSAL HEALTH CARE

Perhaps organized labor's repeated failures in securing universal health care in the postwar years signify its growing political impotence and waning relevance in struggles over social policy in the United States. Even prior to the implosion of the health-care reform effort during the first term of the Clinton administration, doubt was widespread about whether organized labor, even a radically reorganized labor movement, could provide the seeds for its own renewal, let alone engineer a major transformation of U.S. politics.[22] It is hard to see the collapse of yet another effort to achieve universal health care as anything but a defeat for organized labor in the United States. It is not obvious, however, that this was one of the final nails in the political coffin of U.S. unions.

A closer look at the history of labor's triumphs and setbacks in the United States and elsewhere, notably Canada, reveals that the seeds of renewal for organized labor may come from within. And, furthermore, that failure may ironically serve as the soil that nurtures them. For example, the emergence and spread of industrial unionism in the United States, which is associated with the birth of the Congress of Industrial Organizations (CIO) in the 1930s, fundamentally transformed the character of the U.S. labor movement and the character of American politics in important ways. Although the CIO was a new organization, it did not emerge out of political thin air. A vigorous debate over industrial unionism took place for many years within the more conservative American Federation of Labor (AFL), long before the CIO was officially established.[23] On a related point, the Canadian case illustrates how the rebirth of labor can take place in the wake of major defeats at the bargaining table and in national politics. Canada's long history of strident social unionism can be traced back to Ottawa's failure to enact comparable New Deal-type legislation during the Depression in Canada in the 1930s. Unable to achieve a New Deal-style settlement until the 1940s, the Canadian labor movement harbored a deep mistrust of the two major political parties and subsequently set off on the path of social unionism rather than business unionism.[24] This deep-seated commitment to social unionism helped Canadian unions to weather the massive economic restructuring of the last two decades and keep growing while the membership rolls of U.S. unions contracted.[25]

After the latest health-care debacle, organized labor in the United States did not immediately resume business as usual. On September 26, 1994, the same day that Senate majority leader George Mitchell (D-Maine) announced the demise of comprehensive health-care reform, AFL-CIO president Lane Kirkland told a meeting of the federation's health-care committee that escalating medical costs "will continue to be the monster that ate the world." Although Kirkland put health-care costs at the root of many of the economic evils visited upon the U.S. worker, he indicated that the AFL-CIO might consider making major shifts in its stance on health policy. He asked the committee to focus on two areas in particular: a careful assessment of what can be done at the state level to usher in acceptable reform measures; and a reexamination of labor's overall strategy with an eye toward renewing labor's commitment to national health insurance based on a single-payer system.[26]

Although Kirkland appeared ready to concede some political ground, it was not enough. The 1993–94 debacle and the dismal performance of labor and the Democrats in the 1994 midterm elections fortified the resolve of AFSCME and other key unions not to support Kirkland for another term as president. When Kirkland remained noncommittal about staying on or stepping aside, an insurgent movement emerged that was centered around SEIU president John J. Sweeney, the architect of organized labor's doomed health-care strategy. By the time Kirkland read the writing on the wall and stepped aside in June 1995, the insurgent forces had gathered so much steam that Kirkland's handpicked successor, AFL-CIO secretary-treasurer Thomas R. Donahue, was no longer a shoo-in, and the race was on in the federation's first contested election.

Sweeney's "New Voice" ticket, which included United Mine Workers president Richard Trumka for secretary-treasurer and AFSCME vice president Linda Chavez-Thompson for the newly created post of executive vice president, rode to victory in October 1995 on a platform not all that different from Donahue's. Both promised to put more resources into organizing new members, especially women, younger workers, and minorities. Both vowed to mobilize and train a hard core of dedicated organizers who could be counted on to recruit new members and form the nucleus of labor's stepped-up political activities at the grass-roots level. Both promised to revitalize the central labor councils and state labor federations. And both nixed the idea of a labor party. Where they differed was over whether to enlist labor's minions to participate in acts of civil disobedience and to be more confrontational in their struggles against employers and the new conservative agenda articulated in the Republicans' "Contract With America." Donahue contended that workers are reluctant to participate in more militant action.[27] Sweeney, on the other hand, argued that workers must strike the right balance between blocking bridges and building bridges if they are to make any significant economic or political gains. Sweeney was hailed as the great reformer who successfully shook up labor's old guard and challenged the gerontocracy of the AFL-CIO.

This simple picture of an AFL-CIO divided between its old guard and its reformers is misleading, as is the image of Sweeney as a crusading reformer. Over the years, Sweeney resisted efforts to democratize the SEIU, his home base within organized labor.[28] As demonstrated in the preceding chapters, Sweeney was a true labor insider. As head of the federation's health-care committee, his fingerprints were all over the AFL-CIO's doomed health-care strategy. Moreover, other so-called reformers, like Gerald McEntee of AFSCME, shifted back and forth between both sides of the aisle, between accommodation and confrontation on the question of health-care reform and other pressing issues.

As he geared up to contest the presidency of the AFL-CIO, Sweeney appeared ready to be more critical of the Clinton administration and the business sector. After Clinton vowed in his State of the Union address in 1995 that the era of big government was over, Sweeney acerbically remarked:

> But when Clinton said, "Our job is to get rid of yesterday's government so that our people can meet today's and tomorrow's needs," a questioning chill no doubt ran down the spines of millions of Americans who depend on federal laws, regulations and assistance for their very survival.

He then suggested that Clinton was "edging dangerously close to the slimy center line of the Republican leadership's 'Contract With America.' "[29] By the time of the AFL-CIO's historic convention in October 1995, Sweeney had rediscovered the voice of moderation, at least as far as Clinton was concerned. Indeed, Clinton was a featured guest at the convention that elevated Sweeney to the federation presidency.[30] Sweeney continues to express a desire to return to a golden era of harmonious labor-management relations that, in his view, existed in the immediate postwar years. On a number of occasions, he has called for a renewal of the "social compact" that purportedly guided the country during a period in which "[b]usiness, labor, and government all agreed that working people were entitled to a fair share of the wealth they produced" and were willing to uphold that compact.[31]

Yet, in other respects the federation has sought to sharpen the partisan edge of its political activities since 1994. In a major address to a gathering of business and civic leaders in New York City soon after he became president of the AFL-CIO, Sweeney attempted to present a more comprehensive and multidimensional understanding of the U.S. political economy than the picture on which organized labor staked its health-care strategy. Instead of simply blaming escalating medical costs for pricing U.S. workers out of the international market and hurting their economic livelihoods, he castigated U.S. firms for taking the low road and for believing that "the best way to compete in the global economy was by driving down labor costs." He also took corporations to task for not trying to be more competitive through other means—for example, more innovation, improvements in the climate of labor-management relations, and insistence on international social standards and rights for all workers. He charged that U.S. firms chose to respond to intensified economic pressures from abroad by "squeezing the last possible ounce of productivity out of American workers and then throwing them on the scrap heap of unemployment or old age with reduced pensions and health-insurance coverage."[32]

This more encompassing view of the U.S. political economy and more critical view of business is one that the AFL-CIO says it is committed to imparting to its membership in the aftermath of the health-care battle. After extensively polling its rank and file in the wake of the health-care defeat, the AFL-CIO concluded that workers lacked an "economic context" by which "to evaluate where their interests lie," according to Gerald M. Shea, Sweeney's right-hand man. It also discovered that workers resented organized labor telling them whom to vote for. The federation is now more committed to educating its members about economic questions, providing them with information about where various candidates stand on the issues, and then letting them decide.[33] To that end, the AFL-CIO is attempting to develop an independent understanding of the U.S. political economy. It recently created a department that will focus on public policy questions and take a long-range view of economic and social issues like Social Security, international investment, health care, and family issues. Whereas in the past the AFL-CIO directed research at specific legislative proposals, the new department is expected to operate more like a think tank, generating original research and policy prescriptions of its own. The federation also created the Office of Investment to investigate how organized labor can become a more activist investor and use its billions of dollars in pension funds to exert real pressure on business.[34]

Organized labor's new political strategy racked up several impressive victories following the defeat of Clinton's Health Security Act in 1994. In the months prior to the 1996 election, the AFL-CIO waged a media-savvy grass-roots campaign targeted at key Congressional districts that secured a 90–cent increase in the minimum wage, the first hike since 1989. The victory was all the more impressive because labor faced Republican majorities in the House and Senate.[35] In the year prior to the 1996 election, the federation also mounted a $35 million campaign to attack Republican members of the House who supported drastic cutbacks in Medicare and other social programs.[36] Because the Republican Party retained both the House and the Senate in the 1996 elections, business and Republican leaders, and the public generally, dismissed labor's efforts as nothing more than the thrashing about of a paper tiger with money to burn.[37] Although the AFL-CIO's electoral effort was insufficient to return the House and Senate to Democratic control, it did have a substantial effect on the elections. By Gary C. Jacobson's calculations, "targeted incumbents, freshmen or otherwise, lost much more frequently than those who were not targeted" by organized labor.[38]

Unlike in the past, organized labor's electoral apparatus did not hibernate following the 1996 election only to awaken two years later in the midst of another campaign. In early 1997, unions began another targeted blitz, this time against a Republican proposal that would permit workers to take compensation time in lieu of overtime pay. The effectiveness of this campaign, coupled with some of labor's other recent political victories, prompted some Republicans "to refer, in their darker moments, to AFL-CIO honcho John Sweeney as the real speaker of the House."[39] In a major and unexpected victory in November 1997, organized labor defeated "fast-track" trade legislation that would have prevented Congress from amending trade agreements negotiated by the president.[40] After the defeat of the fast-track proposal, *New York Times* columnist William Safire warned of the emergence of the "Demo-Labor Party."[41] In another major victory, in the spring of 1998 unions successfully mobilized against Proposition 226, a California referendum that would have forced unions to get explicit permission from individual members before using their dues for political activities. Early polls indicated that 70 percent of voters were in favor of the proposal.[42] And in the 1998 midterm elections, organized labor provided the margin of victory in a number of close and key races. That year union households accounted for 22 percent of the votes cast, compared to just 14 percent in 1994.[43]

The most dramatic display of labor's strength and new stance on economic issues was the massive demonstations it helped to organize against the World Trade Organization (WTO) in Seattle in late 1999. These protests put the Clinton administration and WTO on the defensive and contributed to a collapse in the global trade negotiations. Labor, environmental, consumer, and other groups forcefully challenged the idea that economic competitiveness and growth demanded the worldwide wholesale deregulation of labor, environmental, and other standards. Although the AFL-CIO was actively involved in planning the demonstrations, some of the leadership was once again out of step with the rank and file. The AFL-CIO emphasized reforming the WTO, while many activists called for scrapping it altogether.[44] Just weeks before the WTO meeting, Sweeney joined a group of business leaders, including Monsanto and Proctor & Gamble executives, in signing a letter endorsing the Clinton administration's agenda in the upcoming trade negotiations, which sparked an angry response from other labor leaders.[45]

It is not obvious that labor's new political activism, and its greater willingness to embed its social and economic policies in a more nuanced and comprehensive understanding of the U.S. political economy, will result in the establishment of universal and affordable health care in the United States. First, labor's new political activism has ignited a fierce and concerted backlash from the Republican leadership and from some of labor's old guard.[46] Furthermore, the AFL-CIO leadership remains congenitally unable to step out of the shadow of Clinton and the Democratic Party despite the NAFTA, health care, and other setbacks. At the AFL-CIO biennial convention in the fall of 1999, Sweeney secured an early endorsement for Vice President Al Gore in his race against former Senator Bill Bradley for the Democratic presidential nomination. Sweeney pushed hard for Gore despite deep concerns amongst the rank and file and some labor leaders about what unions could expect from Gore in return. They also questioned the wisdom of making such an early commitment to the vice president considering his poor performance in the presidential race thus far. Despite organized labor's newfound political feistiness and independence in the wake of the health-care defeat, unions remain highly constrained not only by their political imaginations but also by the institutional context. There are many indications that organized labor's attachment to the private welfare state is intensifying, and that the institutional context continues to be a severe impediment to the development and enactment of any health-care proposal that severs the tie between health benefits and employment status once and for all.

After the Health Security Act went down in flames, some unions retraced their steps and returned to the single-payer path. The departure of Sweeney at the SEIU opened the way for reformer Andrew Stern, head of the union's organizing department, to defeat the old guard and secure the presidency.[47] At the SEIU's April 1996 convention, delegates passed a resolution proposed from the floor by the reform faction that committed the union to a Canadian-style, single-payer system.[48] However, for all the talk about renewing labor's commitment to a single-payer solution and about assuming a more confrontational stance vis-à-vis employers, organized labor has yet to develop a long-term strategy to achieve universal health care.

In the wake of the Health Security Act defeat, organized labor's primary focus shifted to the future of health maintenance organizations.[49] It is deja vu all over again as the AFL-CIO works side-by-side with a new group of business and consumer groups whose aim is to ensure that managed-care insurance plans deliver quality health care. The recently established Foundation for Accountability (also known as Facct) counts among its supporters the AFL-CIO, the AARP, and large health-care purchasers, including American Express and General Motors.[50] Paradoxically, at the center of this effort stands Paul Ellwood, a seminal figure in developing and popularizing the concept of managed care in the first place. Ellwood was the force behind the Jackson Hole Group, a health policy group dominated by insurers that led the charge for managed competition in the early 1990s and that some argue helped bring down Clinton's Health Security Act.[51]

By the late 1990s, the centerpiece of labor's health-care efforts was legislation to establish a "patient's bill of rights" to curb the prerogatives of HMOs and other types of managed care, which altogether insure 85 percent of workers with health benefits. All the political brouhaha that this proposal generated obscures the fact that this measure amounted to little more than a Band-Aid on a health-care system that remains in critical condition. At the close of the decade, health-insurance premiums were escalating at a rate unmatched since the early 1990s. Meanwhile, employers shifted more of the costs of medical care onto workers, and many businesses were dropping coverage altogether, thus consigning more people in the United States to the ranks of the uninsured.[52] In early 1999, the blue-ribbon National Bipartisan Commission on the Future of Medicare narrowly missed securing the votes necessary to recommend to Congress a radically revamped Medicare system. The changes included largely privatizing the government's health-care system for the elderly, raising the eligibility age for Medicare, and essentially eliminating the federal guarantee of low-cost health-care for older Americans.[53]

Meanwhile, organized labor moved to become a more significant health provider in its own right. This will further strengthen its attachment to the private welfare state and to private-sector solutions for health-care reform. Following the defeat of Clinton's Health Security Act, the National Health and Human Service Employees Union, better known as Local 1199, began developing its own managed-care health plan to market to New York's 2.5 million union members.[54] The union, which represents 150,000 health-care workers in the state, also made an unsuccessful attempt in conjunction with the region's hospitals to take over Empire Blue Cross and Blue Shield, the largest insurer in New York state.[55] Today the union runs its own $400 million comprehensive health plan.[56] During the 1995 battle over the draconian cuts to Medicare included in the Medicare Preservation Act proposed by the Republicans, Gingrich shrewdly courted unions that had extensive Taft-Hartley commitments. The Republicans floated proposals that would permit unions to provide health benefits for Medicare-eligible retirees through a new set of funds administered by unions and modeled on the

Taft-Hartley arrangements. The NCCMP, the main lobbying organization for the Taft-Hartley funds, warmly received these proposals.[57] Attempting to address the needs of the contingent workforce, labor is experimenting with new health-insurance arrangements that promise to bolster the shadow welfare state. In Silicon Valley, it created a nonprofit temp agency that offers affordable health-care coverage to temporary workers. The AFL-CIO also is investigating how unions can attract high-tech workers by providing them with portable health and pension benefits that follow them over the course of their career. Here labor explicitly has in mind the Taft-Hartley model of health and welfare funds that proliferated in the building and construction trades and other sectors since World War II.[58] If the past tells us anything, as unions invest heavily in HMOs that they create, seize opportunities to expand Taft-Hartley-style arrangements, and enter the health-insurance market in other ways, they will be less likely to embrace calls for national health insurance that would do away with commercial insurers and make the government the primary payer.[59]

Today the boldest initiatives in health policy come from politicians not organized labor. In his quest for the presidency, Bill Bradley designated universal health care as a pillar of his campaign and declared good health care for all a basic right. In response, Vice President Al Gore proposed a series of incremental steps to expand coverage for poor and low-income families. To his credit, Bradley forced the plight of the uninsured back into the national limelight and conscience. But his proposal perpetuates many problems of the shadow welfare state of job-based benefits. His plan to subsidize coverage for the poorest families and offer tax credits for health insurance on a sliding scale for others gives employers an incentive to shred coverage and continue their assault on the private-sector safety net. Permitting all Americans to buy into the same group health plan that provides private health insurance to federal employees encourages employers and insurers to cherry-pick the healthy and leave the sicker, high-cost patients in the government plan. This raises health-insurance premiums and prices less healthy people out of the market. The Bradley plan also does not address the exorbitant administrative costs of the private health-care system in the United States.[60] Bradley's plan shares some striking similarities with a plan introduced by the health-insurance industry to address the problem of the growing number of uninsured. In May 1999, health-insurance companies proposed new federal subsidies and tax credits to subsidize insurance for the uninsured that would amount to a giant new government subsidy for the insurance industry.[61]

In short, the institutions of the private welfare state discussed in detail in this book are likely to mold the politics of organized labor and of health policy for the foreseeable future. The institutional context continues to provide the facts on the ground that severely constrain reformers who are

Need sever connectin'
health care b
aploy state

committed to bolstering the public welfare state and finally severing the connection between health benefits and employment status.

The foregoing analysis about unions and health-care reform does at times put the national leadership of organized labor under a harsh light. However, this is not meant to suggest that the labor bureaucracy is so diseased from the head down that salvation can only come by throwing everything into local efforts at renewal. Disgusted at organized labor's failure to devote more resources to organizing new members, and its obsequiousness to business and the Democratic Party, some critics have suggested that renewal can only come from the bottom up as workers develop new alliances with the wider community.[62] Thus, they have applauded tales like that of the Local P-9 workers in Austin, Minn., who in the mid-1980s took on the Hormel Meatpacking Company in defiance of the leadership of the international of the United Food and Commercial Workers.[63] They also applauded the Mexican-American copper miners who challenged the Phelps-Dodge Copper Corporation in Arizona in 1983.[64] These local rebellions are amazing tales of heroism, idealism, and courage in the face of incredible odds. They also are good stories about how political consciousness gets raised and how communities of solidarity form. In each of these instances, the sad fact is that these workers made great personal sacrifices and yet ultimately failed to secure good jobs at decent pay and with decent benefits.

Success for organized labor in both the workplace and in the wider political arena must depend on a simultaneous revitalization at both the top and within the ranks. The grass roots just do not have the resources to do it on their own. As Adolph Reed has noted on a number of occasions, there is an inevitable tension between institutional and popular action in political movements, and the labor movement is no exception. However, that tension does not necessarily have to be fatal. Properly channeled, it can be creative. In any case, that tension "certainly isn't reducible to a formula like 'the people, good, the bureaucracy, bad'."[65] Thus, although the reform slate that Sweeney led to victory in October 1995 in the first contested AFL-CIO presidential election was not a leap in the right direction, perhaps it was an important first step for organized labor.

Almost five decades ago, Sumner Slichter posed the question: "Are we becoming a 'laboristic' state?" Today it admittedly "takes an act of historical imagination to retrieve the sense of awe at labor's power and vitality that lay behind Professor Slichter's question."[66] Organized labor is indeed highly constrained by the institutional contours of the private welfare state and broader changes in the U.S. political economy. Organized labor also has been constrained by a lack of political imagination. It missed an opportunity to use the campaign for universal health care as a platform on which to develop a more encompassing and durable political movement committed to "reassert[ing] broader social aims in order to challenge the primacy of narrowly defined budget and economic goals."[67] Thus it may have forfeited the chance to link up its health-care campaign to the inchoate efforts of other groups that challenge corporate America on a number of fronts. To the extent that missed opportunities and a failure of political imagination do not inevitably flow from labor's constrained circumstances, obituaries about the withering away of organized labor in the United States may be premature.

Notes

Chapter 1: Introduction

1 Under a single-payer plan, the government provides health insurance for everyone. Although this would largely eliminate commercial health insurers, the health-care delivery system would remain primarily private with a free choice of provider. Single-payer proposals can vary enormously on issues like financing, budgeting, taxation, and the role of individual states.

2 Cathie Jo Martin, "Inviting Business to the Party: The Corporate Response to Social Policy," in *The Social Divide: Political Parties and the Future of Activist Government*, ed. Margaret Weir (Washington, D.C. and New York: Brookings Institution Press and Russell Sage Foundation, 1998), 233.

3 Beth Stevens, *Complementing the Welfare State: The Development of Private Pension, Health Insurance and Other Employee Benefits in the United States* (Geneva: International Labour Office, 1986), 2.

4 Paul Pierson, "The New Politics of the Welfare State," *World Politics* 48, no. 2 (January 1996): 143–79; Goran Therborn and Joop Roebroek, "The Irreversible Welfare State: Its Recent Maturation, Its Encounter with the Economic Crisis, and Its Future Prospects," *International Journal of Health Services* 16, no. 3 (1986): 319–38; and John Myles and Paul Pierson, "Friedman's Revenge: The Reform of 'Liberal' Welfare States in Canada and the United States," *Politics and Society* 25, no. 4 (December 1997): 443–72.

5 Pierson, "The New Politics of the Welfare State," 151.

6 Pierson, "The New Politics of the Welfare State," 170.

7 The United States spends nearly 14 percent of its GNP on health care—or nearly $1 trillion in 1994. By comparison, Canada, Sweden, and France spend just 9 percent of their GNP on health care; Germany spends 8 percent; and Great Britain and Japan spend 7 percent. Paul A. Lamarche, "Our Health Paradigm in Peril," *Public Health Reports* 110, no. 5 (September–October 1995): 556–60; and Robert Pear, "Health Care Costs Are Growing More Slowly," *The New York Times* (May 28, 1996): A-13.

8 Robert Pear, "More Americans Were Uninsured in 1998, U.S. Says," *The New York Times* (October 4, 1999): A-1.

9 Pear, "More Americans Were Uninsured in 1998, U.S. Says."

By all accounts, the uninsured problem worsened over the course of the 1980s and 1990s. In 1977, an estimated 26.2 million people (or about 14 percent of the nonaged population) did not have health insurance. See Lawrence D. Brown, "The Medically Uninsured: Problems, Policies, and Politics," *Journal of Health Politics, Policy and Law* 15, no. 2 (Summer 1990): 413–14; and Emily Friedman, "The Threat of Time," *Frontiers of Health Services Management* 12, no. 2 (Winter 1995): 35–39.

These figures understate the extent of the uninsured problem. An estimated 20 percent of the nation, or about 50 million Americans, is without health insurance for some portion of any given year. Healthline, "Health Insurance: Interruptions in Coverage Getting Shorter" (June 24, 1996): electronic database.

[10] Bob Hancke, "The Crisis of National Unions: Belgian Labor in Decline," *Politics & Society* 19, no. 4 (1991): 465.

[11] Douglas Fraser, "Inside the 'Monolith'," in *The State of the Unions*, ed. George Strauss, Daniel G. Gallagher, and Jack Fiorito (Madison, Wisc.: Industrial Relations Research Association, 1991), 413.

[12] Here I build on Huntington and Dominguez's classic definition of what constitutes a "political institution." Samuel P. Huntington and Jorge I. Dominguez, "Political Development," in *Handbook of Political Science* 3, ed. Fred I. Greenstein and Nelson W. Polsby (Reading, Mass.: Addison-Wesley, 1975), 47.

[13] Huntington and Dominguez, "Political Development," 47; and Rogers M. Smith, "Political Jurisprudence, the 'New Institutionalism,' and the Future of Public Law," *American Political Science Review* 82, no. 1 (March 1988): 91.

[14] See, for example, Margaret Weir, Ann Shola Orloff, and Theda Skocpol, ed. *The Politics of Social Policy in the United States* (Princeton, N.J.: Princeton University Press, 1988).

[15] Lawrence R. Jacobs, "Politics of America's Supply State: Health Reform and Technology," *Health Affairs* (Summer 1995): 143–57; James A. Morone, "Elusive Community: Democracy, Deliberation, and the Reconstruction of Health Policy," in *The New Politics of Public Policy*, ed. Marc K. Landy and Martin A. Levin (Baltimore: The Johns Hopkins University Press, 1995); and Ellen M. Immergut, "Institutions, Veto Points, and Policy Results: A Comparative Analysis of Health Care," *Journal of Public Policy* 10, no. 4 (1990): 391–416. For a critical view of Immergut that stresses not just how political institutions are organized, but also how interest groups are configured, see David Wilsford, *Doctors and the State: The Politics of Health Care in France and the United States* (Durham, N.C.: Duke University Press, 1991).

[16] Sven Steinmo and Jon Watts, "It's the Institutions, Stupid! Why Comprehensive National Health Insurance Always Fails in America," *Journal of Health Politics, Policy and Law* 20, no. 2 (Summer 1995): 329–72. See also David Brian Robertson, "The Bias of American Federalism: The Limits of Welfare-Sate Development in the Progressive Era," *Journal of Policy History* 1, no. 3 (1989): 261–91.

[17] See, for example, Miriam Golden and Jonas Pontusson, ed. *Bargaining for Change: Union Politics in North America and Europe* (Ithaca, N.Y.: Cornell University Press, 1992); Lowell Turner, *Democracy at Work: Changing World Markets and the Future of Labor Unions* (Ithaca, N.Y.: Cornell University Press, 1992); Andrei S. Markovits, *The Politics of the West German Trade Unions: Strategies of Class and Interest Representation in Growth and Crisis* (Cambridge: Cambridge University Press, 1986); and Bo Rothstein, "Labor-Market Institutions and Working-Class Strength," in *Structuring Politics: Historical Institutionalism in Comparative Analysis*, ed. Sven Steinmo, Kathleen Thelen, and Frank Longstreth (Cambridge: Cambridge University Press, 1992).

[18] The one main exception to this is the widespread interest in the development of U.S. labor law and its impact on unions. Christopher L. Tomlins, *The State and the Unions: Labor Relations, Law, and the Organized Labor Movement in America, 1880–1960* (Cambridge: Cambridge University Press, 1985); William E. Forbath, *Law and the Shaping of the American Labor Movement* (Cambridge, Mass.: Harvard University Press, 1991); Sheldon Friedman et al., ed. *Restoring the Promise of American Labor Law* (Ithaca, N.Y.: ILR Press, 1994); Joel Rogers, "Don't Worry, Be Happy: The Postwar Decline of Private-Sector Unionism in the United States," in *The Challenge of Restructuring: North American Labor Movements Respond*, ed. Jane Jenson and Rianne Mahon (Philadelphia: Temple University Press, 1993); and Victoria C. Hattam, *Labor Visions and State Power: The Origins of Business Unionism in the United States* (Princeton, N.J.: Princeton University Press, 1993).

[19] Cathie Jo Martin, "Together Again: Business Government, and the Quest for Cost Control," *Journal of Health Politics, Policy and Law* 18, no. 2 (Summer 1993): 359–93; Linda A.

Bergthold, "American Business and Health Reform," in *Health Care Reform in the Nineties*, ed. Pauline Vaillancourt Rosenau (Thousand Oaks, Calif.: Sage, 1994); Lawrence D. Brown, "Dogmatic Slumbers: American Business and Health Policy," in *The Politics of Health Care Reform: Lessons From the Past, Prospects for the Future*, ed. James A. Morone and Gary S. Belkin (Durham, N.C.: Duke University Press, 1994); and John B. Judis, "Abandoned Surgery: Business and the Failure of Health Reform,*" The American Prospect* (Spring 1995): 65–73.

    [20] Frances Fox Piven, ed. *Labor Parties in Postindustrial Societies* (Cambridge: Polity Press, 1991), especially Frances Fox Piven, "Structural Constraints and Political Development: The Case of the American Democratic Party"; and Melvyn Dubofsky, *The State and Labor in Modern America* (Chapel Hill: The University of North Carolina Press, 1994); and Rogers, "Don't Worry, Be Happy."

    [21] Alan Derickson, "Health Security for All? Social Unionism and Universal Health Insurance, 1935–1958,*" The Journal of American History* 80, no. 4 (March 1994): 1333–56; and Beth Stevens, "Labor Unions, Employee Benefits, and the Privatization of the American Welfare State," *Journal of Policy History* 2, no. 3 (1990): 233–60. See also Colin Gordon, "Why No National Health Insurance in the U.S.? The Limits of Social Provision in War and Peace, 1941–1948," *Journal of Policy History* 9, no. 3 (1997): 277–310.

    [22] Sanford M. Jacoby, *Modern Manors: Welfare Capitalism Since the New Deal* (Princeton, N.J.: Princeton University Press, 1997). Another notable exception is Laurence A. Weil, "Organized Labor and Health Reform: Union Interests and the Clinton Plan," *Journal of Public Health Policy* 18, no. 1 (1997): 30–48.

    [23] Douglass C. North, *Institutions, Institutional Change and Economic Performance* (Cambridge: Cambridge University Press, 1990): 23 and 22, respectively.

    [24] Sheri Berman, *The Social Democratic Moment: Ideas and Politics in the Making of Interwar Europe* (Cambridge: Harvard University Press, 1998), 18. Emphasis removed from the original.

    [25] Berman, *The Social Democratic Moment*, 25.

    [26] For more on the impediments to reform coalitions, see Weir, ed. *The Social Divide*.

    [27] For more on how policy outcomes vary with the ability of business to define the relevant issues in ways that favor or disfavor business, see Gary Mucciaroni, *Reversals of Fortune: Public Policy and Private Interests* (Washington, D.C.: The Brookings Institution, 1995).

    [28] For a view that stresses the importance of budget deficit politics in defining the parameters of the 1993–94 health-care debate, see Theda Skocpol, *Boomerang: Clinton's Health Security Effort and the Turn Against Government in U.S. Politics* (New York: W.W. Norton & Co., 1996).

    [29] Sheryl R. Tynes, *Turning Points in Social Security: From 'Cruel Hoax' to Sacred Entitlement* (Stanford, Calif.: Stanford University Press, 1996), 17–18.

    [30] Organized labor's recent setbacks in health policy at the national level have helped to unleash a flurry of political action at the state level that could warrant a book-length examination in its own right.

    [31] The UAW collection at the Reuther Library, for example, contains a number of revealing exchanges of letters and memos between automobile executives and labor officials about health and other social and economic policies.

Chapter 2: The Missing Millions

    [1] Rein suggests using an alternative like "welfare economy," whereas Esping-Andersen prefers the term "welfare-state regime" to reflect both the public and private dimensions of social welfare provision. Martin Rein, "The Social Policy of the Firm," *Policy Sciences* 14 (1982): 117–35; Martin Rein and Lee Rainwater, "From Welfare State to Welfare Society," *Stagnation and Renewal in Social Policy: The Rise and Fall of Policy Regimes*, ed. Gosta Esping-

Andersen, Martin Rein, and Lee Rainwater (Armonk, N.Y.: M.E. Sharpe, 1987); and Gosta Esping-Andersen, *The Three Worlds of Welfare Capitalism* (London: Polity, 1990).

[2] Eric Patashnik, "A New Look in Welfare State Research," *Policy Currents* 7, no. 3 (September 1997): 2.

[3] Monte M. Poen, *Harry S. Truman versus the Medical Lobby: The Genesis of Medicare* (Columbia, Mo.: University of Missouri Press, 1979); Martha Derthick, *Policymaking for Social Security* (Washington, D.C.: The Brookings Institution, 1979); Theodore R. Marmor, *The Politics of Medicare* (Chicago: Aldine Publishing Co., 1973); Lawrence D. Brown, *Politics and Health Care Organization: HMOs as Federal Policy* (Washington, D.C.: The Brookings Institution, 1983); Ivana Krajcinovic, *From Company Doctors to Managed Care: The United Mine Workers' Noble Experiment* (Ithaca, N.Y.: Cornell University Press, 1997); and Alan Derickson, *Workers' Health, Workers' Democracy: The Western Miners' Struggle, 1891–1925* (Ithaca, N.Y.: Cornell University Press, 1988).

[4] Donna Allen, *Fringe Benefits: Wages or Social Obligation?* (Ithaca, N.Y.: Cornell University Press, 1964); Joseph W. Garbarino, *Health Plans and Collective Bargaining* (Berkeley: University of California Press, 1960); Raymond Munts, *Bargaining for Health: Labor Unions, Health Insurance, and Medical Care* (Madison: University of Wisconsin Press, 1967); Beth Stevens, "Labor Unions, Employee Benefits, and the Privatization of the American Welfare State," *Journal of Policy History* 2, no. 3 (1990): 233–60; and David Rosner and Gerald Markowitz, "Hospitals, Insurance, and the American Labor Movement: The Case of New York in the Postwar Decades," *Journal of Policy History* 9, no. 1 (1997): 74–95.

[5] Between 1986 and 1989, the number of strikes caused by health-care disputes increased by 300 percent, according to a study by the SEIU cited in Polly Callaghan, "1990 Contract Innovations Address Family Security," *AFL-CIO News* (April 15, 1991): 8. See also "News Brief," *Business and Health* (April 1990): 10; and Michael Byrne, "Health Care, Strikebreaker Ban: Ties That Bind" *AFL-CIO News* (June 10, 1991): 1.

[6] Graham K. Wilson, *Unions in American National Politics* (New York: St. Martin's Press, 1979); J. David Greenstone, *Labor in American Politics* (Chicago: Chicago University Press, 1977); Richard B. Freeman and James L. Medoff, *What Do Unions Do?* (New York: Basic Books, 1984); Dudley W. Buffa, *Union Power and American Democracy: The U.A.W. and the Democratic Party, 1935–72* (Ann Arbor: The University of Michigan Press, 1984); Jill Quadagno, *The Transformation of Old Age Security: Class and Politics in the American Welfare State* (Chicago: University of Chicago Press, 1988); Kevin Boyle, "Little More Than Ashes: The UAW and American Reform in the 1960s," in *Organized Labor and American Politics, 1894–1994: The Labor-Liberal Alliance*, ed. Kevin Boyle (Albany, N.Y.: SUNY Press, 1998); and Alex Hicks, Roger Friedlander, and Edwin Johnson, "Class Power and State Policy: The Case of Large Business Corporations, Labor Unions, and Governmental Redistribution in the American States," *American Sociological Review* 43 (June 1978): 302–15.

[7] Karen Orren, "Union Politics and Postwar Liberalism in the United States," *Studies in American Political Development* 1 (1986): 215–52; Karen Orren, "Organized Labor and the Invention of Modern Liberalism in the United States," *Studies in American Political Development* 2 (1987): 317–36; Joseph A. McCartin, *Labor's Great War: The Struggle for Industrial Democracy and the Origins of Modern American Labor Relations, 1912–1921* (Chapel Hill: University of North Carolina Press, 1997); and David Plotke, *Building a Democratic Political Order: Reshaping American Liberalism in the 1930s and 1940s* (Cambridge: Cambridge University Press, 1996), esp. chaps. 4–8.

[8] Derek C. Bok and John T. Dunlop, *Labor and the American Community* (New York: Simon & Schuster, 1970), 465; Melvyn Dubofsky, *The State and Labor in Modern America* (Chapel Hill: The University of North Carolina Press, 1994); and Vernon Coleman, "Labor Power and Social Equality: Union Politics in a Changing Economy," *Political Science Quarterly* 103, no. 4 (1988): 687–705.

This is not to deny that labor's commitment to expanding the welfare state is not a consistent one or to ignore its uneven record on such issues as civil rights, feminism, and poverty alleviation. See, for example, Philip S. Foner, *Organized Labor and the Black Worker, 1619–1973* (New York: Praeger Publishers, 1974); August Meier and Elliott Rudwick, *Black Detroit and the Rise of the UAW* (Oxford: Oxford University Press, 1979); Linda M. Blum, *Between Feminism and Labor: The Significance of the Comparative Worth Movement* (Berkeley: University of California Press, 1991); Nancy Gabin, *Feminism in the Labor Movement: Women and the United Auto Workers, 1935–75* (Ithaca, N.Y.: Cornell University Press, 1990); and Philip S. Foner, *Women and the American Labor Movement: From World War I to the Present* (New York: The Free Press, 1980). On how labor helped to give a conservative cast to Social Security, see Jerry R. Cates, *Insuring Inequality: Administrative Leadership in Social Security, 1935–54* (Ann Arbor: University of Michigan Press, 1983), esp. 142–43.

⁹ For a review of this literature, see Edwin Amenta and Theda Skocpol, "States and Social Policies," *Annual Review of Sociology* 12 (1986): 131–57.

¹⁰ See Theda Skocpol, *Boomerang: Clinton's Health Security Effort and the Turn Against Government in U.S. Politics* (New York: W.W. Norton & Co., 1996), chap. 3, especially 84–88; John B. Judis, "Abandoned Surgery: Business and the Failure of Health Reform," *The American Prospect* (Spring 1995): 71–72; and Cathie Jo Martin, "Stuck in Neutral: Big Business and the Politics of National Health Reform," *Journal of Health Politics, Policy and Law* 20, no. 2 (Summer 1995): 433.

¹¹ Paul Starr, *The Social Transformation of American Medicine* (New York: Basic Books, 1982).

¹² See Edward Berkowitz and Kim McQuaid, *Creating the Welfare State: The Political Economy of Twentieth-Century Reform* (New York: Praeger, 1988); and Stuart D. Brandes, *American Welfare Capitalism, 1880–1940* (Chicago: University of Chicago Press, 1976).

¹³ Beth Stevens, "In the Shadow of the Welfare State: Corporate and Union Development of Employee Benefits" (Ph.D. dissertation, Harvard University, 1984), 197–98 and 200.

¹⁴ Martin Rein and Lee Rainwater, "The Institutions of Social Protection," in *Public/Private Interplay in Social Protection: A Comparative Study*, ed. Martin Rein and Lee Rainwater (Armonk, N.Y.: M.E. Sharpe, 1986), 41.

¹⁵ Paul D. Pierson, *Dismantling the Welfare State? Reagan, Thatcher, and the Politics of Retrenchment* (New York: Cambridge University Press, 1994); and Pierson, "The New Politics of the Welfare State," *World Politics* 48, no. 2 (January 1996): 143–79.

¹⁶ David Laycock, "Reforming Canadian Democracy? Institutions and Ideology in the Reform Party Project," *Canadian Journal of Political Science* 27, no. 2 (June 1994): 213–47; Janine Brodie, *Politics on the Margins: Restructuring and the Canadian Women's Movement* (Halifax, Nova Scotia: Fernwood Publishing, 1995); and Andrew Gamble, *The Free Economy and the Strong State: The Politics of Thatcherism*, 2nd ed. (London: Macmillan, 1994).

¹⁷ Martin Rein and Lee Rainwater, "The Public/Private Mix," in *Public/Private Interplay in Social Protection*, 18–19.

¹⁸ Indeed, "[n]one of the social science disciplines has played a smaller role in the study of industrial relations than political science." Likewise, specialists in industrial relations pay little attention to politics. Peter Gourevitch, Peter Lange, and Andrew Martin, "Industrial Relations and Politics: Some Reflections," in *Industrial Relations in International Perspective: Essays in Research and Policy*, ed. Peter B. Doeringer (New York: Holmes & Meier, 1981): 401.

¹⁹ See Rein and Rainwater, "The Institutions of Social Protection," 35–36.

²⁰ See Gourevitch et al., "Industrial Relations and Politics," on this point. See also John T. Dunlop, *Industrial Relations Systems* (New York: Holt, 1958). For a fuller discussion of Dunlop's views, see also chapter 5 below.

²¹ Gourevitch et al., "Industrial Relations and Politics."

²² Harry Braverman, *Labor and Monopoly Capital: The Degradation of Work in the Twentieth Century* (New York: Monthly Review Press, 1975); Reinhard Bendix, *Work and Authority in Industry: Ideologies of Management in the Course of Industrialization* (Berkeley: University of California Press, 1974); David M. Gordon, Richard Edwards, and Michael Reich, *Segmented Work, Divided Workers: The Historical Transformation of Labor in the United States* (Cambridge: Cam-

bridge University Press, 1982); David Montgomery, *Workers' Control in America: Studies in the History of Work, Technology, and Labor Struggles* (Cambridge: Cambridge University Press, 1979); Richard Edwards, *Contested Terrain: The Transformation of the Workplace in the Twentieth Century* (New York: Basic Books, 1979); and Dan Clawson, *Bureaucracy and the Labor Process: The Transformation of U.S. Industry, 1860–1920* (New York: Monthly Review Press, 1980).

For more recent works in this genre that stress the impact of management innovations like quality circles and the spread of computers and other high technology on the micro-level politics of labor-management relations, see Mike Parker and Jane Slaughter, *Choosing Sides: Unions and the Team Concept* (Boston: South End Press, 1988); Guillermo J. Grenier, *Inhuman Relations: Quality Circles and Anti-Unionism in American Industry* (Philadelphia: Temple University Press, 1988); Shoshana Zuboff, *In the Age of the Smart Machine: The Future of Work and Power* (New York: Basic Books, 1988); Harley Shaiken, *Work Transformed: Automation and Labor in the Computer Age* (New York: Holt, Rinehart and Winston, 1984); and Robert Howard, *Brave New Workplace* (New York: Viking, 1985).

[23]   Esping-Andersen, *The Three Worlds of Welfare Capitalism,* 70–71.

[24]   Calculated from Rein and Rainwater, "The Public/Private Mix," 17.

[25]   Rein and Rainwater, "The Institutions of Social Protection," 51. This figure is equal to about 7.5 percent of the gross domestic product (GDP). Martin Rein, "Is America Exceptional? The Role of Occupational Welfare in the United States and the European Community," in *The Privatization of Social Policy? Occupational Welfare and the Welfare State in America, Scandinavia and Japan,* ed. Michael Shalev (London: MacMillan Press, 1996), 41. See also Jacob S. Hacker, "Between Welfare Capitalism and the Welfare State: The Politics of Public and Private Pensions in the United States" (paper presented at the annual meetings of the American Political Science Association, Atlanta, Ga., September 2–5, 1999).

[26]   Christopher Howard, "The Hidden Side of the American Welfare State," *Political Science Quarterly* 108, no. 3 (1993): 403–36; Christopher Howard, *The Hidden Welfare State: Tax Expenditures and Social Policy in the United States* (Princeton, N.J.: Princeton University Press, 1997); Michael K. Brown, "Bargaining for Social Rights: Unions and the Reemergence of Welfare Capitalism," *Political Science Quarterly* 112, no. 4 (1997–98): 645–74; Beth Stevens, "Blurring the Boundaries: How the Federal Government Has Influenced Welfare Benefits in the Private Sector," in *The Politics of Social Policy in the United States,* ed. Margaret Weir, Ann Shola Orloff, and Theda Skocpol (Princeton, N.J.: Princeton University Press, 1988); *Masters to Managers: Historical and Comparative Perspectives on American Employers,* ed. Sanford M. Jacoby (New York: Columbia University Press, 1991); Andrea Tone, *The Business of Benevolence: Industrial Paternalism in Progressive America* (Ithaca, N.Y.: Cornell University Press, 1997); and Daniel P. Gitterman, "Redistributing Earnings? The American System of Shared Powers and the Fair Labor Standards Act, 1938–1998" (Ph.D. dissertation, Brown University, 1999).

[27]   Linda Bergthold, *Purchasing Power in Health: Business, the State, and Health Care Politics* (New Brunswick, N.J.: Rutgers University Press, 1990), 30–36. For further discussion of the business press in the 1970s and the corporate push for HMOs, see Jack Warren Salmon, "Corporate Attempts to Reorganize the American Health System," ch. 1 and 3, respectively (Ph.D. dissertation, Cornell University, 1978).

[28]   Bergthold, *Purchasing Power in Health,* 51–58; *Private Sector Coalitions: A Fourth Party in Health Care,* ed. B. Jon Jaeger (Durham, N.C.: Department of Health Administration, 1983); Peter D. Fox, Willis B. Goldbeck, and Jacob J. Spies, *Health Care Cost Management: Private Sector Initiatives* (Ann Arbor, Mich.: Health Administration Press, 1984). The essays in *Private Sector Coalitions* are generally enthusiastic about the potential of business coalitions to contain costs. For one of the few skeptical contributions, see Howard N. Newman, "Other Perspectives on Private Sector Activities."

[29]   See Bergthold, *Purchasing Power in Health,* 49–52.

[30]   Bergthold, *Purchasing Power in Health,* 44; and Linda E. Demkovich, "On Health Issues, This Business Group Is a Leader, But Is Anyone Following?," *National Journal* (June 18, 1983): 1278.

[31] Julie Kosterlitz, "Bottom-Line Pain," *National Journal* (September 9, 1989): 2201.

[32] William Schneider, "Business Warming to National Health," *National Journal* (June 10, 1989): 1546.

[33] John Inglehart, "Health Care and American Business," *New England Journal of Medicine* 306, no. 2 (1982): 120–24; Linda E. Demkovich, "Businesses Drive to Curb Medical Costs Without Much Help From Government," *National Journal* (August 11, 1984): 1508–12; Cathie Jo Martin, "Together Again: Business Government, and the Quest for Cost Control," *Journal of Health Politics, Policy and Law* 18, no. 2 (Summer 1993): 360; and Lawrence D. Brown, "Dogmatic Slumbers: American Business and Health Policy," in *The Politics of Health Care Reform: Lessons From the Past, Prospects for the Future*, ed. James A. Morone and Gary S. Belkin (Durham, N.C.: Duke University Press, 1994), 221. For a more skeptical view, see H.M. Sapolsky et al., "Corporate Attitudes Toward Health Care Costs," *Milbank Memorial Fund Quarterly* 59, no. 4 (1981): 561–85.

[34] Starr does not claim that the private sector necessarily holds the key to a satisfactory reform of the medical system. He is more ambiguous on this point, merely indicating that the private sector is the only one poised to mount the first real challenge to the medical profession's domination of the health-care system. Starr, *The Social Transformation of American Medicine*, 421–45. Alford likewise draws attention to the need to break the choke hold that medical providers are said to have on health policy in the United States. But Alford decidedly does not view business, per se, as a potential savior. Robert R. Alford, *Health Care Politics: Ideological and Interest Group Barriers to Reform* (Chicago: University of Chicago Press, 1975).

[35] See Kosterlitz, "Bottom-Line Pain"; Gary Silverman, "Executives Oppose National Health Insurance," United Press International wire service (March 26, 1990); and Humphrey Taylor, Robert Leitman, and Robert J. Blendon, "Large Employers and Managed Care," and Jennifer N. Edwards et al., "Will Small Business Reform Improve Access in the 1990s," both in *Reforming the System: Containing Health Care Costs in an Era of Universal Coverage*, ed. Robert J. Blendon and Tracey Stelzer Hyams (New York: Faulkner & Gray, 1992).

[36] Susan A. Goldberger, "The Politics of Universal Access: The Massachusetts Health Security Act of 1988," *Journal of Health Politics, Policy and Law* 15, no. 4 (Winter 1990): 857–85; Richard Kronick, "The Slippery Slope of Health Care Finance: Business Interests and Hospital Reimbursement in Massachusetts," *Journal of Health Politics, Policy and Law* 15, no. 4 (Winter 1990): 887–913. For an early skeptical view of the possibilities for reform at the state level, see Frank J. Thompson, "New Federalism and Health Care Policy: States and the Old Questions," in *Health Policy in Transition: A Decade of Health Politics, Policy and Law*, ed. Lawrence D. Brown (Durham, N.C.: Duke University Press, 1987). In some of her later works, Bergthold appears more doubtful about whether business can be counted on to play a constructive role in reform. See Bergthold, "The Frayed Alliance: Business and Health Care in Massachusetts," *Journal of Health Politics, Policy and Law* 15, no. 4 (Winter 1990): 915–28; and Bergthold, "American Business and Health Reform," in *Health Care Reform in the Nineties*, ed. Pauline Vaillancourt Rosenau (Thousand Oaks, Calif.: Sage, 1994).

[37] Gaston V. Rimlinger, *Welfare Policy and Industrialization in Europe, America, and Russia* (New York: John Wiley & Sons, 1971), 112–13. At the time, the chancellor held no illusions about what to expect from the private sector in the way of social welfare. "Belief in a harmony of interests has been made bankrupt by history. No doubt the individual can do much good, but the social problem can only be solved by the state," he declared at one point. Quoted in Hans Rothfels, "Bismarck's Social Policy and the Problem of State Socialism in Germany," Part I, *Sociological Review* 30 (1938): 92, as cited in Rimlinger, *Welfare Policy and Industrialization*, 113.

[38] For a sum, friendly society members were guaranteed that a general practitioner would treat them during times of illness. Many of the physicians were under contract with these workingmen's associations. This account of the friendly societies and national health insurance in England is based on J. Rogers Hollingsworth, *A Political Economy of Medicine: Great Britain and the United States* (Baltimore: The Johns Hopkins University Press, 1986), ch. 1.

[39] Public indignation soared when it became known that nearly half of the eligible recruits during the Boer War (1899–1902) were medically unfit to serve in the British army. Carol Sakala, "The Development of National Medical Care Programs in the United Kingdom and Canada: Applicability to Current Conditions in the United States," *Journal of Health Politics, Policy and Law* 15, no. 4 (Winter 1990): 709–53.

[40] Hollingsworth, *A Political Economy of Medicine*, 46–63; and John Stewart, *The Battle for Health: A Political History of the Socialist Medical Association, 1930–51* (Abindgon, England: Ashgate, 1999).

[41] Divisions between hospital-based and non-hospital physicians helped neutralize the medical profession's opposition to national health insurance in Great Britain. Daniel M. Fox, *Health Politics: The British and American Experience, 1911–1965* (Princeton, N.J.: Princeton University Press, 1986); Hollingsworth, *A Political Economy of Medicine*, 124; and Vicente Navarro, *The Politics of Health Policy: The U.S. Reforms* (Cambridge, Mass.: Blackwell, 1994): 143–44.

[42] His close understanding of the British case prompted Hollingsworth to speculate that the U.S. business sector's spreading disillusionment with the medical providers in the 1980s would not necessarily result in a desirable transformation of the U.S. medical system because the wider public was comparatively disorganized on health-care matters. Hollingsworth, *A Political Economy of Medicine*, 124. On the failed attempts to provide American consumers with meaningful ways to participate in health policy, see James A. Morone and Theodore R. Marmor, "Representing Consumer Interests: The Case of American Health Planning," in Marmor's *Political Analysis and American Medical Care: Essays* (Cambridge: Cambridge University Press, 1983); and James A. Morone, *The Democratic Wish: Popular Participation and the Limits of American Government* (New York: Basic Books, 1990), ch. 7.

[43] Sakala, "The Development of National Medical Care Programs," 743.

[44] Malcolm G. Taylor, *Health Insurance and Canadian Public Policy: The Seven Decisions that Created the Canadian Health Insurance System* (Montreal: McGill-Queen's University Press, 1978). For the abridged version, see Malcolm G. Taylor, *Insuring National Health Care: The Canadian Experience* (Chapel Hill: University of North Carolina Press, 1990).

[45] "There seems never to have been any other thought than that the program should be universal and compulsory" on the part of the CCF. Taylor, *Health Insurance and Canadian Public Policy*, 91. Taylor also underscores the importance of an infusion of more progressive and dynamic blood into the Liberal Party after it suffered major electoral setbacks in the late 1950s at the hands of the Progressive Conservatives, Canada's other major political party.

[46] Antonia Maioni, *Parting at the Crossroads: The Emergence of Health Insurance in the United States and Canada* (Princeton, N.J.: Princeton University Press, 1998); and Maioni, "Parting at the Crossroads: The Development of Health Insurance in Canada and the United States, 1940–65," *Comparative Politics* 29, no. 4 (July 1997): 411–31. See also William M. Chandler, "Canadian Socialism and Policy Impact: Contagion From the Left?" *Canadian Journal of Political Science* 10, no. 4 (December 1977): 755–80. For a broader discussion of the critical role of labor in Canadian social policy, see Jane Jenson and Rianne Mahon, "Legacies for Canadian Labour of Two Decades of Crisis," in *The Challenge of Restructuring: North American Labor Movements Respond*, ed. Jane Jenson and Rianne Mahon (Philadelphia: Temple University Press, 1993).

[47] In 1950, 29 percent of nonagricultural workers in Canada were union members, compared to 32 percent in the United States. Ten years later, both countries stood at 31 percent. Maioni, *Parting at the Crossroads*, 19. Beginning in the 1970s and continuing to the present, the union membership figures diverged greatly as the unionized labor force shrank in the United States while Canadian unions continued to grow. Edward Ian Robinson, "Organizing Labour: Explaining Canada–U.S. Union Diversity in the Post-War Period" (Ph.D. dissertation, Yale University, 1992).

[48] In a submission to the Royal Commission created in 1960 to study the health-care issue, the Canadian Labour Congress said: "We look to a system of health care that will be re-

garded as a public service and not as an insurance mechanism. We consider that the public health care program is one of the remaining major gaps in our social security system." Taylor, *Health Insurance and Canadian Public Policy*, 358.

⁴⁹ This discussion of the CCF and universal health care is based primarily on Maioni, *Parting at the Crossroads*, 120–21 and 129–30.

⁵⁰ "By 1965, the Saskatchewan example was, like Banquo's ghost, a constant spectre at every Liberal Cabinet meeting when medicare was discussed." Taylor, *Health Insurance and Canadian Public Policy*, 353.

⁵¹ David Coburn et al., "Medical Dominance in Canada in Historical Perspective: The Rise and Fall of Medicine?" *International Journal of Health Services* 13, no. 3 (1983): 407–32; D. Swatz, "The Politics of Reform: Conflict and Accommodation in Canadian Health Policy," in *The Canadian State: Political Economy and Political Power*, ed. Leo Panitch (Toronto: University of Toronto Press, 1977); and Harley D. Dickinson, "The Struggle for State Health Insurance: Reconsidering the Role of Saskatchewan Farmers," *Studies in Political Economy* 41 (Summer 1993): 133–56. For one of the few accounts that puts business at the center of its analysis, see V. Walters, "State, Capital, and Labour: The Introduction of Federal-Provincial Insurance for Physician Care in Canada," *Canadian Review of Sociology and Anthropology* 19, no. 2 (1982): 157–72.

⁵² Delfi Mondragon and Barry B. Schweig, "Enactment of Mandated Health Insurance in Hawaii," *Review of Social Economy* 53, no. 2 (Summer 1995): 243–59; Deane Neubauer, "Hawaii: The Health State," in *Health Policy Reform in America: Innovations from the States*, ed. H.M. Leichter (Armonk, N.Y.: M.E. Sharpe, 1992); and John C. Lewin, "The Implementation of Health Care Reform: Lessons From Hawaii," in *Implementation Issues and National Health Care Reform*, ed. Charles Brecher (Washington, D.C.: Josiah Macy, Jr. Foundation, 1992).

⁵³ Deborah A. Stone, "Drawing Lessons From Comparative Health Research," in *Critical Issues in Health Policy*, ed. Ralph A. Straetz, Marvin Lieberman, and Alice Sardell (Lexington, Mass.: Lexington Books, 1981). By contrast, many other countries looked outward as they reformed their medical systems. Sakala, "The Development of National Medical Care Programs," 725; and Taylor, *Health Insurance and Canadian Public Policy*, ch. 1. Even Bismarck kept one eye on the experience of France and England as he devised his social welfare policies for Germany in the 1880s. Rimlinger, *Welfare Policy and Industrialization*, 90–92.

⁵⁴ Sven Steinmo and Jon Watts, "It's the Institutions, Stupid! Why Comprehensive National Health Insurance Always Fails in America," *Journal of Health Politics, Policy and Law* 20, no. 2 (Summer 1995): 334.

⁵⁵ John D. Stephens, *The Transition from Capitalism to Socialism* (New Jersey: Humanities Press, 1980); Walter Korpi, "Social Policy and Distributional Conflict in the Capitalist Democracies," *West European Politics* 3 (1980): 296–316; Gosta Esping-Andersen, "Power and Distributional Regimes," *Politics and Society* 14, no. 2 (1985): 223–56; David R. Cameron, "Social Democracy, Corporatism, Labour Quiescence, and the Representation of Economic Interests in Advanced Capitalist Society," in *Order and Conflict in Contemporary Capitalism: Studies in the Political Economy of Western European Nations*, ed. John H. Goldthorpe (New York: Oxford University Press, 1984); and David R. Cameron, "The Politics and Economics of the Business Cycle," in *The Political Economy: Readings in the Politics and Economics of American Public Policy*, ed. Thomas Ferguson and Joel Rogers, (Armonk, N.Y.: M.E. Sharpe, 1984).

⁵⁶ Kathleen Thelen, "Beyond Corporatism: Toward a New Framework for the Study of Labor in Advanced Capitalism," *Comparative Politics* 27, no. 1 (October 1994): 107.

⁵⁷ They emphasize various political factors, such as the willingness of employers to maintain corporatist arrangements and institutional factors that include shop-floor institutions and the industrial relations and vocational education systems. For an overview of this scholarship, see Thelen, "Beyond Corporatism"; and Jill Quadagno, "Theories of the Welfare State," *Annual Review of Sociology* 13 (1987): 109–28. For some representative works, see *Bargaining for Change: Union Politics in North America and Europe*, ed. Miriam Golden and Jonas

Pontusson (Ithaca, N.Y.: Cornell University Press, 1992); and Peter Swenson, "Bringing Capital Back In; or Social Democracy Reconsidered: Employer Power, Cross-Class Alliances, and Centralization of Industrial Relations in Denmark and Sweden," *World Politics* 43, no. 4 (July 1991): 513–44.

[58] Two notable recent exceptions are Taylor Dark, *The Unions and the Democrats: An Enduring Alliance* (Ithaca, N.Y.: Cornell University Press, 1999); and some of the contributors to *Organized Labor and American Politics, 1894–1994: The Labor-Liberal Alliance*, ed. Kevin Boyle (Albany, N.Y.: SUNY Press, 1998).

[59] On organized labor's membership decline and its possible causes, see Michael Goldfield, *The Decline of Organized Labor in the United States* (Chicago: The University of Chicago Press, 1987); Paul Weiler, "Who Will Represent Labor Now?," *American Prospect* (Summer 1990): 78–92; Richard Edwards and Michael Podgursky, "The Unraveling Accord: American Unions in Crisis," in *Unions in Crisis and Beyond: Perspectives from Six Countries*, ed. Richard Edwards (Dover, Mass.: Auburn House Publishing Co., 1986); *Unions in Transition: Entering the Second Century*, ed. Seymour Martin Lipset (San Francisco: ILR Press, 1986); *The State of the Unions*, ed. George Strauss, Daniel G. Gallagher, and Jack Fiorito (Madison, Wisc.: Industrial Relations Research Association, 1991); and Jack Fiorito and Charles R. Greer, "Determinants of U.S. Unionism: Past Research and Future Needs," *Industrial Relations* 21, no. 1 (1982): 1–32.

[60] This is the mantra of some scholars as well. See Robert H. Zieger, *American Workers, American Unions*, 2nd ed. (Baltimore: The Johns Hopkins University Press, 1994), ch. 7. Shortly after his election, John J. Sweeney, who succeeded Lane Kirkland as president of the federation, committed $20 million, or nearly one-third of the federation's $65 million budget, to organizing new members and launched "Union Summer" in 1996 to train 1,000 workers and students at the AFL-CIO's revamped Organizing Institute. David Moberg, "The New Union Label," *The Nation* (April 1, 1996): 13.

[61] Steven Greenhouse, "Despite Efforts to Organize, Union Rosters Have Declined," *The New York Times* (March 22, 1998): sec. 1, 21.

[62] For the current figures, see Robert L. Rose, "New AFL-CIO President Seeks to Revitalize Old Federation," *The Wall Street Journal* (October 29, 1996): B-1. For the eve of the Depression, see Irving Bernstein, *The Lean Years* (Boston: Houghton, Mifflin, 1960), 84.

[63] Calculated from Jelle Visser, "The Strength of Union Movements in Advanced Capitalist Democracies: Social and Organizational Variations," in *The Future of Labour Movements*, ed. Marino Regini (London: Sage, 1992), 19.

[64] Michael Shalev, "The Resurgence of Labor Quiescence," in *The Future of Labour Movements* (London: Sage, 1992); and Bruce Western, *Between Class and Market: Postwar Unionization in the Capitalist Democracies* (Princeton, N.J.: Princeton University Press, 1997), 21 and 145. See also Miriam A Golden, Michael Wallerstein, and Peter Lange, "Postwar Trade-Union Organization and Industrial Relations," in *Continuity and Change in Contemporary Capitalism*, ed. Herbert Kitschelt et al. (Cambridge: Cambridge University Press, 1999), 194–230.

[65] Visser, "The Strength of Union Movements in Advanced Capitalist Democracies," 237; and Richard M. Locke, *Remaking the Italian Economy* (Ithaca, N.Y.: Cornell University Press, 1995), 99–102.

[66] *Working Under Different Rules*, ed. Richard Freeman (New York: Russell Sage Foundation, 1994), 16.

[67] The fiery words and personalities of labor leaders like Walter Reuther of the UAW and John L. Lewis of the United Mine Workers, household names at the time, belie the widespread quiescence within the ranks of organized labor during this period. Many union officials deliberately sought to politically demobilize their rank and file in the aftermath of the massive strike wave of the late 1940s and to bureaucratize labor-management relations to tame the radicals and insurgents within their swollen ranks. Nelson Lichtenstein, *Labor's War at Home: The C.I.O. in World War II* (Cambridge: Cambridge University Press, 1982); Martin

Halpern, *U.A.W. Politics in the Cold War Era* (Albany, N.Y.: SUNY Press, 1988); Judith Stepan-Norris and Maurice Zeitlin, "Insurgency, Radicalism, and Democracy in America's Industrial Unions," *Social Forces* 75, no. 1 (September 1996); and Howell John Harris, *The Right to Manage: Industrial Relations Policies of American Business in the 1940s* (Madison: The University of Wisconsin Press, 1982).

⁶⁸ Sar A. Levitan, "Union Lobbyists' Contributions to Tough Labor Legislation," *Labor Law Journal* 10, no. 10 (October 1959): 675–82; Alan K. McAdams, *Power and Politics in Labor Legislation* (New York: Columbia University Press, 1959); R. Alton Lee, *Eisenhower and Landrum-Griffin: A Study in Labor-Management Politics* (Lexington: University Press of Kentucky, 1990); Harry A. Millis and Emily Clark Brown, *From the Wagner Act to Taft-Hartley; A Study of National Labor Policy and Labor Relations* (Chicago: Chicago University Press, 1950); and James Gross, *Broken Promises: The Subversion of U.S. Labor Relations Policy, 1947–1994* (Philadelphia: Temple University Press, 1995).

⁶⁹ As of 1990, the UAW had 868,000 active dues-paying members and 450,000 retirees, or about one retiree for every two working members. "U.A.W. Finances, 1990," *Solidarity* (November–December 1991): 20.

Membership figures for the Christian Coalition come from Skocpol, *Boomerang*, 154–55. The Christian Coalition collects $15 in annual dues from each of its members, much less than the annual dues of a regular member of the UAW, or a UAW retiree who chooses to stay active in the union.

⁷⁰ "Partners for Life: The UAW and Retired Workers," *Solidarity* (December 1987): 12–16; and Dave Elsila, "Retirees Who Won't Quit," *Solidarity* (September 1990): 9–14.

⁷¹ For the Gallup poll, see "More Americans Say Yes to Unions," *AFL-CIO News* (August 27, 1988): 1. For postwar trends, Lipset, "Labor Unions in the Public Mind," in *Unions in Transition.*

⁷² "Americans Look at Unions, and They Like What They See," *Solidarity* (May–June 1988): 7.

⁷³ Grace Budrys, *When Doctors Join Unions* (Ithaca, N.Y.: ILR Press/Cornell University Press, 1996). As of 1992, opposition to union membership stood at 38 percent among executives and professionals, down 10 percent from a decade earlier. Among white-collar workers, opposition stood at 23 percent, down 14 percent from 1981. See the 1992 Roper Organization survey cited in "Perception of Labor Swings Toward the Positive, Survey Shows," *AFL-CIO News* (February 1, 1993). See also *Not Your Father's Union Movement: Inside the AFL-CIO*, ed. Jo-Ann Mort (London and New York: Verso, 1998), 75–77.

⁷⁴ Steven Greenhouse, "In Shift to Labor, Public Supports U.P.S. Strikers," *The New York Times* (August 17, 1997): A-1.

⁷⁵ It is important to note that five of the major unions hold almost two-thirds of that wealth, and that public-sector unions generally do not hold wealth comparable to private-sectors ones. Moreover, even though organized labor's wealth holds steady, operating income has plummeted in many unions, compelling significant reductions in expenditures. Marick F. Masters, "Unions at the Crossroads," *WorkingUSA* (January/February 1998): 14–15.

⁷⁶ Marick F. Masters, *Unions at the Crossroads: Strategic Membership, Financial, and Political Perspectives* (Westport, Conn.: Quorum Books, 1997), 73.

⁷⁷ Richard Rothstein, "Toward a More Perfect Union: New Labor's Hard Road," *The American Prospect* (May–June 1996): 51; and Masters, "Unions at the Crossroads," 15.

⁷⁸ Masters, "Unions at the Crossroads," 16; and Masters, *Unions at the Crossroads*, 121–24.

⁷⁹ Jonathan Tasini, *The Edifice Complex: Rebuilding the American Labor Movement to Face the Global Economy* (New York: Labor Research Association, 1995), 19. By comparison, the AFL-CIO's Organizing Institute received just $365,000 in 1990, the year of its first full budget. Tasini, *The Edifice Complex*, 25.

⁸⁰ Harold Meyerson, "Labor's Risky Plunge Into Politics: From Top-Down to Bottom-Up," *Dissent* (Summer 1984): 286–87.

[81] Tasini, *The Edifice Complex*, 21; and Larry Makinson and Joshua Goldstein, *Open Secrets: The Encyclopedia of Congressional Money and Politics*, 4th ed. (Washington, D.C.: Congressional Quarterly Press, 1996), 84–85.

[82] Jill Abramson and Steven Greenhouse, "Labor Victory on Trade Bill Reveals Power," *The New York Times* (November 12, 1997): A-1.

[83] Mike Davis, *Prisoners of the American Dream* (London: Verso, 1986), 265–66. For more on labor and the Democrats, see ch. 5 below.

[84] Kevin Sack, "Differences Aside, Labor Embraces the Democrats," *The New York Times* (August 26, 1996): A-9.

[85] Taylor E. Dark, "Organized Labor and the Congressional Democrats: Reconsidering the 1980s," *Political Science Quarterly* 111, no. 1 (1996): 90.

[86] Dark, "Organized Labor and the Congressional Democrats," 91–92.

[87] Robin Toner, "Battered by Labor's Ads, Republicans Strike Back," *The New York Times* (July 15, 1996): A-1. The surcharge was equal to 15 cents per month for each worker belonging to a union affiliated with the AFL-CIO. Glenn Burkins, "Labor's Bid to Aid Democrats Faces One Hurdle: Many of Its Members Often Vote for Republicans," *The Wall Street Journal* (April 9, 1996): A-20.

[88] James T. Bennett, "Private Sector Unions: The Myth of Decline," *Journal of Labor Research* 12, no. 1 (Winter 1991): 1–12. In the 1995–96 campaign cycle, corporate PAC, individual, and "soft money" contributions totaled $653.4 million compared to $58.1 million in labor contributions, or a ratio of 11:1, up from 10:1 in 1994 and 9:1 in 1992. Figures from Center for Responsive Politics, "The Big Picture," http://www.crp.org/crpdocs/bigpicture/default.htm and http://www.crp.org/crpdocs/bigpicture/blio/bpbliotot.html. See also Makinson and Goldstein, *Open Secrets*, 24–26.

[89] David Brody, "Labor's Crisis in Historical Perspective," in *The State of the Unions;* David Milton, *The Politics of U.S. Labor: From the Great Depression to the New Deal* (New York: Monthly Review Press, 1982); Robert H. Zieger, *The C.I.O., 1935–1955* (Chapel Hill: The University of North Carolina Press, 1995); Alan Draper, *A Rope of Sand: The AFL-CIO Committee on Political Education, 1955–1967* (New York: Praeger, 1989); *The C.I.O.'s Left-Led Unions*, ed. Steve Rosswurm (New Brunswick, N.J.: Rutgers University Press, 1992); Kevin Boyle, *The U.A.W. and the Heyday of American Liberalism* (Ithaca, N.Y.: Cornell University Press, 1995); Stephen Amberg, *Union Inspiration in American Politics: The Autoworkers and the Making of a Liberal Industrial Order* (Philadelphia: Temple University Press, 1994); Julie Greene, *Pure and Simple Politics: The American Federation of Labor and Political Activism, 1881–1917* (Cambridge and New York: Cambridge University Press, 1998); and Plotke, *Building a Democratic Political Order*.

[90] For a critique of this trend in history, see the introduction to Dubofsky, *The State and Labor in Modern America*.

[91] Marick F. Masters and John Thomas Delaney, "Union Political Activities: A Review of the Empirical Literature," *Industrial and Labor Relations Review* 40, no. 3 (April 1987): 336–53; David J. Sousa, "Organized Labor in the Electorate, 1960–1988," *Political Research Quarterly* 46, no. 4 (1993): 741–58; and James T. Bennett and John T. Delaney, "Research on Unions: Some Subjects in Need of Scholars," *Journal of Labor Research* 14, no. 2 (Spring 1993): 95–110.

[92] For an elaboration on this point, see Daniel B. Cornfield, "The U.S. Labor Movement: Its Development and Impact on Social Inequality," *Annual Review of Sociology* 17 (1991): 27–49; and John T. Delaney and Marick F. Masters, "Unions and Political Action," in *The State of the Unions*.

[93] Labor's relationship with the New Left was complex, variable, and not always antagonistic. Peter Levy, *The New Left and Labor in the 1960s* (Urbana: University of Illinois Press, 1994).

[94] Seymour Martin Lipset, "America's Changing Unions," *The New York Times* (December 11, 1983): sec. 7, 3.

[95] Extrapolated from Paul R. Abramson, John H. Aldrich, and David W. Rohde, *Change and Continuity in the 1996 Elections* (Washington, D.C.: Congressional Quarterly Press, 1998), Fig. 5–3, 107.

[96] These figures come from, "Portrait of the Electorate," *The New York Times* (November 10, 1996): 28.

Other surveys of union electoral behavior indicate even wider spreads between the union vote for the Democratic and Republican presidential candidates. In 1984, 64 percent of union members in Pennsylvania voted for Democrat Walter Mondale in the presidential race compared to 35 percent for Ronald Reagan. The AFL-CIO claims that 61 percent of union members nationwide stuck with Mondale that year. Tom Juravich and Peter R. Shergold, "The Impact of Unions on the Voting Behavior of Their Members," *Industrial and Labor Relations Review* 41, no. 3 (April 1988): 374–85. The *New York Times* survey found the Mondale-Reagan split to be a more modest 46–53.

[97] "Portrait of the Electorate," *The New York Times.* See also Sousa, "Organized Labor in the Electorate."

[98] David Sousa, "Union Politics in an Era of Decline" (Ph.D. dissertation, University of Minnesota, 1991), 283, cited in Dark, "Organized Labor and the Congressional Democrats," 96; and Sousa, "Organized Labor in the Electorate," 745.

[99] "Portrait of the Electorate," *The New York Times.* Families in the next highest income bracket ($12,001 to $20,000 in 1976, the equivalent of $30,000 to $49,999 in 1996) vote more consistently for Republican candidates. Whereas the Republican edge for this category of voters was 2 percent in the 1976 presidential contest, it widened to 27 percent in 1980, but has been shrinking ever since. It was 19 percent and 13 percent, respectively, in 1984 and 1988. In 1992 and 1996, Clinton won this category of voters by 3 percent and 8 percent, respectively.

[100] Calculated from Frances Fox Piven, "Structural Constraints and Political Development," in *Labor Parties in Postindustrial Societies*, ed. Frances Fox Piven (Cambridge: Polity Press, 1991), Table 11.1, 236. These figures are based on whites who voted for major party candidates. See also Michael Hout, Clem Brooks, and Jeff Manza, "The Democratic Class Struggle in the United States, 1948–1992," *American Sociological Review* 60 (December 1995): 805–28.

[101] Burkins, "Labor's Bid to Aid Democrats Faces One Hurdle."

[102] Robin Gerber, "Changing the Way Unions Do Politics," *WorkingUSA* (January–February 1999): 66; and Steven Greenhouse, "Republicans Credit Labor for Success by Democrats," *The New York Times* (November 6, 1998): A-28.

[103] Michael Goldfield, "Race and Labor Organization in the United States," *Monthly Review* 49, no. 3 (July–August 1997): 80–97.

[104] Indeed, some contend that the public-sector unions could serve as the fulcrum of a new style of social unionism that will "build new alliances that defend and assert public needs." See Paul Johnston, *Success Where Others Fail: Social Movement Unionism and the Public Workplace*, 13. See also Deborah E. Bell, "Unionized Women in State and Local Govern ment," in *Women, Work and Protest: A Century of U.S. Women's Labor History*, ed. Ruth Milkman (Boston: Routledge & Kegan Paul, 1985); Norma H. Riccucci, *Women, Minorities, and Unions in the Public Sector* (New York: Greenwood Press, 1990); Mark H. Maier, *City Unions: Managing Discontent in New York City* (New Brunswick, N.J.: Rutgers University Press, 1987); *When Public Sector Workers Unionize*, ed. Richard B. Freeman and Casey Ichniowski (Chicago: Chicago University Press, 1988); Leon Fink and Brian Greenberg, *Upheaval in the Quiet Zone: A History of Hospital Workers' Union 1199* (Urbana and Chicago: University of Illinois Press, 1989); and Leo Troy, *The New Unionism in the New Society: Public Sector Unions in the Redistributive State* (Fairfax, Va.: George Mason University Press, 1994).

[105] A combination of factors explain this development, in particular declines in union membership and electoral turnout among union and nonunion whites during a period

when black electoral participation increased dramatically. Abramson et al., *Change and Continuity in the 1996 Elections*, 106; Robert Axelrod, "Presidential Election Coalitions in 1984," *American Political Science Review* 80 (March 1986): 281–84; and "1988–92: National Election Studies," cited in Nelson W. Polsby and Aaron Wildavsky, *Presidential Elections: Strategies and Structures in American Politics*, 9th ed. (Chatham, N.J.: Chatham House Publishers, 1996). See also William Form, *Segmented Labor, Fractured Politics: Labor Politics in American Life* (New York and London: Plenum Press, 1995), 270.

[106] For an overview of the rise in scholarly interest in business-government relations, see Stephen Wilks, "Government-Industry Relations: A Review Article," *Policy and Politics* 14, no. 4 (1986): 491–505.

[107] Charles E. Lindblom, *Politics and Markets: The World's Political-Economic Systems* (New York: Basic Books, 1977).

[108] Beth Mintz and Michael Schwartz, "Capital Flows and the Process of Financial Hegemony," in *Structures of Capital: The Social Organization of the Economy*, ed. Sharon Zukin and Paul DiMaggio (Cambridge: Cambridge University Press, 1990); Cathie Jo Martin, "Business and the New Economic Activism: The Growth of Corporate Lobbies in the Sixties," *Polity* 27, no. 1 (Fall 1994): 49–76; Mark S. Mizruchi, *The Structure of Corporate Political Action: Interfirm Relations and Their Consequences* (Cambridge: Harvard University Press, 1992); Michael Useem, *The Inner Circle: Large Corporations and the Rise of Business Political Activity in the U.S. and U.K.* (New York: Oxford University Press, 1984); Sharon Zukin and Paul DiMaggio, "Introduction," in *Structures of Capital;* and David Vogel, *Fluctuating Fortunes: The Political Power of Business in America* (New York: Basic Books, 1989).

[109] Vogel, *Fluctuating Fortunes;* David Vogel, "The Power of Business in America: A Reappraisal," *British Journal of Political Science* 13, no. 1 (1983): 19–43; and Michael W. McCann, *Taking Reform Seriously: Perspectives in Public Interest Liberalism* (Ithaca, N.Y.: Cornell University Press, 1986). See also Steven M. Gillon, *Politics and Vision: The A.D.A. and American Liberalism, 1947–1985* (New York: Oxford University Press, 1987). This study of the leading liberal lobbying organization in the postwar era devotes just a few pages to organized labor.

[110] Vogel, *Fluctuating Fortunes*, ch. 9.

[111] Thomas Byrne Edsall, *The New Politics of Inequality* (New York: W.W. Norton & Co., 1984); Benjamin Ginsberg, "Money and Power: The New Political Economy of American Elections," in *The Political Economy;* Kevin Phillips, *The Politics of Rich and Poor: Wealth and the American Electorate in the Reagan Aftermath* (New York: Random House, 1990); William Greider, *Who Will Tell the People? The Betrayal of American Democracy* (New York: Simon & Schuster, 1992); and Thomas Ferguson and Joel Rogers, *Right Turn: The Decline of the Democrats and the Future of American Politics* (New York: Hill and Wang, 1986).

[112] See *Bringing the State Back In*, ed. Peter B. Evans, Dietrich Rueschemeyer, and Theda Skocpol (Cambridge: Cambridge University Press, 1985).

[113] For a development of this point, see Ira Katznelson, "The State to the Rescue? Political Science and History Reconnect," *Social Research* 59, no. 4 (Winter 1992): 719–37.

[114] Theda Skocpol, "Political Response to Capitalist Crisis: Neo-Marxist Theories of the State and the Case of the New Deal," *Politics & Society* 10, no. 2 (1980): 155–201; Colin Gordon, "New Deal, Old Deck: Business and the Origins of Social Security," *Politics & Society* 19, no. 2 (1991): 165–207; and Peter Swenson, "Arranged Alliance: Business Interests in the New Deal," *Politics & Society* 25, no. 1 (March 1997): 66–116.

[115] A few scholars accord labor an important, if not central, role in the politics of the New Deal. See Michael Goldfield, "Worker Insurgency, Radical Organization, and New Deal Labor Legislation," *American Political Science Review* 83, no. 4 (1989): 1257–82; Plotke, *Building a Democratic Political Order;* Quadagno, *The Transformation of Old Age Security;* Jill Quadagno and Madonna Meyer, "Organized Labor, State Structures, and Social Policy Development: A Case Study of Old Age Assistance in Ohio, 1916–1940," *Social Problems* 36, no. 2 (1989): 181–96; Theda Skocpol and Edwin Amenta, "Did Capitalists Shape Social Security? Com-

ment on Quadagno," *American Sociological Review* 50, no. 4 (1985): 572–75; and Jill Quadagno, "Two Models of Welfare State Development: Reply to Skocpol and Amenta," *American Sociological Review* 50, no. 4 (1985): 575–78.

Chapter 3: The Institutional Straightjacket of the Private Welfare State

¹ Uwe E. Reinhardt, "How the Devil Subverted the Nation's Soul: An Allegory About American Health Policy," in *Social Insurance Issues for the Nineties, Proceedings of the Third Conference of the National Academy of Social Insurance*, ed. Paul N. Van De Water (Dubuque, Iowa: Kendall/Hunt, 1992), 77.

² Joseph W. Garbarino, *Health Plans and Collective Bargaining* (Berkeley: University of California Press, 1960), 249–51; and Raymond Munts, *Bargaining for Health: Labor Unions, Health Insurance, and Medical Care* (Madison: University of Wisconsin Press, 1967), ch. 12.

³ Gerald Markowitz and David Rosner, "Seeking Common Ground: A History of Labor and Blue Cross," *Journal of Health Politics, Policy and Law* 16, no. 4 (Winter 1991): 695–718; Munts, *Bargaining for Health*, ch. 10; Rickey L. Hendricks, "Liberal Default, Labor Support, and Conservative Neutrality: The Kaiser Permanente Medical Care Program After World War II," *Journal of Policy History* 1, no. 2 (1989): 156–80; and David Rosner and Gerald Markowitz, "Hospitals, Insurance, and the American Labor Movement: The Case of New York in the Postwar Decades," *Journal of Policy History* 9, no. 1 (1997): 74–95.

⁴ Munts, *Bargaining for Health*, 3–5; Daniel B. Cornfield, "Labor Unions, Corporations, and Families: Institutional Competition in the Provision of Social Welfare," *Marriage and Family Review* 15, no. 3/4 (1990): 38–46; and Julie Greene, "Negotiating the State: Frank Walsh and the Transformation of Labor's Political Culture in Progressive America," in *Organized Labor and American Politics, 1894–1994: The Labor-Liberal Alliance*, ed. Kevin Boyle (Albany: SUNY Press, 1998).

⁵ Beth Stevens, "Labor Unions, Employee Benefits, and the Privatization of the American Welfare State," *Journal of Policy History* 2, no. 3 (1990): 233–60; and Alan Derickson, "Health Security for All? Social Unionism and Universal Health Insurance, 1935–1958," *The Journal of American History* 80, no. 4 (March 1994): 1353–56. On the importance of ethnic mutual benefit societies in the early provision of social welfare, see Lizabeth Cohen, *Making a New Deal: Industrial Workers in Chicago, 1919–1939* (Cambridge: Cambridge University Press, 1990), especially 64–75 and 227–30.

⁶ Donna Allen, *Fringe Benefits: Wages or Social Obligation?* (Ithaca, N.Y.: Cornell University Press, 1964), 25; and Steven A. Sass, *The Promise of Private Pensions: The First Hundred Years* (Cambridge, Mass.: Harvard University Press, 1997), 121.

⁷ Raymond Munts and Mary Louise Munts, "Welfare History of the ILGWU," *Labor History* 9, special supplement (Spring 1968): 95. See also Beth Stevens, "In the Shadow of the Welfare State: Corporate and Union Development of Employee Benefits" (Ph.D. dissertation, Harvard University, 1984).

⁸ Allen, *Fringe Benefits*, 67.

⁹ Opinions differ widely over why U.S. companies initially adopted social welfare schemes and why these programs expanded in the 1920s and 1930s. Analysts ascribe various motivations to employers, including a desire to keep unions at bay; increase productivity and efficiency; instill moral uplift in workers; reduce employee turnover; and address social problems associated with rapid industrialization. For a good survey of the contending views, see Stuart D. Brandes, *American Welfare Capitalism, 1880–1940* (Chicago: University of Chicago Press, 1976), 1–19 and ch. 14; Stevens, "In the Shadow of the Welfare State," preface and ch. 1. See also Irving Bernstein, *The Lean Years* (Boston: Houghton, Mifflin, 1960); Edward Berkowitz and Kim McQuaid, *Creating the Welfare State: The Political Economy of Twentieth-Century Reform* (New York: Praeger, 1988); David Brody, *Workers in Industrial America*, 2nd ed.

(New York: Oxford University Press, 1993); Sanford M. Jacoby, *Modern Manors: Welfare Capitalism Since the New Deal* (Princeton, N.J.: Princeton University Press, 1997); and Andrea Tone, *The Business of Benevolence: Industrial Paternalism in Progressive America* (Ithaca, N.Y.: Cornell University Press, 1997). For a view that stresses the importance of the insurance industry in expanding welfare capitalism, see Frank R. Dobbin, "The Origins of Private Social Insurance: Public Policy and Fringe Benefits in America, 1920–1950," *American Journal of Sociology* 97, no. 5 (1992).

[10] Jill Quadagno, *The Transformation of Old Age Security: Class and Politics in the American Welfare State* (Chicago: University of Chicago Press, 1988); and Beth Stevens, "Blurring the Boundaries: How the Federal Government Has Influenced Welfare Benefits in the Private Sector," in *The Politics of Social Policy in the United States*, ed. Margaret Weir, Ann Shola Orloff, and Theda Skocpol (Princeton, N.J.: Princeton University Press, 1988). Dobbin takes issue with the emphasis that Stevens and Quadagno put on changes in the tax code and wage controls to explain the explosion of benefits during World War II. He contends that the 1939 amendments to the Social Security Act were critical in encouraging employers to develop and expand private insurance programs. See Dobbin, "The Origins of Private Social Insurance," 1438.

[11] Michael K. Brown, "Bargaining for Social Rights: Unions and the Reemergence of Welfare Capitalism," *Political Science Quarterly* 112, no. 4 (1997–98): 653.

[12] Nelson Lichtenstein, *The Most Dangerous Man in Detroit: Walter Reuther and the Fate of American Labor* (New York: Basic Books, 1995), 282.

[13] Brown, "Bargaining for Social Rights," 665.

[14] Nelson Lichtenstein, "Labor in the Truman Era: Origins of the 'Private Welfare State'," in *The Truman Presidency*, ed. Michael J. Lacey (Cambridge: Cambridge University Press, 1989), 151; and Stevens, "Labor Unions, Employee Benefits," 234–35.

[15] Brown, "Bargaining for Social Rights," 653.

[16] Garbarino, *Health Plans and Collective Bargaining*, 249. One should not necessarily view this increase as a net increase in health-insurance coverage because many workers who received health insurance through collective bargaining were previously enrolled in other coverage. Garbarino, *Health Plans and Collective Bargaining*, 19.

[17] Lichtenstein, "Labor in the Truman Era," 152.

[18] Brown, "Bargaining for Social Rights," 653.

[19] Derickson, "Health Security for All?"; Martha Derthick, *Policymaking for Social Security* (Washington, D.C.: The Brookings Institution, 1979), 121–27; and Edwin E. Witte, "Organized Labor and Social Security," in *Labor and the New Deal*, ed. Milton Derber and Edwin Young (Madison: University of Wisconsin Press, 1957), 270–71.

[20] Derickson, "Health Security for All?" 1351–52.

[21] National Coordinating Committee of Multiemployer Plans (NCCMP), "Taft-Hartley, Multiemployer Health and Welfare Plans and National Health Care Reform," report (Washington, D.C.: NCCMP, n.d.); and NCCMP, "Multiemployer Plans: A Basic Guide," pamphlet (Washington, D.C.: NCCMP, n.d.).

[22] NCCMP, "Characteristics of Multiemployer Plans," *Employee Benefits Basics* (International Foundation of Employee Benefit Plans) (2nd Quarter 1996): 1.

[23] NCCMP, "Multiemployer Trust Funds," *Employee Benefits Basics* (July 1988): 1; NCCMP, "Taft-Hartley, Multiemployer Health and Welfare Plans and National Health Care Reform"; and NCCMP, "Multiemployer Plans: A Basic Guide."

[24] John T. Dunlop, "Health Care Coalitions," in *Private Sector Coalitions: A Fourth Party in Health Care*, ed. B. Jon Jaeger (Durham, N.C.: Department of Health Administration, 1983), 10.

[25] NCCMP, "Characteristics of Multiemployer Plans."

[26] Harry A. Millis and Emily Clark Brown, *From the Wagner Act to Taft-Hartley: A Study of National Labor Policy and Labor Relations* (Chicago: Chicago University Press, 1950), 283–332; Robert H. Zieger, *American Workers, American Unions*, 2nd ed. (Baltimore: The Johns Hopkins

University Press, 1994), 108–14; James Gross, *Broken Promises: The Subversion of U.S. Labor Relations Policy, 1947–1994* (Philadelphia: Temple University Press, 1995), 57; and Arthur F. McClure, *The Truman Administration and the Problems of Postwar Labor, 1945–48* (Rutherford, N.J.: Fairleigh Dickinson University Press, 1969).

[27] The Wagner Act merely states that business had to bargain on "wages and conditions of employment."

[28] Munts, *Bargaining for Health*, 10.

[29] For a detailed history of the rise and demise of the welfare and retirement fund of the United Mine Workers, see Ivana Krajcinovic, *From Company Doctors to Managed Care: The United Mine Workers' Noble Experiment* (Ithaca, N.Y.: Cornell University Press, 1997).

[30] Supplemental views of Senators Taft, Ball, Donnell, and Jenner, U.S. Senate, Committee on Labor and Public Welfare, "Federal Labor Relations Act of 1947," Report no. 105, 80th Cong., 1st Sess. (April 17, 1947), 52.

[31] About one-third of the plans established prior to the Taft-Hartley Act were administered jointly by employers and unions, another third by the insurance companies, and the rest solely by labor unions. U.S. Congress, Joint Committee on Labor-Management Relations, "Labor-Management Relations," U.S. Senate, Report no. 986, 80th Cong., 2nd Sess. (March 15, 1948), pt. 1:41.

[32] U.S. Senate, Committee on Labor and Public Welfare, "National Relations Act of 1949," Report no. 99, 81st Cong., 1st. Sess., Minority Views (May 4, 1949), pt. 2:49.

[33] U.S. House of Representatives, Committee on Education and Labor, "Labor-Management Relations Act, 1947," Report no. 245, 80th Cong., 1st Sess. (April 11, 1947), 29–30. A business executive charged at the time that these funds would permit unions "to build up enormous sums of tax-free money which could be administered, invested and distributed as union leaders saw fit." Testimony of mining executive Rolla D. Campbell, U.S. House, Committee on Education and Labor, "Amendments to the National Labor Relations Act," vol. 2, 80th Congress, 1st Sess. (February–March 1947), 634–35.

[34] Supplemental views of Senators Taft et al., "Federal Labor Relations Act of 1947," 52.

[35] See Munts, *Bargaining for Health*, ch. 1; Fred A. Hartley, Jr., *Our New National Labor Policy* (New York: Funk & Wagnalls, 1948); Millis and Brown, *From the Wagner Act to Taft-Hartley*, 564; and Susan M. Hartmann, *Truman and the 80th Congress* (Columbia: University of Missouri Press, 1971).

[36] Supplemental Views of Senator Taft et al., "Federal Labor Relations Act of 1947," 52.

[37] Millis and Brown, *From the Wagner Act to Taft-Hartley*, 567.

[38] U.S. Senate, Committee on Labor and Public Welfare, "Federal Relations Act of 1947," Report no. 105, Minority Views, 80th Cong., 1st Sess. (April 22, 1947), pt. 2:23.

[39] Ibid. See also "Labor-Management Relations Act, 1947," Report no. 245, Minority Report, 80th Cong., 1st Sess. (April 11, 1947), 79.

[40] George Meany, letter to National and International Unions, State Federations, City Central Bodies, Federal Labor Unions, and Regional Organizers, January 7, 1953, AFL, AFL-CIO Department of Legislation, 1906–78 (hereafter, AFL-CIO Department of Legislation Collection), George Meany Memorial Archives, Silver Spring, Md., Box 24, Folder 39, "Health."

[41] See U.S. Congress, Joint-Committee on Labor-Management Relations, "Labor-Management Relations," U.S. Senate Report no. 374, 81st Cong., 1st Sess. (May 13, 1949), especially 5 and 39.

[42] In his State of the Union Address, Truman made no specific recommendations for amendments to the Taft-Hartley Act. R. Alton Lee, *Truman and Taft-Hartley: A Question of Mandate* (Lexington: University of Kentucky Press, 1966), 108–109.

[43] *Public Papers of the Presidents of the United States: Harry S. Truman, 1950* (Washington, D.C.: U.S. Government Printing Office, 1965), 72.

[44] Munts, *Bargaining for Health*, 10.

[45] Munts, *Bargaining for Health*, chs. 5 and 6; and Lawrence S. Root, *Fringe Benefits: Social Insurance in the Steel Industry* (Beverly Hills, Calif.: Sage, 1982).

[46] See the testimony of Raymond S. Smethurst, counsel of the National Association of Manufacturers, and other business representatives in U.S. Congress, Joint Committee on Labor-Management Relations, "Operation of the Labor-Management Relations Act," 80th Cong., 2nd Sess. (May–June, 1948), pts. 1 and 2.

[47] Stevens, "In the Shadow of the Welfare State," 129.

[48] That year the steelworkers also won life insurance benefits, an increase in disability benefits, and company-paid health insurance during layoffs. For an account of the development of fringe benefits in the steel industry, see Munts, *Bargaining for Health*, ch. 5; and Root, *Fringe Benefits*.

[49] Munts, *Bargaining for Health*, ch. 6.

[50] Jacoby, *Modern Manors;* and H.M. Sapolsky et al., "Corporate Attitudes Toward Health Care Costs," *Milbank Memorial Fund Quarterly* 59, no. 4 (1981): 561–85.

[51] The NAM suggested that the provision of retiree benefits could serve as an important public relations tool because it presents "businessmen with an excellent opportunity to participate in a humanitarian service." NAM Employee Health and Benefits Committee, "On the Horizon: Medical Care Protection for Retired Employees," pamphlet at Hagley Library, Wilmington, Del. (New York: NAM, 1961), 5.

[52] Andrew J. Biemiller, memorandum Re: Additional subject to discuss with President Meany, January 13, 1954, AFL-CIO Department of Legislation Collection, Box 25, File 14, "Health, Education, and Welfare, Department of"; and Andrew J. Biemiller, memorandum to George Meany Re: Proposed Legislation on Health and Welfare Funds, January 28, 1954, AFL-CIO Department of Legislation Collection, Box 85, Folder 8, "Memoranda to George Meany, 1954." For more about the corruption associated with some of these funds, see Munts, *Bargaining for Health*, ch. 8.

[53] "In fact, once jointly administered health and welfare funds are liberated from the tyranny of escalating health-insurance costs they may develop broad new programs of significant value for their membership," AFL-CIO officials told trustees of the numerous Taft-Hartley funds. Bert Seidman, memorandum to Al Barkan et al. Re: Health and Welfare Trusts and National Health Insurance, May 21, 1970, attachment, 2, AFL-CIO Department of Legislation Collection, Box 25, Folder 24, "Health Insurance"; and Bert Seidman, former director of the department of social security, AFL-CIO, Interview, Washington, D.C., June 13, 1996.

[54] One 1994 survey concluded that 25 percent of contributions to health and welfare funds were used to cover the costs of providing care to people without health insurance (up from 15 percent in 1987) as health-care providers overcharged those with insurance to make up for the expense of treating the uninsured. Laborers' Health and Security Fund of America, "Cost Shifting: Who Shoulders the Burden of the Health Care Crisis," report (Washington, D.C.: Laborers' Health and Safety Fund, n.d.); and "Health Care 'Reform' Should NOT Come at the Expense of the Building Trades!!!," mimeo, n.d., received from James S. Ray, legislative representative, NCCMP.

[55] NCCMP, "Taft-Hartley, Multiemployer Health and Welfare Plans," 2; and U.S. General Accounting Office, "Employer-Based Health Plans; Issues, Trends, and Challenges Posed by ERISA" (Washington, D.C.: GAO, 1995), 39.

[56] NCCMP, "Taft-Hartley, Multiemployer Health & Welfare Plans," 2.

[57] Leo J. Purcell, letter to Robert Georgine, January 28, 1991, Personal Files of Robert McGarrah, AFSCME headquarters, Washington, D.C. (hereafter, McGarrah Papers).

[58] Employers' contributions to Taft-Hartley funds are typically calculated based on the number of hours worked by a covered worker.

[59] On the development of nonunion beachheads in traditionally unionized sectors, see Thomas A. Kochan, Harry C. Katz, and Robert B. McKersie, *The Transformation of American Industrial Relations* (New York: Basic Books, 1986), ch. 3.

⁶⁰ As of 1988, over one-third of those working in the construction industry were employed by firms that did not offer health benefits. The only other sector with a higher percentage of workers employed by firms that did not offer health insurance was agriculture (56 percent). The figures for other sectors are: business/repair (34 percent), retail (32 percent), personal/professional service (18 percent), wholesale (12 percent), financial/insurance (11 percent), transportation (9 percent), manufacturing (8 percent), and public administration (3 percent). Stephen H. Long and M. Susan Marquis, "Gaps in Employer Coverage: Lack of Supply or Lack of Demand?" *Health Affairs* Supplement (1993): 287.

⁶¹ "Now, the tables are turning. The crisis in health costs is of sufficient magnitude that many of our local union officers and fund administrators see the funds as an albatross around their necks," he said. Leo J. Purcell, letter to Robert Georgine, January 28, 1991, McGarrah Papers.

⁶² Howard S. Berliner, "Payment for Uncompensated Hospital Care in New Jersey: Impact on Union Health and Welfare Funds," report (Washington, D.C.: Laborers' National Health and Safety Fund, March 1989), 5.

⁶³ For example, the building trades in Massachusetts were at the center of one of the most high profile and successful campaigns against the perceived corporate excesses of the Reagan years, the 1988 battle to preserve a state law governing wages on publicly-funded construction sites. Mark Erlich, *Labor at the Ballot Box: The Massachusetts Prevailing Wage Campaign of 1988* (Philadelphia: Temple University Press, 1990).

⁶⁴ Albert B. Crenshaw, "The Aim to Be Letter Perfect; ULLICO Repositions for Growth and 'A' Insurance Rating," *The Washington Post* (July 11, 1994): F-1; and "Ullico Inc.," *The Washington Post* (April 18, 1995): F-47.

⁶⁵ Merrill Goozner, "Health Care Debate Splits Union Ranks," *Chicago Tribune* (February 18, 1991): 1

⁶⁶ Robert McGarrah, director of public policy, AFSCME, interview, Washington, D.C., June 5, 1996.

⁶⁷ McGarrah, interview; and James S. Ray, legislative representative, NCCMP, interview, Washington, D.C., June 13, 1996.

⁶⁸ Ray, interview.

⁶⁹ Ray notes that because many AFSCME members are employed by public hospitals funded by tax money that "comes out of the pockets of our members," the public-employee union naturally is more sympathetic than the building and construction trades to a single-payer plan. Ray, interview.

⁷⁰ Ray, interview; J. Peter Nixon, senior policy analyst, SEIU, interview, Washington, D.C., June 3, 1996; Claudia Bradbury St. John, former senior health policy specialist, AFL-CIO, interview, Washington, D.C., June 7, 1996; and J. Peter Nixon, memorandum to Hal Alpert, president of Local 531 of the Service Employees International Union, Re: Health Care Reform, March 2, 1994, Personal Files of J. Peter Nixon (hereafter, Nixon Papers), SEIU headquarters, Washington, D.C.

⁷¹ After Clinton was elected president in 1992, the ILGWU qualified its support of national health insurance and indicated its willingness to support health-care proposals based on the employer mandate and the preservation of the Taft-Hartley arrangements. See ch. 7 below.

⁷² Munts and Munts, "Welfare History," 96.

⁷³ Sar A. Levitan and Martha R. Cooper, *Business Lobbies: The Public Good and the Bottom Line* (Baltimore: Johns Hopkins University Press, 1984), ch. 5.

⁷⁴ Daniel M. Fox and Daniel C. Schaffer, "Health Policy and ERISA: Interest Groups and Semipreemption," *Journal of Health Politics, Policy and Law* 14, no. 2 (Summer 1989): 240; and Sass, *The Promise of Private Pensions*, ch. 8.

⁷⁵ Margaret G. Farrell, "ERISA Preemption and Regulation of Managed Care: The Case for Managed Federalism," *American Journal of Law & Medicine* 23, no. 2 and 3 (1997): 251–89.

[76] The "Health Insurance Portability and Accountability Act of 1996," commonly known as the Kennedy-Kassebaum bill, subjects self-insured plans, which were protected from state oversight due to ERISA, to new broad federal regulations regarding medical underwriting practices. It also forbids self-insured and non-self-insured group health plans from limiting the health coverage they offer to new employees with pre-existing conditions. The HIPAA did not significantly alter the ERISA preemption. Reforming States Group, "Balanced Federalism and Health System Reform," *Health Affairs* (May/June 1998): 181–91.

[77] Fox and Schaffer, "Health Policy and ERISA," 243.

[78] See the testimony of George J. Pantos of the ERISA Industry Committee (ERIC), U.S. Senate, Committee on Labor and Human Resources, "E.R.I.S.A. Improvements Acts of 1979," 96th Cong., 1st Sess. (February 1979), 522. ERIC, which counts dozens of firms among its members, is the main vehicle among employers to defend an expansive ERISA preemption.

[79] Mary Ann Chirba-Martin and Troyen A. Brennan, "The Critical Role of ERISA in State Health Reform," *Health Affairs* 13, no. 2 (Spring 1994): 142–56; and Wendy Parmet, "Regulation and Federalism: Legal Impediments to State Health Care Reform," *American Journal of Laws and Medicine* 19, no. 1 and 2 (1993): 132–40. For a slightly different view, see Colleen M. Grogan, "Hope in Federalism? What Can the States Do and What Are They Likely To Do?" *Journal of Health Politics, Policy and Law* 20, no. 2 (Summer 1995): 477–84.

[80] By the early 1990s, nearly 60 percent of Americans insured through their employers were covered by such plans. Malcolm Gladwell, "When Health Plan Changes Leave Employees Vulnerable; AIDS Case Targets Federal Self-Insurance Law," *The Washington Post* (August 20, 1992): A-1.

[81] Testimony of Robert Georgine, president of the building and construction trades department of the AFL-CIO, U.S. House, Subcommittee on Health and the Environment of the Committee on Energy and Commerce, "Health Care Reform," 103rd Cong., 1st Sess. (November 1993): pt. 5, 103–105.

[82] *EBRI Databook on Employee Benefits*, 3rd ed., ed. Carolyn Pemberton and Deborah Holmes (Washington, D.C.: Employee Benefit Research Institute, 1995), 291; Milt Freudenheim, "Employers Winning Wide Leeway to Cut Medical Insurance Benefits," *The New York Times* (March 29, 1992): A-1; and Joseph B. Treaster, "Protecting Against the Little Risks," *The New York Times* (December 31, 1996): D-1.

Recently, small businesses lobbied fiercely for controversial legislation that would in effect greatly extend the ERISA umbrella by permitting national membership organizations, such as trade associations, to band together to set up self-insured plans called multiple employer welfare associations (MEWAs). MEWAs would not be subject to state-level insurance regulations. Harris W. Fawell, "Squeezing Small Business," *The Washington Post* (April 16, 1997): A-17. See also Reforming States Group, "Balanced Federalism."

[83] Research Institute of America, Inc., *Executive Compensation Alert* (May 15, 1991): electronic database.

[84] In its 1987 *Pilot Life* decision, the Supreme Court held that state laws setting standards for the processing of health benefits claims by insurance companies were preempted by ERISA. States had attempted to use the laws to provide employees with legal recourse for what was seen as an unfair denial of claims. Research Institute of America, Inc., *Executive Compensation Alert;* and Freudenheim, "Employers Winning Wide Leeway."

[85] Linda Greenhouse, "Managed Care Challenge to Be Heard by Supreme Court," *The New York Times* (September 29, 1999): A-22; Robert Pear, "Series of Rulings Eases Constraints on Suing HMOs," *The New York Times* (August 15, 1999): sec. 1, 1; Pear, "H.M.O.'s Using Federal Law to Deflect Malpractice Suits," *The New York Times* (November 17, 1996): sec. 1, 24; and Farrell, "ERISA Preemption and Regulation of Managed Care."

[86] Employers used the ERISA preemption to mount successful challenges to prevailing wage laws, state standards for the certification or training of apprentices, and state mandates

in the area of workers' compensation coverage. "Businesses Await Ruling on Unified Self-Insured Plans," *HR Focus* (electronic database) (April 1993): 1.

Robert Georgine of the AFL-CIO testified in 1991 that federal legislation was needed to restrict ERISA's preemption of state laws in three specific areas unrelated to health benefits. He did not advocate scrapping the ERISA preemption altogether and was forced to concede that the AFL-CIO was a longtime defender of a broad ERISA preemption. Research Institute of America, Inc., *Executive Compensation Alert.*

[87] Testimony of Robert Georgine, U.S. Senate, Committee in Labor and Human Resources, "ERISA Improvements Act of 1979," 96th Cong., 1st Sess. (February 1979), 281; and Fox and Schaffer, "Health Policy and ERISA."

[88] Robert Pear, "Court Approves Cuts in Benefits in Costly Illness," *The New York Times* (November 27, 1991): A-1; Robert Pear, "U.S. to Argue Employers Can Cut Health Coverage," *The New York Times* (October 16, 1992): A-18; and Thomas D. Stoddard, "Now You're Insured, Now You're Not," *The New York Times* (May 23, 1992): A-23.

[89] Jonathan Goldberg-Hiller, "The Limits to Union: Labor, Gays and Lesbians, and Marriage in Hawai'i," paper presented at the annual meetings of the American Political Science Association, Boston, Mass., September 3–6, 1998.

[90] Alex Michelini, "Union's $1 M AIDS Penalty," *New York Daily News* (December 15, 1995): 16; and Richard A. Oppel, Jr., "Health-Benefits Ruling Poses Risk for Small Firms; EEOC Decision Would Not Allow Discriminatory Coverage," *The Dallas Morning News* (June 11, 1993): D-1.

[91] I am indebted to Professor Alan Draper of St. Lawrence University for this metaphor.

[92] Duncan M. MacIntyre, *Voluntary Health Insurance and Rate Making* (Ithaca, N.Y.: Cornell University Press, 1962), 111.

[93] MacIntyre, *Voluntary Health Insurance and Rate Making*, 39–42.

[94] In 1946, some 32 million Americans had some form of health insurance. Just two years later, the figure stood at 53 million. By 1951, 77 million Americans were covered. Rashi Fein, *Medical Care, Medical Costs: The Search for Health Insurance Policy* (Cambridge, Mass.: Harvard University Press, 1986), 23.

[95] Garbarino, *Health Plans and Collective Bargaining*, 228.

[96] MacIntyre, *Voluntary Health Insurance and Rate Making*, 237 and 252.

[97] MacIntyre, *Voluntary Health Insurance and Rate Making*, 234–35.

[98] Indeed, Lichtenstein claims that Reuther "was becoming a prisoner of the institutions he had done so much to construct." Lichtenstein, *The Most Dangerous Man in Detroit* (New York: Basic Books, 1995), 295 and 281–82. See also Colin Gordon, "Why No National Health Insurance in the U.S.? The Limits of Social Provision in War and Peace, 1941–1948," *Journal of Policy History* 9, no. 3 (1997): 302.

[99] Garbarino, *Health Plans and Collective Bargaining*, 228–32.

[100] Gordon, "Why No National Health Insurance in the U.S.?", 287.

[101] A 1956 study by the New York State Department of Insurance described the rating practices of some insurance carriers as "arbitrary," "capricious," and involving "discriminatory opportunism." MacIntyre, *Voluntary Health Insurance and Rate Making*, 103. See also Deborah A. Stone, "The Struggle for the Soul of Health Insurance," *Journal of Health Politics, Policy and Law* 18, no. 2 (Summer 1993): 287–317.

[102] Stone, "The Struggle for the Soul of Health Insurance." An advertisement that insurance companies ran in major magazines in 1990 epitomizes this view. It asks, "Why should women pay more for health insurance than men?" and notes that women visit doctors more often than men. The ad then goes on to say: "If you don't group people with similar risks, people with low risks [read: healthy people] would subsidize people with high risks [read: sick people], and that wouldn't be fair." See Reinhardt, "How the Devil Subverted the Nation's Soul," 85. For another example of this sort of reasoning, see David F. Bradford and Derrick A. Max, *Intergenerational Transfers Under Community Rating* (Washington, D.C.: The

AEI Press, 1996). The authors contend that a switch to a pure community-rated system would be tantamount to a substantial transfer of income "toward older generations, at the expense of younger and future birth cohorts." See page 36.

[103] This is 40 times more than administrative costs consume in the Canadian health system and 18 times higher than Medicare spends on administration. Overhead and marketing costs are included in the figures for administrative costs. Citizens Fund, "Premiums Without Benefits: The Decade-Long Growth in Commercial Health Insurance Industry Waste and Inefficiency" (Washington, D.C.: Citizens Fund, April 1992), 1.

[104] Deborah A. Stone, "AIDS and the Moral Economy of Insurance," *The American Prospect* (Spring 1990): 72.

[105] Dean C. Coddington, David J. Keen, and Keith D. Moore, "Cost Shifting Overshadows Employers' Cost-Containment Efforts," *Business and Health* (January 1991): 45–46.

[106] John Judis, "Abandoned Surgery: Business and the Failure of Health Reform," *The American Prospect* (Spring 1995): 66.

[107] The Tax Reform Act of 1986 modified the situation somewhat by allowing a 25 percent tax deduction for health-insurance premiums paid by unincorporated businesses. In 1990, the tax deduction taken by corporations for employee health benefits totaled $36.5 billion, a figure nearly equal to the government expenditures for Medicaid that year. Christopher Howard, "The Hidden Side of the American Welfare State," *Political Science Quarterly* 108, no. 3 (1993): 413.

[108] Congressional Research Service, *Cost and Effects of Extending Health Insurance Coverage* (Washington, D.C.: Education and Labor Serial No. 100–EE, 1988), 46, cited in *Reforming the System*, ed. Blendon and Hyams, Fig. 1–2, 11. Experience rating alone does not account for the differences in administrative costs. What should also be considered is the difference in costs between marketing and servicing dozens of plans each covering a handful of people and those associated with administering a single plan covering hundreds or thousands of employees.

[109] Haynes Bonner Johnson and David S. Broder, *The System: The American Way of Politics at the Breaking Point* (Boston: Little, Brown, 1996). For a view that stresses the important but not necessarily decisive role of small business groups, see Theda Skocpol, *Boomerang: Clinton's Health Security Effort and the Turn Against Government in U.S. Politics* (New York: W.W. Norton & Co., 1996). For a more detailed discussion of business, labor, and the Clinton plan, see ch. 7 in this text.

[110] Figures comparing the availability of health-insurance benefits at small and large firms may overstate the effect of size on the likelihood that a firm will offer benefits. Once unionization is factored in, the gap between fringe benefits in small and large firms evaporates. Charles Brown, James Hamilton, and James Medoff, *Employers Large and Small* (Cambridge, Mass.: Harvard University Press, 1990), 41–43 and 47. Another survey appears to contradict this conclusion. However, it is based on data from an earlier period, the late 1970s, which may account for discrepancies in the findings. Louis F. Rossiter and Amy K. Taylor, "Union Effects on the Provision of Health Insurance," *Industrial Relations* 21, no. 2 (Spring 1982): 167–77.

[111] Jennifer Edwards et al., "Will Small Business Reform Improve Access in the 1990s," in *Reforming the System*, 127–28.

[112] Cathie Jo Martin, "Inviting Business to the Party: The Corporate Response to Social Policy," in *The Social Divide: Political Parties and the Future of Activist Government*, ed. Margaret Weir (Washington, D.C., and New York: Brookings Institution Press and Russell Sage Foundation, 1998); Skocpol, *Boomerang;* and Johnson and Broder, *The System.*

[113] What is less well known and recognized is that the NFIB clashed not only with the Clinton administration, legislators, and large corporations over health-care reform, but with other representatives of the small business community who fiercely dissented from their "just say no" approach to health-care reform. The Small Business Coalition for Health Care Reform (SBCHCR) created in May 1994 took direct aim at the NFIB by questioning its

claims about the degree to which an employer mandate would hurt small business. The SBCHCR pulled together 29 national organizations comprised of 626,000 small businesses, a total that rivaled the stated membership of the NFIB. Charles A. Riley II, *Small Business, Big Politics: What Entrepreneurs Need to Know to Use Their Growing Political Power* (Princeton, N.J.: Pacesetter Books, 1995), ch. 5.

[114] A 1991 Harris survey found that 54 percent of small employers said they did not provide health insurance because the cost was too high. Edwards et al., "Will Small Business Reform Improve Access in the 1990s," 128.

[115] A Louis Harris poll in early 1991 of 501 small business owners found that half of firms with one to five employees offer health insurance to all or some of their employees; three-quarters of firms with six to 25 employees did; and nine out of ten firms with 26 to 100 employees did. Most small firms pay at least half the cost. Edwards et al., "Will Small Business Reform Improve Access in the 1990s," 126–28. See also Stephen H. Long and M. Susan Marquis, "Gaps in Employer Coverage: Lack of Supply or Lack of Demand?", *Health Affairs* supplement (1993): 286–87.

[116] John J. Motley III, vice president, federal governmental relations, NFIB, prepared statement, U.S. House, Subcommittee on Small Business, "The Small Business Community's Recommendations for National Health Reform," 103rd Cong., 1st Sess. (August 4, 1993), 90.

[117] Edwards et al., "Will Small Business Reform Improve Access in the 1990s," 128–29. By contrast, just 31 percent of senior business executives of large corporations characterized their company's health-care costs as "somewhat out of control" and a mere 3 percent described them as "totally out of control." See the 1992 Harris poll cited in Taylor et al., "Large Employers and Managed Care," 91.

[118] Three out of 10 small business respondents said they believed the medical system was so flawed that it needed to be completely rebuilt. About half reported wanting to see fundamental change, while just 16 percent thought only minor changes were needed. Edwards et al., "Will Small Business Reform Improve Access in the 1990s," 130–31.

[119] Motley, "The Small Business Community's Recommendations," 34; and Michael O. Roush, director of federal governmental relations, Senate, NFIB, interview, Washington, D.C., June 3, 1996. Another survey found that nearly half of small business owners preferred some version of a single-payer system. Edwards et al., "Will Small Business Reform Improve Access in the 1990s," 130–32. This figure may be on the high end because the poll was taken without direct reference to what tax burden small firms were willing to shoulder to finance a single-payer system.

[120] It should be noted that this poll was commissioned by the Health Insurance Association of America. Gary Silverman, "Executives Oppose National Health Insurance," United Press International wire service (March 26, 1990): electronic database. There also appear to be great regional variations on the issue of national health insurance. A 1990 poll of business executives found that 38 percent of those in the East favored a government-sponsored health program compared to just 31 percent in the South and 25 percent in the Midwest. "The 1990 National Executive Poll on Health Care Costs and Benefits," *Business and Health* (April 1990): 36–37.

[121] U.S. House, Committee on Ways and Means, "Employer Mandate and Related Provisions of the Administration's Health Security Act," 103rd Cong., 2nd Sess. (February 3, 1994), 132.

[122] William T. Archey, senior vice president for policy and Congressional affairs, U.S. Chamber of Commerce, cited this survey from the September/October 1993 issue of *Journal of Health Policy* in testimony before Congress. U.S. House, Subcommittee on Health of the Committee on Ways and Means, "Health Care Reform," vol. 10, 103rd Cong., 1st Sess. (October 1993), pt. 1:20.

[123] Cathie Jo Martin, "Nature or Nurture? Sources of Firm Preference for National Health Reform," *American Political Science Review* 89, no. 4 (1995): 898–913.

[124] One of the most comprehensive surveys of small business attitudes on health matters found that firms not offering health insurance were more likely to prefer an all-government system (56 percent) to those who already offer their employees medical benefits (45 percent). Edwards et al., "Will Small Business Reform Improve Access in the 1990s," 132.

[125] Edwards et al., "Will Small Business Reform Improve Access in the 1990s," 130–32.

[126] Deborah A. Stone, "The Resistible Rise of Preventive Medicine," in *Health Policy in Transition: A Decade of Health Politics, Policy and Law*, ed. Lawrence D. Brown (Durham, N.C.: Duke University Press, 1987), 115. A 1991 poll of leading business executives found that 50 percent of the respondents favored pre-screening job applicants and hiring only those thought to be less likely to incur large medical costs. "The 1991 National Executive Poll on Health Care Costs and Benefits," *Business and Health* (September 1991): 71.

[127] A 1991 report by the U.S. Congress Office of Technology Assessment found that 42 percent of companies surveyed considered a job applicant's health-insurance risks as factors in determining his or her employability. Ellen E. Schultz, "Advantages of Employer Health Plans Are Disappearing," *The Wall Street Journal* (June 17, 1994): C-1.

[128] For instance, the Coors Brewing Co. of Colorado administers a health assessment program in which it mails out surveys to employees and their spouses with more than 100 routine questions about such things as smoking and seat-belt use. But the surveys also ask respondents questions about such sensitive and personal matters as whether they are having "sexual difficulties" and whether they had had a "stressful Christmas." Nancy Madlin, "Wellness Incentives: How Well Do They Work?" *Business and Health* (April 1991): 70–74; and Schultz, "Advantages of Employer Health Plans."

[129] In late 1992, a federal appeals court in Denver ruled that employers are allowed to require their employees to provide medical information. Schultz, "Advantages of Employer Health Plans Are Disappearing." A subsequent ruling by a Colorado district court in a different case found that the Americans With Disabilities Act bars employers from demanding to know what prescription drugs employees take. Julie Gannon Shoop, "Employers Can't Ask About Prescription Drug Use, Court Holds," *Trial* 32, no. 4 (April 1996): 14.

[130] Thomas C. Buchmueller, "Health Risk and Access to Employer-Provided Health Insurance," *Inquiry* 32, no. 1 (1995): 75–86.

[131] Meg Bryant, "Comeback for the Company Doc?" *Business and Health* (February 1991): 44. For more on the early history of the company doctor, see Brandes, *American Welfare Capitalism*, ch. 10.

[132] Anne Ghislaine Oopay, "Welfare Organization: The Case of Worksite Health Promotion" (Ph.D. dissertation, University of Illinois at Urbana–Champaign, 1991); and John Riley, "Can't Keep a Secret: Insurers' Cost-Cutters Demand Your Medical Details," *Newsday* (April 1, 1996): A-7.

[133] For more on pre-existing clauses and redlining, see Cynthia B. Sullivan and Thomas Rice, "The Health Insurance Picture in 1990," *Health Affairs* (Summer 1991): 112; Milt Freudenheim, "Insurers, to Reduce Losses, Blacklist Dozens of Occupations," *The New York Times* (February 5, 1990): A-1; and Paul Cotton, "Pre-Existing Conditions 'Hold Americans Hostage' to Employers and Insurers," *Journal of the American Medical Association* 265, no. 19 (May 15, 1991): 2451–53.

Chapter 4: Labor Embraces a New Idea

[1] Bill Clinton, "State of the Union," *Vital Speeches* 60, no. 9 (February 15, 1994): 258.

[2] Margaret Weir, *Politics and Jobs: The Boundaries of Employment Policy in the United States* (Princeton, N.J.: Princeton University Press, 1992), 15; and Peter A. Hall, "Conclusion: The Politics of Keynesian Ideas," in *The Political Power of Economic Ideas: Keynesianism Across Nations*, ed. Peter A. Hall (Princeton, N.J.: Princeton University Press, 1989), esp. 369.

³ Theda Skocpol, *Boomerang: Clinton's Health Security Effort and the Turn Against Government in U.S. Politics* (New York: W.W. Norton & Co., 1996).

⁴ For more on "carriers" and the fit between ideas and their environment, see Sheri Berman, *The Social Democratic Moment: Ideas and Politics in the Making of Interwar Europe* (Cambridge: Harvard University Press, 1998), 25–26 and 209–10.

⁵ For more on "focal points," see Geoffrey Garrett and Barry R. Weingast, "Ideas, Interests, and Institutions: Constructing the European Community's Internal Market," in *Ideas and Foreign Policy: Beliefs, Institutions, and Political Change*, ed. Judith Goldstein and Robert O. Keohane (Ithaca, N.Y.: Cornell University Press, 1993), 173–231; and John Kurt Jacobsen, "Much Ado About Ideas: The Cognitive Factor in Economic Policy," *World Politics* 47 (January 1995): 283–310.

⁶ Sheri Berman, "Ideas and Culture in Political Analysis," paper presented at workshop on "Ideas, Culture and Political Analysis," Princeton University, May 15–16, 1998, 4.

⁷ When Sen. Edward M. Kennedy (D-Mass.) reintroduced legislation based on an employer mandate, a health economist tweaked Kennedy's top aide for health policy by asking him whether the senator planned on footnoting Richard Nixon in the bill. Mark A. Peterson, "Report from Congress: Momentum Toward Health Care Reform in the U.S. Senate," *Journal of Health Politics, Policy and Law* 17, no. 3 (Fall 1992): 560.

⁸ In the summer of 1994, the First Lady said to Packwood: "Senator, introduce the Nixon bill. We can live with that." To which Packwood did not reply. Haynes Bonner Johnson and David S. Broder, *The System: The American Way of Politics at the Breaking Point* (Boston: Little, Brown, 1996), 500 and 521–22.

⁹ Tom Wicker, "The Health Insurance Minefield," *The New York Times* (December 20, 1977): 35; Max W. Fine, letter to George Hardy, May 30, 1978, UAW Washington Office: Stephen Schlossberg Collection (hereafter, UAW Schlossberg Collection), Walter P. Reuther Library, Wayne State University, Detroit, Mich., Box 56, Folder 43, "S.E.I.U., George Hardy"; and CNHI, report sent to members of the technical committee, April 13, 1978, Committee for National Health Insurance Collection (hereafter, CNHI Collection), Walter P. Reuther Library, Wayne State University, Detroit, Mich., Box 15, Folder 20, "Technical Committee, memos, 1975–9."

¹⁰ *Congress and the Nation, 1969–1972*, vol. 3 (Washington, D.C.: Congressional Quarterly Press, 1973): 551.

¹¹ Unlike Medicaid, which is administered jointly by the states and the federal government, the new program proposed for low-income families would be paid for and run primarily by the federal government. While the poorest families would pay nothing, better-off low-income families would be required to pay the premiums based on a sliding scale. The proposal did not include any measure to provide health-care coverage to low-income people without children. *Congress and the Nation, 1969–1972*, 564; and U.S. Department of Health, Education, and Welfare, "Toward a Comprehensive Health Policy for the 1970s; A White Paper" (May 1971), submitted to U.S. House, Committee on Ways and Means, "National Health Insurance Proposals," 92nd. Cong., 1st Sess. (October–November 1971).

¹² Richard Nixon, "Message From the President of the United States Relative to Building a National Health Strategy," *National Health Insurance Proposals* (February 18, 1971), pt. 1, 232.

¹³ Richard Lyons, "Nixon's Health Care Plan Proposes Employers Pay $2.5-Billion More A Year," *The New York Times* (February 19, 1971): 1; and Sen. Edward M. Kennedy, "National Health Insurance Proposals," pt. 13, 2959.

¹⁴ *Congress and the Nation, 1969–1972*, 564.

¹⁵ Leonard Woodcock, U.S. Senate, Subcommittee on Health of the Committee on Labor and Public Welfare, "Health Care Crisis in America, 1971," 92nd Cong., 1st Sess. (March 1971), pt. 1, 103–25.

¹⁶ Louis B. Knecht, executive vice-president, Communications Workers of America, "National Health Insurance Proposals," pt. 7, 1467.

¹⁷ "National Health Insurance Proposals," pt. 8, 1802–804; and "National Health Insurance Proposals," pt. 11, 2495–508. In a referendum held early that year on whether to support a federal requirement that all employers provide their workers with a minimum basic health insurance package, the vote was 61 percent in favor. U.S. Chamber of Commerce, press release (June 7, 1971), CNHI Collection, Box 61, Folder 22, "U.S. Chamber of Commerce."

¹⁸ James A. Gavin, "National Health Insurance Proposals," pt. 1, 322–24.

¹⁹ Although both the NAM and the Chamber count among their members corporate giants, mom-and-pop shops, and everything in-between, these organizations tend to reflect the interests of big business. Robert H. Wiebe, *Businessmen and Reform: A Study of the Progressive Movement* (Cambridge: Harvard University Press, 1962); James Weinstein, *The Corporate Ideal in the Liberal State: 1900–1918* (Boston: Beacon Press, 1968); Philip H. Burch, Jr., "The NAM as an Interest Group," *Politics and Society* 4, no. 1 (Fall 1973): 97–130; and Robert M. Collins, *The Business Response to Keynes, 1929–1964* (New York: Columbia University Press, 1981), ch. 5. The U.S. Chamber of Commerce has tilted more consistently than the NAM toward the needs of big business over the years. Sar A. Levitan and Martha R. Cooper, *Business Lobbies: The Public Good and the Bottom Line* (Baltimore: Johns Hopkins University Press, 1984), 18–19. On the political revitalization of the Chamber in the 1970s and its efforts to cater more to small business, see Thomas Byrne Edsall, *The New Politics of Inequality* (New York: W.W. Norton & Co., 1984), 123–25.

²⁰ Arch N. Booth, letter to William R. Clark, April 10, 1970, Statements, Speeches, Etc., Arch N. Booth, Accession 1960, Chamber of Commerce of the United States Records, Hagley Library, Wilmington, Del., Box 27, "Welfare" folder. See also *Washington Report* (April 20, 1970, and December 16, 1970) in the same folder.

²¹ In announcing the results of the poll, the NFIB remarked that "the nation's independent and small businessmen generally considered to be innately conservative, are apparently in support. Even more significant is the heavy support being cast by these independent businessmen in areas generally considered to be bastions of rock-ribbed conservatism." It also noted that in South Carolina, "which has long been mirrored to the nation as living in the 19th century insofar as social outlook is concerned," a whopping 81 percent of small business owners polled supported the family assistance plan. National Federation of Independent Business, press release (n.d.), Statements, Speeches, Etc., Arch N. Booth, Accession 1960, Chamber of Commerce of the United States Records, Hagley Library, Wilmington, Del., Box 27, "Welfare" folder.

²² In 1972, the Senate approved one feature of the administration's package—a $5.2 billion allocation for the establishment of HMOs to encourage the spread of prepaid comprehensive health-care programs. This measure, which was many times over what the administration had requested, died at the end of the 92nd Congress.

²³ For a detailed examination of the early legislative history of HMOs, including a discussion of organized labor's waxing and waning enthusiasm for prepaid health plans, see Lawrence D. Brown, *Politics and Health Care Organization: HMOs as Federal Policy* (Washington, D.C.: The Brookings Institution, 1983). On one union's efforts to establish an HMO, see Dominique M. Colon, "Labor's Dilemma in Providing Health Care Benefits and Services to American Workers: A Study of a Union's Approach to Health Planning in the 1980s" (master's thesis, Yale University, 1983).

²⁴ As with the earlier proposal, employers would be required to cover 75 percent of the insurance costs at the end of a three-year phase-in period. The proposal also called for federally subsidized health coverage for the poor and a revamped Medicare program for the aged. *Congress and the Nation, 1973–1976*, vol. 4 (Washington, D.C.: Congressional Quarterly Press, 1977): 334 and 338–39. For more on the legislative struggle for national health insurance in the 1970s, see Rashi Fein, *Medical Care, Medical Costs: The Search for Health Insurance Policy* (Cambridge: Harvard University Press, 1986), chs. 7 and 8.

25 Caspar W. Weinberger, U.S. House Committee on Ways and Means, "National Health Insurance," 93rd Cong., 2nd Sess (April–July 1974), 564 and 600–609.

26 Rep. Claude Pepper (D-Fla.), U.S. House Committee on Ways and Means,"National Health Insurance," 93rd Cong., 2nd Sess. (April–July 1974), 3511.

27 "National Health Insurance," 893–906.

28 "National Health Insurance," 2699–708.

29 "National Health Insurance," 1426–44. During the 1974 hearings on health insurance, as during the 1971 hearings, it was rare for an individual corporation that was not a major health-care provider or insurer to testify. One exception was DuPont, whose executives testified that an employer mandate was unlikely to have any major impact on its bottom line or hiring practices. In later debates over health care, individual corporations appeared more frequently on Capitol Hill to express their views. U.S. House, Subcommittee of Public Health and the Environment of the Committee on Interstate and Foreign Commerce, "National Health Insurance, Implications," 93rd Cong., 2nd. Sess. (February 1974), 367–70.

30 *AFL-CIO Executive Council Statements and Reports, 1956–1975*, ed. Gary M. Fink (Westport, Conn.: Greenwood Press, 1978), 2480, 2481, and 2489. People considered poor health risks would have the option to pay 150 percent of the average insurance rate to secure coverage. If insurance companies refused to cover these high-risk individuals even at the higher rate, an employee would have to do without health insurance unless she or he qualified for the administration's new means-tested federal health plan. For more on the history and practice of experience rating, see ch. 3.

31 Nelson Cruikshank, "National Health Insurance," 3041–42.

32 In 1974, median household income was $11,200. *Statistical Abstract of the United States*, 107th ed. (Washington, D.C.: U.S. Department of Commerce, 1987), 431.

33 The AFL-CIO calculated that fewer than 2 percent of those covered by the new program would have medical expenses in excess of $1,500 per year and therefore be eligible to receive full coverage. *AFL-CIO Executive Council Statements and Reports*, ed. Fink, 2485. See also "Summary of Mills-Kennedy Bill: The Comprehensive National Health Insurance Act of 1974," AFL, AFL-CIO Department of Legislation, 1906–78 (hereafter, AFL-CIO Department of Legislation Collection), George Meany Memorial Archives, Silver Spring, Md., Box 25, Folder 36, "Health Insurance, 1974."

34 "National Health Insurance," 1361–68.

35 "National Health Insurance Implications," 363–70.

36 Woodcock, "National Health Insurance," 1144.

37 Ibid.

38 AFL-CIO, "Summary of Mills-Kennedy Bill," 24. Although the AFL-CIO continued to voice its disappointment with the Mills-Kennedy bill in public, in private labor officials apparently indicated that they were willing to settle for Mills-Kennedy, but that they feared a final compromise would fall short of that legislation. They also expressed concern about how to explain to their membership a public retreat from the Health Security Act. *Washington Report on Medicine & Health*, no. 1042 (May 13, 1974), AFL-CIO Department of Legislation Collection, Box 25, Folder 36, "Health Insurance 1974."

39 Under the Mills-Kennedy plan, families would shoulder a reduced—but still hefty—amount of their medical expenses due to a $300 deductible and a requirement that families earning $8,800 or more annually lay out $1,000 a year in the form of deductibles and copayments before full coverage kicked in. A 3 percent payroll tax on employers and a 1 percent payroll tax on employees would finance the plan. Families of four earning less than that amount would be subject to a sliding scale for deductibles and copayments. Those with an annual income of $4,800 or less would not be required to pay any deductible or coinsurance. AFL-CIO, "Summary of Mills-Kennedy Bill," 3–4.

⁴⁰ Rep. Claude Pepper (D-Fla.), "National Health Insurance," 3511; and Caspar W. Weinberger, "National Health Insurance," 600.

⁴¹ Under this proposal, the federal government would function as the primary insurer and a new board set up within the Department of Health, Education and Welfare would run the program, which would be financed by a combination of a new payroll tax for employers and employees and general revenues. *Congress and the Nation, 1973–1976*, 339.

⁴² Leonard Woodcock, letter to Nelson Cruikshank, August 31, 1973, CNHI Collection, Box 28, Folder 39, "Cruikshank, correspondence."

⁴³ Ralph Nader, "National Health Insurance," 3318 and 3337. See also Elizabeth Langer, legislative director, Consumer Federation of America, "National Health Insurance," 2322–28.

⁴⁴ See testimony by representatives of organized labor in "National Health Insurance," 1361–68, 1421–23, and 3031–41; and Sven Steinmo and Jon Watts, "It's the Institutions, Stupid! Why Comprehensive National Health Insurance Always Fails in America," *Journal of Health Politics, Policy and Law* 20, no. 2 (Summer 1995): 353.

⁴⁵ Frank Carlucci, Memorandum for the President (August 29, 1974), Re: Health Insurance Legislation, AFL-CIO Department of Legislation Collection, Box 25, Folder 39, "Health Insurance, 1974."

⁴⁶ *Congress and the Nation, 1973–1976*, 335.

⁴⁷ Michael Foley and John E. Owens, *Congress and the Presidency: Institutional Politics in a Separated System* (Manchester: Manchester University Press, 1996), 313.

⁴⁸ David C. Jacobs, "The U.A.W. and the Committee for National Health Insurance: The Contours of Social Unionism," in *Advances in Industrial and Labor Relations* 4, ed. David Lewin, David B. Lipsky, and Donna Sockell (Greenwich, Conn.: JAI Press, 1987), 119–40.

⁴⁹ *Medical World News* (December 20, 1974), 58, AFL-CIO Department of Legislation Collection, Box 25, Folder 39, "Health Insurance 1974."

⁵⁰ The account of this meeting is based on Bert Seidman memorandum to George Meany and Lane Kirkland, December 16, 1974, Re: Meeting of Executive Committee, Committee for National Health Insurance, AFL-CIO Department of Legislation Collection, Box 25, Folder 39, "Health Insurance, 1974." Despite his expressed misgivings about national health insurance, Kennedy eventually agreed to cosponsor the Health Security Act with Rep. James C. Corman (D-Calif.) at the start of the new Congress.

⁵¹ The one exception was spending on energy-related programs. George J. Lankevich, *Gerald R. Ford, 1913–: Chronology, Documents, Biographical Aids* (Dobbs Ferry, N.Y.: Oceana Publications, Inc., 1977), 126–31.

⁵² See "National Health Insurance," pt. 1; "Health Care Crisis in America, 1971," pt. 6; and "National Health Insurance Implications."

⁵³ See the remarks by Leonard Woodcock in CNHI Collection, Box 20, Folder 20, "Executive Committee Minutes and Members."

⁵⁴ Leonard Woodcock, U.S. House, Subcommittee on Health of the Committee on Ways and Means, "Health Insurance for the Unemployed and Related Legislation," 94th Cong., 1st Sess. (March 1975), 90–110.

⁵⁵ Roger C. Sonnemann, "Health Insurance for the Unemployed and Related Legislation," 127; and Roger C. Sonnemann, U.S. House, Subcommittee on Health and the Environment of the Committee on Interstate and Foreign Commerce, "National Health Insurance, Major Proposals," 94th Cong., 1st Sess. (December 8–10, 1975), 203–15. See also, U.S. House, Subcommittee on Health of the Ways and Means Committee, "National Health Insurance," 94th Cong., 1st Sess. (November–December 1975), pt. 3:2.

⁵⁶ For the administration's view, see Caspar W. Weinberger, "Health Insurance for the Unemployed and Related Legislation," 317–26; for NAM's view, see 389–90.

⁵⁷ *Congress and the Nation, 1973–76*, 353–54.

⁵⁸ For more on how the 1974 Congressional reforms affected health-care legislation, see Steinmo and Watts, "It's the Institutions, Stupid!" 354–61.

⁵⁹ Roger C. Sonnemann, "National Health Insurance, Major Proposals," 203–15. See also, "National Health Insurance," Subcommittee on Health of the Ways and Means Committee, U.S. House, 94th Cong., 1st Sess. (November–December 1975), pt. 3:2.

⁶⁰ Melvin A. Glasser, U.S. House, Subcommittee on Health and the Environment of the Committee on Interstate and Foreign Commerce, "National Health Insurance: Major Issues," 94th Cong., 2nd. Sess. (February 1976), 241–46, and 254–55. Emphasis in the original.

⁶¹ Wilbur J. Cohen, U.S. House, Subcommittee on Health and the Environment of the Committee on Interstate and Foreign Commerce, "Maternal and Child Health Care Act," 94th Cong., 2nd Sess. (June 16, 1976), 187.

⁶² Victor M. Zink, U.S. Senate, Subcommittee on Health of the Committee on Labor and Public Welfare, "Inflation of Health Care Costs, 1976," 94th Cong., 2nd Sess. (April–May 1976), 127. See also the testimony by executives from Goodyear, Ford, and the Aluminum Company of America.

⁶³ Taylor Dark, *The Unions and the Democrats: An Enduring Alliance* (Ithaca, N.Y.: Cornell University Press, 1999), 102.

⁶⁴ Wicker, "The Health Insurance Minefield"; Martin Halpern, "Jimmy Carter and the UAW: Failure of an Alliance," *Presidential Studies Quarterly* 26, no. 3 (Summer 1996): 764–66; Burton I. Kaufman, *The Presidency of James Earl Carter, Jr.* (Lawrence: University Press of Kansas, 1993), 99–116; and David Jacobs, "Labor and the Strategy of Mandated Health Benefits," *Labor Studies Journal* 14, no. 3 (Fall 1989): 23–33.

⁶⁵ Max W. Fine, letter to George Hardy, May 30, 1978; and CNHI, report sent to members of the technical committee, April 13, 1978.

⁶⁶ Steven Schlossberg, memorandum to Douglas A. Fraser, April 5, 1978, UAW President's Office: Douglas A. Fraser Collection (hereafter, UAW Fraser Collection), Wayne State University, Walter P. Reuther Library, Detroit, Mich., Box 2, Folder 24, "C.N.H.I., 1977–78."

⁶⁷ The account of this White House meeting is based on, "Notes on White House Meeting on National Health," April 10, 1978, UAW Fraser Collection, Box 2, Folder 24, "C.N.H.I., 1977–78."

⁶⁸ "Notes on White House Meeting on National Health." Emphasis in the original.

⁶⁹ Martha Derthick, *Policymaking for Social Security* (Washington, D.C.: The Brookings Institution, 1979), 111. Years later, Nelson Cruikshank of the AFL-CIO fondly reminisced about holding Medicare strategy and planning sessions at the White House in the early 1960s to which President John F. Kennedy would periodically drop by in short sleeves to see how it was going. Nelson H. Cruikshank, address to the National Council of Senior Citizens, June 28, 1979, CNHI Collection, Box 2, Folder 33, "Cruikshank, Nelson H., Correspondence."

⁷⁰ Max Fine, memorandum to Douglas A. Fraser and Lane Kirkland, July 5, 1978, Re: National Health Insurance—It's Time to Change Some Players," CNHI Collection, Box 5, Folder 23, "Lane Kirkland, Correspondence, 1971–80."

⁷¹ On the rising importance of the economics profession in formulating economic policy after the shattering of the Keynesian consensus, see Weir, *Politics and Jobs,* 158–62.

⁷² Fine, memorandum to Douglas A. Fraser and Lane Kirkland, July 5, 1978, Re: National Health Insurance—It's Time to Change Some Players. See also, "Executive Committee Meeting Minutes," March 20, 1978, CNHI Collection, Box 20, Folder 30, "Executive Committee Meeting Minutes."

⁷³ Labor contended that high deductibles and copays were self-defeating because they discouraged people from seeking timely medical care. The administration's domestic policymakers reportedly responded by saying, "although *we* don't believe that cost sharing saves

money, the Congress, most economists, academicians and the people do." Max W. Fine, memorandum to Douglas A. Fraser and Lane Kirkland, May 22, 1978, Re: Today's meeting with Eizenstat, May 19, 1978, CHNI Collection, Box 5, Folder 23, "Lane Kirkland, Correspondence, 1971–80." Emphasis in the original.

74 Max Fine, memorandum to Douglas A. Fraser and Lane Kirkland, January 3, 1977, CNHI Collection, Box 5, Folder 23, "Lane Kirkland, Correspondence, 1971–80."

75 Carter's themes of "smaller, cheaper, more efficient government" were troubling to labor leaders not only with respect to health care, but also to a range of other issues. Melvyn Dubofsky, "Jimmy Carter and the End of the Politics of Productivity," in *The Carter Presidency: Policy Choices in the Post–New Deal Era*, ed. Gary M. Fink and Hugh D. Graham (Lawrence: University Press of Kansas, 1998), 95.

76 Melvin Glasser, memorandum to Douglas A. Fraser, March 3, 1978, Re: National Health Insurance and the White House Staff, UAW Fraser Collection, Box 2, Folder 24, "C.N.H.I., 1977–78."

77 Joseph Califano, memorandum to Jimmy Carter, May 22, 1978, CNHI Collection, Box 52, Folder 20, "Califano re: National Health Plan." Emphasis in the original.

78 A key executive branch official reportedly voiced "strong misgivings about community rating on the basis that large corporations' premiums would increase and they would oppose the bill." Max W. Fine, memorandum to Douglas A. Fraser and Lane Kirkland, June 2, 1978, Re: Meeting of June 1, 1978 with Eizenstat on national health insurance, UAW Fraser Collection, Box 2, Folder 22, "C.N.H.I., 1978." For more on experience rating and community rating, see ch. 3.

79 Douglas A. Fraser, memorandum to International Executive Board, October 24, 1978, Re: Health Care for All Americans Act, UAW Fraser Collection, Box 2, Folder 23, "C.N.H.I., 1978."

80 U.S. Senate, Finance Committee, "Presentation of the Major Health Insurance Proposals," 96th Cong., 1st Sess. (June 19 and 21, 1979), 508–509. Kennedy's new stance on health care was also consistent with a broader policy shift at the time as the Massachusetts senator became a proponent of deregulating key industries, notably airlines and trucking. Paul J. Quirk, "Deregulation and the Politics of Ideas in Congress," in *Beyond Self-Interest*, ed. Jane J. Mansbridge (Chicago and London: The University of Chicago Press, 1990), 183–99.

81 Under Carter's proposal, families or individuals would pay up to $2,500 per year in medical bills in addition to the cost of their health insurance premiums. Employers would be obligated to pay 75 percent of the cost of a basic health benefit package, with employees picking up the remaining 25 percent. *Congress and the Nation, 1977–80*, vol. 5 (Washington, D.C.: Congressional Quarterly Press, 1981): 638–39.

82 James C. Corman, letter to Douglas A. Fraser, May 17, 1978, CNHI Collection, Box 70, Folder 33, "Corman, James C., Correspondence, 1978."

83 James C. Corman, letter to Douglas A. Fraser, December 20, 1978, UAW Fraser Collection, Box 2, Folder 23, "C.N.H.I., 1978."

84 Keith W. Johnson, letter to Douglas A. Fraser, January 17, 1979, UAW Fraser Collection, Box 2, Folder 21, "C.N.H.I., 1982–83."

85 "New Kennedy Bill Signals Retreat on National Health Insurance," *Labor Notes* (April 24, 1979): 10.

86 Fraser then noted that a couple of years earlier 13 senators and 78 House members supported the Health Security Act, while only seven senators and 59 representatives came out in support of Kennedy's new proposal. "So you do not seem to have had a great leap forward during this compromise period," Corman dryly noted. U.S. House, Joint Hearing of the Subcommittee on Health and the Environment of the Committee on Interstate and Foreign Commerce and the Subcommittee on Health of the Committee on Ways and Means, "National Health Insurance," 96th Cong., 1st Sess. (November 29, 1979), 565 and 568.

87 For more on the Canadian case, see ch. 2.

Chapter 5: Workers and Managers of the World, Unite

[1] The title of this chapter was inspired by a witty headline that captured the prevailing mood of optimism about the possibilities for labor-management cooperation on the health-care issue. See Nancy N. Bell, "Workers and Managers of the World, Unite!" *Business and Health* (August 1991): 27–34.

[2] Rockefeller was one of the leading figures in the Health Care Reform Project, the major pro-reform coalition. The account of this meeting is based on Alan Reuther, legislative director, UAW, interview, Washington, D.C., June 7, 1996; James Johnston, former vice president of industry-government relations, General Motors, interview, Washington, D.C., June 21, 1996; and William F. Little, health and benefits manager, Ford, interview, Washington, D.C., June 12, 1996. Senator Rockefeller's staff reportedly later accepted the check on his behalf.

[3] Cathie Jo Martin, "Mandating Social Change: The Business Struggle Over National Health Reform" (February 1995), typescript.

[4] Reuther, interview.

[5] Shortly before the unveiling of the Health Security for All Americans Act in 1978, Max Fine, CNHI's executive director, told Douglas A. Fraser of the UAW: "The Corporations don't give a damn, even though the high cost of health care weakens their competitive position internationally." Max W. Fine, memorandum to Douglas A. Fraser, August 7, 1978, CNHI Collection, Box 2, Folder 22, "C.N.H.I., 1978."

[6] Timothy I. Cook, *Governing With the News: The News as a Political Institution* (Chicago: University of Chicago Press, 1998), 66–67. Emphasis removed from the original. See also Rogers M. Smith, "Political Jurisprudence, the 'New Institutionalism,' and the Future of Public Law," *American Political Science Review* 82, no. 1 (March 1988): 91.

[7] Richard B. Freeman and Morris M. Kleiner, "Employer Behavior in the Face of Union Organizing Drives," *Industrial and Labor Relations Review* 43, no. 4 (April 1990): 351–65; Mike Davis, *Prisoners of the American Dream* (London: Verso, 1986); Thomas Geoghegan, *Which Side Are You On? Trying to Be for Labor When It's Flat on Its Back* (New York: Farrer, Straus & Giroux, 1991); Gordon L. Clark, *Unions and Communities Under Siege: American Communities and the Crisis of Organized Labor* (Cambridge: Cambridge University Press, 1989); Roger Keeran and Greg Tarpinian, "Public Policy and the Recent Decline of Strikes," *Policy Studies Journal* 18, no. 2 (Winter 1989–90): 461–70; *The State of the Unions*, ed. George Strauss, Daniel G. Gallagher, and Jack Fiorito (Madison, Wis.: Industrial Relations Research Association, 1991); and David Moberg, "Union Busting, Past and Present," *Dissent* (Winter 1992): 73–80.

[8] For a good discussion of how the given institutional setting in an earlier period—the late 19th and early 20 century—induced certain political strategies that congealed into a particular worldview that molded the preferences of organized labor in the United States, see Victoria C. Hattam, *Labor Visions and State Power: The Origins of Business Unionism in the United States* (Princeton, N.J.: Princeton University Press, 1993).

[9] Davis, *Prisoners of the American Dream*, 102–103.

[10] The views of business that do "receive public attention often appear as extreme and reflect anti-social practices by a few enterprises or sectors" and thus "adversely reflect upon all business." John T. Dunlop, "Business and Public Policy," in *Business and Public Policy*, ed. John T. Dunlop, (Cambridge: Harvard University Press, 1980), 103.

[11] John T. Dunlop, *Dispute Resolution: Negotiation and Consensus Building* (Dover, Mass.: Auburn House, 1984), 258–60.

[12] Nelson Lichtenstein, *The Most Dangerous Man in Detroit: Walter Reuther and the Fate of American Labor* (New York: Basic Books, 1995), 361, esp. ch. 13; and David L. Stebenne, *Arthur J. Goldberg: New Deal Liberal* (New York: Oxford University Press, 1996), esp. ch. 3.

[13] Several scholars who challenge this view of the 1950s contend that the consensus was more apparent than real. They have documented the great lengths business went to in or-

der to marginalize labor and "to reshape the ideas, images, and attitudes through which Americans understood their world, specifically their understanding of their relationships to the corporation and the state." Elizabeth A. Fones-Wolf, *Selling Free Enterprise: The Business Assault on Labor and Liberalism, 1945–60* (Urbana: University of Illinois Press, 1994), 5. See also Howell John Harris, *The Right to Manage: Industrial Relations Policies of American Business in the 1940s* (Madison, Wis.: The University of Wisconsin Press, 1982); Ellen W. Schrecker, "McCarthyism and the Labor Movement: The Role of the State," in *The C.I.O.'s Left-Led Unions*, ed. Steve Rosswurm (New Brunswick, N.J.: Rutgers University Press, 1992); Robert Griffith, "Forging America's Postwar Order: Domestic Politics and Political Economy in the Age of Truman," in *The Truman Presidency*, ed. Michael J. Lacey (Cambridge: Cambridge University Press, 1989); and Thomas A. Kochan, Harry C. Katz, and Robert B. McKersie, *The Transformation of American Industrial Relations* (New York: Basic Books, 1986).

[14] Many unionists opposed this recommendation, fearing that, if enacted, it would open the door to company unions. Jane Slaughter and Ellis Boal, "Unions Slam Dunlop Commission Proposals," *Labor Notes* (February 1995): 1; Steve Early, "Clinton's Commission Opens Door to Company Unions," *Labor Notes* (July 1994): 1; and Stephen Amberg, "The CIO Political Strategy in Historical Perspective: Creating a High-Road Economy in the Post-War Era," in *Organized Labor and American Politics, 1894–1994: The Liberal-Labor Alliance*, Kevin Boyle, ed. (Albany: SUNY Press, 1998), 160.

[15] Davis, *Prisoners of the American Dream*, 133.

[16] William T. Moye, "Presidential Labor-Management Committees: Productive Failures," *Industrial and Labor Relations Review* 34, no. 1 (October 1980): 51–66.

[17] *Common situs* would allow a union to picket an entire building site in a dispute involving a single contractor.

[18] Sar A. Levitan and Martha R. Cooper, *Business Lobbies: The Public Good and the Bottom Line* (Baltimore: Johns Hopkins University Press, 1984), ch. 7; and John T. Dunlop, "Some Recollections of a Brief Tenure," *Monthly Labor Review* (February 1988): 46–49.

[19] Moye, "Presidential Labor-Management Committees."

[20] George Meany and Reginald H. Jones, letter to Joseph A. Califano, Jr., December 2, 1977, UAW President's Office: Douglas A. Fraser Collection, Wayne State University, Walter P. Reuther Library, Detroit (hereafter, UAW Fraser Collection), Box 1, Folder 28, "Labor-Management Group, 1977–78"; and Labor-Management Group, "Policy Issues in Health Care and Six Case Studies" (S.L.: The Group, 1987).

[21] Linda Bergthold, *Purchasing Power in Health: Business, the State, and Health Care Politics* (New Brunswick, N.J.: Rutgers University Press, 1990), 174, f.n. 31, and ch. 4. See also, John T. Dunlop, "Health Care Coalitions," in *Private Sector Coalitions: A Fourth Party for Health Care?* ed. B. Jon Jaeger (Durham, N.C.: Duke University Press, 1983).

[22] Claude Poulin, memorandum to Douglas A. Fraser, July 11, 1977, UAW Fraser Collection, Box 1, Folder 30, "Labor-Management Group, 1977–78."

[23] In one instance, UAW staff members wanted to release publicly some data contained in a paper on international trade prepared by the staff of General Motors for the Dunlop group. They believed the information would be helpful for the union's organizing efforts and its struggles to combat right-to-work legislation if GM was cited as its source. They were told that release of the information would be considered "dirty pool" under the operating rules of the Dunlop group. See the exchange of memos between Howard Young and Steve Schlossberg, June 27 and June 30, 1978, UAW Washington Office: Stephen Schlossberg Collection, Walter P. Reuther Library, Wayne State University, Detroit (hereafter, UAW Schlossberg Collection), Box 18, Folder 17, "Labor-Management Relations, Dunlop Commission."

[24] Kim McQuaid, *Big Business and Presidential Power: From F.D.R. to Reagan* (New York: William Morrow & Co., 1982), 301–302, cited in Davis, *Prisoners of the American Dream*, 135,

f.n. 43. See also Levitan and Cooper, *Business Lobbies*, ch. 7; D. Quinn Mills, "Flawed Victory in Labor Law Reform," *Harvard Business Review* (May–June 1979): 92–102.

[25] Martin Halpern, "Jimmy Carter and the UAW: Failure of an Alliance," *Presidential Studies Quarterly* 26, no. 3 (Summer 1996): 759–63. For a more sympathetic view of Carter's role, see Melvyn Dubofsky, "Jimmy Carter and the End of the Politics of Productivity," in *The Carter Presidency: Policy Choices in the Post-New Deal Era*, ed. Gary M. Fink and Hugh D. Graham (Lawrence: University Press of Kansas, 1998), 105–108; and Taylor Dark, *The Unions and the Democrats: An Enduring Alliance* (Ithaca, N.Y.: Cornell University Press, 1999), 107–14.

[26] For background information on the Business Roundtable and the other major business lobbying organizations, see Levitan and Cooper, *Business Lobbies*, chs. 2 and 3; and McQuaid, *Big Business and Presidential Power*, ch. 9.

[27] Levitan and Cooper, *Business Lobbies*, 131.

[28] Irving Bluestone, letter to Douglas A. Fraser, July 18, 1978, UAW Fraser Collection, Box 78, Folder 13, "Irving Bluestone, 1970–78."

[29] "Everyone in the Group knows there is no chance the business elite will join the fight for national health insurance or even remain neutral, despite the fact that the U.S. is the only industrial country in the world, except for South Africa, without it," he charged. Douglas A. Fraser, Resignation Letter, July 19, 1978, UAW Fraser Collection, Box 1, Folder 27, "Labor-Management Group, DAF's Resignation Letter."

[30] Fraser, Resignation Letter, July 19, 1978.

[31] For a sampling of these letters, see UAW Fraser Collection, Box 15, Folder 29, "Correspondence, Labor-Management Group."

[32] In making his case for sticking with the Democratic Party, Fraser argued that as long as there was a "strong nucleus" within the party "which shares our philosophical point of view, and there is realistic hope of having this nucleus become the majority point of view, we should withhold any action toward starting a third political party." Douglas A. Fraser, letter to Al Gardner, September 6, 1978, UAW Fraser Collection, Box 15, Folder 28, "Labor-Management Group, 1978."

[33] Transcript of press conference held August 7, 1978, AFSCME Office of the President: Jerry Wurf Papers, Walter P. Reuther Library, Wayne State University, Detroit (hereafter, Wurf Papers), Box 79, "AFL-CIO Executive Council Meeting, August 1978" folder. The Wurf Papers were in the midst of being processed at the Reuther Library, so the final box and folder locations will likely be different from those cited here.

[34] S.D. Bechtel, Jr., letter to Douglas A. Fraser, August 10, 1978, UAW Fraser Collection, Box 1, Folder 28, "Labor-Management Group, 1977–78."

[35] "Toward a Progressive Alliance," statement adopted at second meeting, January 15, 1979, Wurf Papers, Box 25, "Progressive Alliance" folder.

[36] Douglas A. Fraser, memorandum to the officers of the Progressive Alliance, May 3, 1979, UAW Schlossberg Collection, Box 5, Folder 23, "Progressive Alliance 1979." See also Ed James, memorandum to Douglas A. Fraser, September 25, 1979, UAW Schlossberg Collection, Box 7, Folder 1, "Progressive Alliance Meeting."

[37] Douglas A. Fraser, memorandum to Progressive Alliance executive committee, May 7, 1979, UAW Schlossberg Collection, Box 5, Folder 22, "Progressive Alliance, 1979." He and his staff came up with two—economic dislocations from plant closings, and health and safety issues, in particular, cancer, lead poisoning, and other environmental threats. Steve Schlossberg et al., memorandum to Douglas A. Fraser, September 5, 1979, Wurf Papers, Box 25, "Progressive Alliance" folder.

[38] Jon Guillory drew parallels to the 1930s and said, "It will be easy to smear corporations and the rich and it will become increasingly necessary to do so as the debate naturally splits into opposing factions and classes. We must recognize these divisions and use them." Jon

Guillory, memorandum to Ed James, September 25, 1979, UAW Schlossberg Collection, Box 7, Folder 1, "Progressive Alliance Meeting."

[39] Frank Cowan, memorandum to Jerry Wurf, June 26, 1979, Wurf Papers, Box 25, "Progressive Alliance" folder; and Edgar James, letter to Jerry Wurf, May 30, 1980, Wurf Papers, Box 15, "Progressive Alliance" folder.

[40] The account of this meeting is based on Frank Cowan, assistant to the president of AFSCME, memorandum to Jerry Wurf, December 5, 1980, Wurf Papers, Box 15, "Progressive Alliance, 1980" folder. William Wynn of the UFCW reportedly had a long conversation with Fraser in which he underscored how important it was for labor to speak in unison. He also encouraged Fraser to bring the autoworkers back into the fold of the AFL-CIO as soon as possible to strengthen the hand of progressive unionists within the federation.

[41] On the Democrats' shift toward business, see Thomas Ferguson and Joel Rogers, *Right Turn: The Decline of the Democrats and the Future of American Politics* (New York: Hill and Wang, 1986); Thomas Byrne Edsall, *The New Politics of Inequality* (New York: W.W. Norton & Co., 1984); and James A. Barnes, "Paying the Piper," *National Journal* (September 23, 1989): 2323–26.

[42] Graham K. Wilson, *Unions in American National Politics* (New York: St. Martin's Press, 1979), 21–23.

[43] Andrew Battista, "Political Divisions in Organized Labor," *Polity* 24 no. 2 (Winter 1991): 173–97.

[44] Byron E. Shafer, *Quiet Revolution: The Struggle for the Democratic Party and the Shaping of Post-Reform Politics* (New York: Russell Sage Foundation, 1983), esp. 55–57, 86–87, 97–98, 108, and 360–62; and Nelson Polsby, *Consequences of Party Reform* (Oxford: Oxford University Press, 1983).

[45] While this may be an accurate reading of the source of the UAW's concerns about the McGovern reforms, it may be too generous to Meany and Kirkland. Kirkland's concerns about the expanded role of women and minorities in the Democratic Party may have been motivated by more than just pragmatic electoral considerations. In a 1985 interview, Kirkland charged that the party was "riddled with factions who . . . drain the resources but who don't put resources in." Asked who these factions were, Kirkland replied, "All of them—except us." He then singled out many of the official caucuses of the Democratic National Committee that, in his view, had brought the party to such a lowly state, including blacks, Hispanics, homosexuals, liberals, progressives, and women. Interview with *The Washington Post,* cited in *Labor Notes* (May 1985): 2.

[46] The Labor Council appears to have functioned primarily as a fund-raising vehicle. Union participation in the Labor Council was contingent on making a suitable donation to the party—either $15,000 to the national coffers or $50,000 to local and state party organizations. Charles T. Manatt, letter to Douglas A. Fraser, July 10, 1981, UAW Fraser Collection, Box 53, Folder 21, "Democratic National Committee." See also Charles T. Manatt, letter to Jack Sheinkman, January 21, 1983, Jack Sheinkman Papers, Amalgamated Clothing Workers of America Records, Labor-Management Documentation Center, Cornell University (hereafter, Sheinkman Papers), Box 38, "Democratic National Committee, 1983–84" folder.

[47] Harold Meyerson, "Labor's Risky Plunge Into Politics: From Top-Down to Bottom-Up," *Dissent* (Summer 1984): 285–94. This account of the McGovern reforms is based in part on Dudley W. Buffa, *Union Power and American Democracy: The U.A.W. and the Democratic Party, 1935–72* (Ann Arbor: The University of Michigan Press, 1984), 192–247. See also Dark, *The Unions and the Democrat,* 83–87.

[48] Jack W. Germond and Jules Witcover, "Liberal Alliance Falls Apart at Strange Time," *The Washington Star* (March 23, 1981).

[49] Davis, *Prisoners of the American Dream,* 265.

[50] Since officeholders must stand for re-election, they were the ones most in contact with the party's various constituencies. Thus they were thought to be best able to "stand above the

competing claims of the single issue groups and help construct the necessary compromises and coalitions essential to a winning campaign." Glenn Watts, president of the CWA, "AFL-CIO Testimony Before the Hunt Commission," November 6, 1981, UAW Fraser Collection, Box 12, Folder 16, "Hunt Commission, 1981–82."

51 Davis, *Prisoners of the American Dream*, 265; and Taylor E. Dark, "Organized Labor and the Presidential Nominating Process: Reconsidering the 1980s," *Presidential Studies Quarterly* 26, no. 2 (Spring 1996): 391–401.

52 The Kamber Group, memorandum to the Progressive Alliance, October 28, 1980, Wurf Papers, Box 15, "Progressive Alliance, 1980" folder; and Hank Lacayo, memorandum to Douglas A. Fraser, Re: Lane Kirkland Meeting, May 6, 1981, UAW Fraser Collection, Box 53, Folder 21, "Democratic National Committee, 1977–83."

53 Between 1978 and 1982, the number of workers employed by the five unionized automakers dropped from 723,000 to 438,000. In 1982–83, 200,000 UAW workers were on indefinite layoff. Davis Dyer, Malcolm S. Salter, and Alan M. Webber, *Changing Alliances* (Boston: Harvard Business School Press, 1987), 184–85.

54 "Labor-Management Climate Continued: Outline of Discussion Points for March 9, 1982 Meeting," UAW Fraser Collection, Box 1, Folder 28, "Labor Management Group, 1977–82"; and John T. Dunlop, letter to Douglas A. Fraser, February 25, 1982, UAW Fraser Collection, Box 1, Folder 28, "Labor-Management Group, 1977–82."

55 Stephen Herzenberg, "Whither Social Unionism? Labor and Restructuring in the U.S. Auto Industry," in *The Challenge of Restructuring: North American Labor Movements Respond*, ed. Jane Jenson and Rianne Mahon (Philadelphia: Temple University Press, 1993), 319–20. For more on the UAW in the 1980s, see Dyer et al., *Changing Alliances;* Christopher J. Singleton, "Auto Industry Jobs in the 1980's: A Decade of Transition," *Monthly Labor Review* (February 1992): 18–27; *North American Auto Unions in Crisis: Lean Production as Contested Terrain*, ed. William C. Green and Ernest J. Yanarella (Albany: State University of New York Press, 1996); and Harry Katz, "Policy Debates Over Work Reorganization in North American Unions," in *New Technology and Industrial Relations*, ed. Richard Hyman and Wolfgang Streeck (Oxford: Basil Blackwell, 1988).

56 For instance, Roger Smith, the chairman of General Motors, reportedly asked for the union's assistance in getting the federal government "off the industry's back with regard to extremely burdensome regulatory provisions," many of which had the support of consumer and environmental groups. "File-Note—April 16, 1980," UAW Fraser Collection, Box 61, Folder 3, "GM 1980."

57 The UAW subsequently agreed to deep concessions for both the Ford and GM workforces. Although Ford lost $1 billion in 1981, GM turned a profit of $333 million, and its share of the market was virtually unaffected by the influx of foreign-made cars. Ruth Milkman, "The Anti-Concessions Movement in the UAW: Interview With Douglas Stevens," *Socialist Review* 12, no. 5 (1982): 25–27 and 38. The day the contract was signed, General Motors sent its stockholders a proxy statement announcing a new plan to increase executive bonuses, which infuriated the UAW rank and file.

58 Members had long feared that the UAW risked being " 'swallowed up' by the sea of conservatism, which characterizes the AFL-CIO" should the union decide to reaffiliate with the federation. Marc Stepp, memorandum to Douglas A. Fraser, Re: UAW Reaffiliation with AFL-CIO, August 24, 1977, UAW Fraser Collection, Box 48, Folder 3, "AFL-CIO 1977." In the months leading to the affiliation vote, members charged that the UAW staff was using "Alexander Haig-type tactics" to undermine democratic discussion about whether to rejoin the federation. Bill Parker, "U.A.W. Dissidents Denounce 'Haig-Type' Tactics as Union Leaders Drive for AFL-CIO Reaffiliation," *Labor Notes* (April 28, 1981): 5.

59 Herzenberg, "Whither Social Unionism?" and Lichtenstein, *The Most Dangerous Man in Detroit*, 311–13. For a discussion of why grass-roots democracy flourished in the Canadian branch of the UAW but not in its U.S. counterpart, see Charlotte Yates, "North American Au-

toworkers' Response to Restructuring," in *Bargaining for Change: Union Politics in North America and Europe*, ed. Miriam Golden and Jonas Pontusson (Ithaca, N.Y.: Cornell University Press, 1992).

[60] At one point the leadership was found guilty of improperly using union funds and tampering with the delegate selection process in an effort to deny Jerry Tucker of the New Directions movement the directorship of Region 5, which covers parts of the Midwest and Southwest. The union was also accused of employing race-baiting tactics against Tucker and other New Directions candidates. The premier source on dissident movements in the UAW and other unions is *Labor Notes*. For coverage of dissidents in the UAW, see the following issues: May 1988, 1; June 1988, 5; October 1988, 1; August 1989, 8; December 1989, 8; June 1990, 3; December 1990, 6; December 1991, 3; and July 1992, 3.

[61] UAW, "Proceedings of the 29th Constitutional Convention," Anaheim, Calif., June 18–23, 1989 (Detroit, Mich.: UAW, 1989), 175.

[62] Herzenberg, "Whither Social Unionism?" 322.

[63] For example, Chrysler's Lee Iacocca called upon Fraser to participate in a labor-industry coalition that would "alert our fellow citizens to the pervasive danger of unchecked, unfair foreign competition," especially from the Japanese. Lee Iacocca, letter to Douglas A. Fraser, April 27, 1983, UAW Fraser Collection, Box 51, Folder 7, "Chrysler." At the time, General Motors was more reluctant to go public about the Japanese import problem. Instead, Chairman Roger Smith urged the UAW to put public pressure on the Japanese auto industry to reduce its imports into the United States and to locate more plants in this country. "File Note—April 16, 1980," UAW Fraser Collection, Box 51, Folder 3, "General Motors, 1980."

[64] "UAW Members Go Back to Washington," *Solidarity* (February 1982): 9–10; "UAW Girds for a Turnaround Year," *Solidarity* (February 1986): 8–9; "Workers Go to Washington," *Solidarity* (February 1988): 6–7; "Bieber: 'It's Companies' Turn to Give,' " *Solidarity* (June 1983): 2–4; and James T. Bennett and Thomas J. DiLorenzo, "Unions, Politics, and Protectionism," *Journal of Labor Research* 5, no. 3 (Summer 1984): 296.

[65] Mike Parker, "The 'Local Content' Law: Wrong Direction," *Labor Notes* (May 26, 1982): 12–13.

[66] At one point the editor of *Solidarity*, the house organ of the UAW, publicly acknowledged that when the magazine covered economic issues, readers regularly responded by sending hate mail to the editor that blamed "Japs" and "niggers" for the nation's economic woes. "Keeping the Dream Alive," *Solidarity* (January–February 1990). *Solidarity* tried to keep the trade campaign on a higher level by denouncing derogatory references to the physical characteristics of the Japanese and other foreigners, and attacking a popular bumper sticker that linked imported automobiles to Pearl Harbor. For months the UAW's national headquarters in Detroit displayed that very bumper sticker on its main gate. Parker, "The 'Local Content' Law."

[67] UAW literature talked about how the Japanese were "savaging our markets" and about "predatory Japanese producers." In his testimony on behalf of domestic content legislation, Fraser refused to attack outsourcing by U.S. auto manufacturers, yet time and again sharply criticized the Japanese. Not surprisingly, when workers were asked who was to blame for their plight, "the Japanese" and "people who buy Japanese cars" were most frequently mentioned. Auto companies placed a distant third. Jane Slaughter, "Japan-Bashing Will Get Us Nowhere," *Labor Notes* (February 1992): 8–9; and Parker, "The 'Local Content' Law."

[68] The group included the heads of the American Medical Association, Blue Cross/Blue Shield, the Health Insurance Association of America, the Business Roundtable, the Pharmaceutical Manufacturers Association, and the American Hospital Association. Mel Glasser, memorandum to Douglas A. Fraser, November 11, 1981, UAW Fraser Collection, Box 2, Folder 17, "Committee for National Health Insurance."

[69] Marc Stepp, memorandum to Douglas A. Fraser, September 1, 1981, UAW Fraser Collection, Box 51, Folder 14, "Chrysler, 1980–83"; and Jake Hurwitz, memorandum to Douglas A. Fraser, August 12, 1981, UAW Fraser Collection, Box 51, Folder 21, "Chrysler, 1979–83."

70 Jack Horne, memorandum to Marc Stepp, August 26, 1981, UAW Fraser Collection, Box 51, Folder 14, "Chrysler, 1980–83."

71 "Under the strategy of 'jointness' the UAW has become increasingly isolated from the local and national coalitions attempting to restrict corporate behavior," one UAW dissenter charged. Quoted in David C. Jacobs, *Collective Bargaining as an Instrument of Social Change* (Westport, Conn.: Quorum Books, 1994), 76.

72 Steffie Woolhandler and David Himmelstein, "A National Health Program: Northern Light at the End of the Tunnel," *Journal of the American Medical Association* 262, no. 15 (1989): 2136.

73 They called for comprehensive and universal health coverage to be financed by a payroll or general tax. This approach would largely eliminate the role of the insurers because all payments for medical care would be handled by a single body—be it the federal government, the state government, or some entirely new creation (hence the name "single-payer" plan).

74 UAW, "UAW President Owen Bieber's Report to the 29th Constitutional Convention" (Detroit, Mich.: UAW, 1989), 197.

75 Jane Slaughter, "UAW's New Directions Movement Plans Campaign Aimed at Top Union Leadership," *Labor Notes* (December 1991): 3; and Slaughter, "Is Labor Movement Reaching a Turning Point?" *Labor Notes* (January 1990): 7.

76 I am deeply grateful to Professor Alan Draper of St. Lawrence University for his comments on this chapter. He helped to refine my argument about what significance rank-and-file militancy in the UAW had for broader social policy questions.

77 Karen Gutloff, "The Making of a Million," *Service Employees Union* (Spring 1992): 9–10.

78 Mary Kay Henry, director of the health-care division, SEIU, interview, Washington, D.C., June 3 and 4, 1996; and J. Peter Nixon, senior policy analyst, SEIU, interview, Washington, D.C., June 3, 1996.

79 Gerald M. Shea, assistant to the president for governmental affairs, AFL-CIO, interview, Washington, D.C., June 13, 1996.

80 John J. Sweeney, "The Union for Professionals," *Service Employee* (June 1986): 2.

81 Social unionism attempts to make more general appeals to workers as members of broader social groups, such as consumers or citizens. By contrast, business unionism appeals "to workers on narrow, particularistic grounds, eschewing any claim to represent interests outside immediate needs." See Michael J. Piore, "Unions and Politics," in *The Shrinking Perimeter: Unionism and Labor Relations in the Manufacturing Sector*, ed. Hervey A. Jurvis and Myron Roomkin (Lexington, Mass.: Lexington Books, 1980), 173. Many analysts characterize American unionism as "business unionism" because of the perceived focus on collective bargaining, inattention to political action and broader social and economic policy questions, and disregard for ideology. See Lloyd G. Reynolds, *Labor Economics and Labor Relations*, 8th ed. (Englewood Cliffs, N.J.: Prentice Hall, 1982).

82 John Mehring, "AIDS at Work: The SEIU AIDS Project," *Labor Research Review* 14, no. 2 (1990): 83–89; John Mehring, "AFL-CIO Meeting Discusses Union Action on HIV/AIDS," *Labor Notes* (March 1994): 4. Passed at the 1983 convention, this resolution committed the labor movement to educating workers about the disease and urged more federal funding for AIDS research and education. The union also successfully battled attempts by Sen. Jesse Helms (R-N.C.) to institute involuntary HIV testing of patients and to make it a criminal penalty for health-care workers who fail to disclose their HIV status to patients.

83 Kathleen M. Skrabut, senior legislative representative, SEIU, interview, Washington, D.C., June 4, 1996.

84 By contrast, declining and/or predominantly white male unions in construction and manufacturing tend to focus their legislative activities on measures that will bolster their unions as organizations. Daniel B. Cornfield, "Union Decline and the Political Demands of Organized Labor," *Work and Occupations* 16, no. 3 (August 1989): 298 and 313.

85 Ellen Cassedy, "A Family Fight," *Service Employees Union* (Spring 1993): 12–15.

[86] Skrabut, interview.

[87] "Fencing in Employers," *Nation's Business* 74, no. 6 (July 1986): 13; "Business Battle Over Parental Leave," *Nation's Business* 74, no. 8 (August 1986): 12; and Harry Bacas, "Mandated Leave: Small Firms' Nightmare," *Nation's Business* 75, no. 8 (August 1987): 33.

[88] "It surprised me more than anything else that they were so viciously opposed to this. A lot of this was symbolic. It was purely about who controlled the workplace," explained Skrabut. Skrabut, interview. A Chamber of Commerce survey published at the time found employers solidly against the proposed legislation by a margin of nearly nine to one. "Where I Stand," *Nation's Business* 74, no. 9 (September 1986): 64. Another survey published just months later on whether the federal government should require all employers to provide medical benefits found that businesses opposed such a mandate by nearly an identical margin, with 13 percent supporting the employer mandate idea for health care and 84 percent opposed. "Where I Stand," *Nation's Business* 75, no. 5 (May 1987): 88.

[89] Anya Bernstein, "Inside or Outside? The Politics of Family and Medical Leave," *Policy Studies Journal* 25, no. 1 (Spring 1997): 95. See also, Ronald D. Elving, *Conflict and Compromise: How Congress Makes the Law* (New York: Simon & Schuster, 1995), 289–90; and Cathie Jo Martin, "Inviting Business to the Party: The Corporate Response to Social Policy," in *The Social Divide: Political Parties and the Future of Activist Government,* ed. Margaret Weir (Washington, D.C. and New York: Brookings Institution Press and Russell Sage Foundation, 1998), 243–47.

[90] Carol Dilks and Nancy L. Croft, "Day Care: Whose Baby Is It?" *Nation's Business* 74, no. 12 (December 1986): cover story; and "Small Business: What's Next," *Nation's Business* 74, no. 10 (October 1986): 48.

[91] After the battle over health policy died down, Roush expressed concern about the longer-term political implications of staking one's legislative strategy time and again on just saying no. He conceded that regular appeals to an organization's "membership on that basis troubles me," and indicated that such appeals may contribute to the growing fragmentation, cynicism, gridlock, and "dangerous" single-issue politics in the United States. Michael O. Roush, director of federal governmental relations, NFIB, interview, Washington, D.C., June 3, 1996.

[92] Many other unions were initially cool to the family leave proposal, dismissing it as the "yuppie bill." Elving, *Conflict and Compromise,* 152–55 and 63–64.

[93] The U.S. Chamber of Commerce charged that the measure represented a "disturbing trend . . . toward accepting the concept that the federal government should mandate and regulate the extent of employer financed benefits to workers." "Why the Federal Bureaucracy Should Stay Out of Employee Benefits Issues," editorial, *Nation's Business* 74, no. 12 (December 1986): 76.

[94] Many unions featured children on the cover of their magazines, participated in a Washington, D.C., rally on behalf of families in the spring of 1988, and argued that the ultimate family value was to allow an employee time off from work to take care of a newborn or an ailing mother or father. "Why Is This Family Going to Washington," *Solidarity* (April 1988): 12–13; "Our Families, Our Futures: The Real Issues in the Election," *Solidarity* (October 1988): 14; and Daniel B. Cornfield, "Labor Unions, Corporations, and Families: Institutional Competition in the Provision of Social Welfare," *Marriage and Family Review* 15, no. 3/4 (1990): 37–57.

[95] Rep. Marge Roukema (R-N.J.), who worked closely with the small business community on this issue, helped break the legislative logjam. The representative, largely at the suggestion of the NFIB, modified the original proposal to exempt businesses with 50 or fewer employees, or essentially half the workforce, from any obligation to provide unpaid family leave. Steve Wilson, chief of staff, Rep. Marge Roukema (R-N.J.), interview by telephone, June 18, 1996; Skrabut, interview.

Although the NFIB was instrumental in developing the 50–employee exemption, it remained opposed to the measure even after the exemption was adopted. Labor lobbyists ultimately accepted this compromise despite their concerns about creating a precedent for a labor standard that exempted employers based on the size of their workforce rather than on alternative criteria, such as asset base or average employee salary.

96 Bernstein, "Inside or Outside?"

97 John J. Sweeney, "Our Families Are Under Attack," *Service Employee* (July 1981): 2.

98 John J. Sweeney, "Democrats Are in Serious Trouble," *Service Employee* (June/July 1985): 2.

99 SEIU, *S.E.I.U. Leadership News Update* (Winter 1985): 5.

100 In the spring of 1983, the SEIU launched a massive drive to organize Beverly Enterprises, the largest nursing home chain in the United States, by attacking its record of poor patient care. That fall the union also sponsored a resolution at the AFL-CIO convention that condemned "the corporate takeover of health care in America," which was adopted unanimously. SEIU, *S.E.I.U. Leadership News Update* (Fall 1983).

101 Robert Kuttner, "Will Unions Organize Again? Why Some Succeed and Others Don't," *Dissent* (Winter 1987): 56. The SEIU worked closely with 100 Baptist churches in the Los Angeles area. Ministers announced union meetings from the pulpit and urged their parishioners to attend. This strategy helped the SEIU reach its target groups, 90 percent of whom were church-going black women. Arthur B. Shostak, *Robust Unionism: Innovations in the Labor Movement* (Ithaca, N.Y.: ILR Press, 1991), 64.

102 Under its plan, employers would be "encouraged"—not required—to provide a minimum package of health benefits to employees. Those who did not would be assessed a special fee to help pay for health care for the uninsured. National Leadership Commission on Health Care, *For the Health of a Nation: A Shared Responsibility* (Ann Arbor, Mich.: Health Administration Press Perspectives, 1989), 32; Margaret M. Rhoades, executive director, National Leadership Coalition on Health Care, interview, Washington, D.C., June 11, 1996.

103 For more on the Pepper Commission (formally known as the U.S. Bipartisan Commission on Comprehensive Health Care), see ch. 6.

104 Shea, interview.

105 John J. Sweeney, "Healthcare Reform," *Service Employees Union* (October–November, 1989): 30.

106 Sweeney, "Healthcare Reform." In an address on health care before the NAM that year, Iacocca asked, "How would you like to compete without this albatross around your neck called runaway health costs?" He went on to say, "For me, it's $700 a car and still going up at twice the rate of inflation. Other countries put their costs in their taxes. We put them in the price of our products." Wilson da Silva, "American Companies Eye Canada's Health System," *The Reuter Business Report* (August 7, 1989). See also Pat Wechsler, "Crying Uncle," *Newsday* (June 11, 1989): business section, 70.

107 Harris, *The Right to Manage*, 33.

108 Ronald W. Schatz, *The Electrical Workers: A History of Labor at General Electric and Westinghouse, 1923–60* (Urbana: University of Illinois Press, 1983), 170–71.

109 Harris, *The Right to Manage*, 37.

110 Harris, *The Right to Manage*, 198–204. Instead, most corporations pursued an approach that was known as "Boulwarism," in honor of Lemuel R. Boulware, the public relations expert who was General Electric's director of employee relations after the 1946 strike, which shut down every plant in the electric industry. Boulware based his new hard-line strategy on reasserting management's ideological supremacy throughout the workplace. Schatz, *The Electrical Workers*, 170–75; and Nelson Lichtenstein, "Labor in the Truman Era: Origins of the 'Private Welfare State'," in *The Truman Presidency*, ed. Michael J. Lacey (Cambridge: Cambridge University Press, 1989), 136.

111 Harris, *The Right to Manage*, 154. For a similar view, see Herman E. Krooss, *Executive Opinion: What Business Leaders Said and Thought on Economic Issues, 1920s–1960s* (Garden City, N.Y.: Doubleday, 1970), ch. 10, esp. 378–81; and Lichtenstein, "Labor in the Truman Era," 136.

112 See Fraser's response to speeches by Iacocca that lampooned Reaganomics and attacked the wave of corporate mergers in the United States. "Remarks by Lee A. Iacocca,"

Toronto, October 29, 1981, UAW Fraser Collection, Box 5, Folder 13, "Chrysler 1980–83"; Douglas A. Fraser, memorandum, November 3, 1981, UAW Fraser Collection, Box 5, Folder 13, "Chrysler 1980–83"; "Prepared Remarks by Lee Iacocca at the 1983 Society of Automotive Engineers International Banquet," March 3, 1981, UAW Fraser Collection, Box 51, Folder 8, "Chrysler 1980–83"; and Douglas A. Fraser, memorandum to international executive board members, March 28, 1983, UAW Fraser Collection, Box 51, Folder 8, "Chrysler 1980–83."

[113] Douglas A. Fraser, letter to Lane Kirkland, October 20, 1981, UAW Fraser Collection, Box 4, Folder 81, "AFL-CIO, 1981."

[114] Howard Paster, memorandum to Douglas A. Fraser, June 29, 1979, UAW Fraser Collection, Box 51, Folder 19, "Chrysler, 1979."

[115] Douglas A. Fraser et al., letter to Lee Iacocca, December 20, 1980, UAW Fraser Collection, Box 15, Folder 18, "Chrysler, 1978–81."

[116] Harris, *The Right to Manage*, 28–31.

[117] Brian Rixner, "Japanese Automobile Transplants: Redefining Relationships in the American Auto Industry" (senior essay, Yale University, 1995); and Johnston, interview.

[118] "Prepared Remarks by Lee Iacocca at the 1983 Society of Automotive Engineers International Banquet," March 3, 1981, UAW Fraser Collection, Box 51, Folder 8, "Chrysler 1980–83."

[119] Ford refused to accept seats made by managers and replacement workers at Johnson Controls, a main supplier, after UAW members went out on strike there in early 1997. Robert L. Rose and Robert L. Simison, "Johnson Controls and UAW Reach Pact," *The Wall Street Journal* (March 21, 1997): A–3. See also Keith Bradsher, "General Motors and UAW Agree on End to Strike," *The New York Times* (July 29, 1998): A-1.

[120] After the bailout, Chrysler was "more inclined to go along with the government," said James Johnston, GM's vice president of industry-government relations until 1994, as he explained why Chrysler was more receptive to a government-led solution to the nation's health-care problems than GM. Johnston, interview.

[121] Mark Green and Andrew Buchsbaum, *The Corporate Lobbies: Political Profiles of the Business Roundtable and the Chamber of Commerce* (Washington, D.C.: Public Citizen, 1980), cited in David Plotke, "The Political Mobilization of Business," in *The Politics of Interests: Interest Groups Transformed*, ed. Mark Petracca (Boulder, Colo.: Westview Press, 1992), 189.

[122] Maher traces Chrysler's interest in health-care issues back to the late 1970s and what he calls the company's "brush with death." The company's precarious finances at that time forced it to put all expenses under a magnifying glass in a way that other companies were not forced to do, and to come to grips earlier with the limits of what corporations could do internally to stem their rising medical costs. Walter B. Maher, director of public policy, Chrysler Corporation, interview, Washington, D.C., June 5, 1996.

[123] Barbara Markham Smith, former legislative aide to Rep. James McDermott (D-Md.), interview, Washington, D.C., June 24, 1996; and Sara Nichols, former staff attorney, Public Citizen, interview, Washington, D.C., June 13, 1996.

[124] "He's gung-ho on government health-care programs. He's not as skeptical as some of the rest of us," explained GM's Johnston. Johnston, interview. Also, G. Lawrence Atkins, coordinator, Corporate Health Care Coalition, interview, Washington, D.C., June 6, 1996.

[125] In 1984, Iacocca's autobiography led the nonfiction bestseller list. That year he was ranked among the 10 most admired men in the United States, the first business executive to make the list in nearly three decades. David Vogel, *Fluctuating Fortunes: The Political Power of Business in America* (New York: Basic Books, 1989), 274.

[126] For instance, in drumming up support for a financing mechanism to cover long-term medical care, Rep. Claude Pepper (D-Fla.) took a jab at Iacocca. "Mr. Iacocca, who's reputed to have made $20 million last year, can pay his 1.45 percent. He'd have about $19,750,000 left—and with a little help from food stamps, I think he can get by." Dan Carmichael, United Press International wire service report (May 19, 1988): electronic database.

[127] Democratic leaders said that Iacocca's reputation was so besmirched by his recent hard-line tactics at Chrysler that he was unlikely to be offered any major position should the Democrats regain the White House. James Risen, " 'I've Taken a Beating': Lee Iacocca Falls From Public Grace," *Los Angeles Times* (May 3, 1988): 1.

[128] "LBOs: Wrecking Havoc from Wall St. to Main St.," *AFL-CIO News* (February 4, 1989): 6–7; "UAW Pushes Restrictions on LBOS," *UAW Washington Report* (March 24–31, 1989): 1; "Congress Pressed to Curb Takeovers," *AFL-CIO News* (February 18, 1989): 1; "LBOs Turn Economy into Giant Board Game," *AFL-CIO News* (April 1, 1989); "Tax Reforms Urged to Curb LBOs," *AFL-CIO News* (May 27, 1989): 8; and Jon A. Zverina, "UAW Blasts Chrysler for Obscene Executive Pay," United Press International wire service (April 20, 1988): electronic database.

[129] Lee Iacocca, "Corporations Warming Up to National Health," *UAW Washington Report* (May 5, 1989): 2, reprinted from *LA Times* Syndicate.

[130] "UAW Blasts 'Pigout' by Auto Execs," *UAW Washington Report* (May 5, 1989): 3.

[131] Faced with a health-care bill of nearly $3 billion, John Butler, GM's director of employee benefits, reportedly said in 1988 that the auto giant was no longer certain that it opposed national health insurance. *Health Security News* 7, no. 2 (April–May 1988): 3. Three years later, when asked whether GM supported a single-payer plan, Gregory E. Lau, its assistant treasurer, did not reject the idea outright. He told legislators, "we would again be concerned about the details of exactly how single-payer system was written into the legislation." U.S. Senate, Finance Committee, "Comprehensive Health Care Reform and Cost Containment," 102nd Cong, 2nd Sess. (May 6 and 7, 1992), pt. 1, 153.

[132] Employees in firms with no union members were six times more likely to work for a firm that did not provide health insurance. Craig Renner and Vicente Navarro, "Why is Our Population of Uninsured and Underinsured Persons Growing? The Consequences of 'Deindustrialization' of the United States," *International Journal of Health Services* 19, no. 3 (1989): 435–37. Unionized firms consistently spend about twice as much of their payroll on benefits as nonunion ones. Beth Stevens, *Complementing the Welfare State: The Development of Private Pension, Health Insurance and Other Employee Benefits in the United States* (Geneva: International Labour Office, 1986), 26.

[133] See ch. 6 for a more detailed discussion of cost-shifting and the plight of retired workers.

[134] GM, the largest private purchaser of health insurance, spent $3.6 billion in 1995 on health care for more than 1.6 million people, including workers, retirees, and their families. GM health coverage is so far-flung that there are only three major Zip Codes in the United States where the auto giant does not have a person covered. Rebecca Blumenstein, "Auto Makers Attack High Health-Care Bills With a New Approach," *The Wall Street Journal* (December 9, 1996): A-1.

[135] According to one estimate, by the early 1990s cost-shifting added 25 percent or more to the cost of health insurance. Medicare patients receive an estimated $1.15 in physician and hospital services for every dollar spent by the patient and federal government. Dean C. Coddington, David J. Keen, and Keith D. Moore, "Cost Shifting Overshadows Employers' Cost-Containment Efforts," *Business and Health* (January 1991): 45–46. To curtail the widespread practice of cost-shifting, Sweeney of the SEIU proposed that every payer be required to pay the same amount for each procedure. Joyce Frieden, "Pricing: All for One and One for All," *Business and Health* (March 1991): 66.

[136] The steel companies and their union representatives comprised one-third of the signatories of the agreement. Julie Kosterlitz and Rowena Daly, "A Tattered 'Consensus' on Health Care," *National Journal* (December 14, 1991): 3032. On support within the steel sector, see also "A.I.S.I. Backs Health Care Reform Package," *Iron Age* (January 1992): 8.

[137] Susan B. Garland, "Already, Big Business' Health Plan Isn't Feeling So Hot," *Business Week* (November 18, 1991): 48.

[138] Little, interview.

[139] J.J. Barry, "Long-term Solution Necessary," *Business and Society Review* 72 (Winter 1990); and Gerald Markowitz and David Rosner, "Seeking Common Ground: A History of Labor and Blue Cross," *Journal of Health Politics, Policy and Law* 16, no. 4 (Winter 1991): 695–718. At the time, the CWA had hoped to get a stronger commitment from the phone companies. The union's original proposal called for annual contributions from the phone companies to "be used to build coalitions with other groups from labor, business and the community to work for progressive health care reform" financed by progressive corporate and individual taxes. A copy of the original proposal was included in a May 9, 1990 letter from Louise Novotny of the CWA to Robert McGarrah of AFSCME, Personal Files of Robert McGarrah, AFSCME headquarters, Washington, D.C. (hereafter, McGarrah Papers), "Health Care, 1990."

[140] Kosterlitz and Daly, "A Tattered 'Consensus' on Health Care."

[141] Louis Uchitelle, "Insurance as a Job Benefit Shows Signs of Overwork," *The New York Times* (May 1, 1991): A-1.

[142] Atkins, interview.

[143] One other competing interest that should be mentioned here, and probably warrants a more detailed examination, is the close financial connections between the insurance companies and other Fortune 500 companies. Insurance companies, as major stock and bond holders for leading corporations, are among the biggest institutional investors on Wall Street. In 1989, the investment income of the top 50 insurance firms topped $58 billion. More than half of that came from the eight leading insurance companies. *Fortune* (June 5, 1989), as cited in "Is Iacocca for Real? Labor Should Not Depend on It," *Economic Notes* (July–August, 1989): 4.

[144] J. David Greenstone, *Labor in American Politics* (Chicago: Chicago University Press, 1977).

[145] On labor's disarray and newfound unity, see Dark, *The Unions and the Democrats*, 84–113 and 141–59.

[146] J.G. March, "The Business Firm as a Political Coalition," *Journal of Politics* 24 (1962): 662–78, as cited in Steven Tolliday and Jonathan Zeitlin, "Employers and Industrial Relations Between Theory and History," in *The Power to Manage? Employers and Industrial Relations in Comparative-Historical Perspective*, ed. Steven Tolliday and Jonathan Zeitlin (London: Routledge, 1991).

[147] Tolliday and Zeitlin, "Employers and Industrial Relations Between Theory and History," 2.

Chapter 6: Taking Care of Business

[1] Deborah Stone, "Causal Stories and the Formulation of Agendas," *Political Science Quarterly* 104, no. 2 (1989): 282.

[2] For more on problem definition, see Frank R. Baumgartner and Bryan D. Jones, *Agendas and Instability in American Politics* (Chicago: Chicago University Press, 1993), especially ch. 2; David A. Rochefort and Roger W. Cobb, "Problem Definition, Agenda Access, and Policy Choice," *Policy Studies Journal* 21, no. 1 (1993): 56–71, and John W. Kingdon, *Agendas, Alternatives, and Public Policies* (Boston: Little, Brown, 1984), 115–19.

[3] The First Lady told legislators: "It is a uniquely American solution to an American problem. It is the *least disruptive option* that we could consider because we have used this system for 50 years or more and most Americans are familiar with it." U.S. House, Committee on Education and Labor, "The President's Health Care Reform Proposal," vol. 1, 103rd Cong., 1st Sess. (October 7 and 14, 1993), 5. Emphasis added.

⁴ Max W. Fine, memorandum to Douglas A. Fraser and Lane Kirkland, June 2, 1978, Re: Meeting of June 1, 1978, with Eizenstat on national health insurance, Fraser Collection, Box 2, Folder 22, "CNHI, 1978."

⁵ For example, when the concept of an employer mandate resurfaced in 1987 with the introduction of the Minimum Health Benefits for All Workers Act, Sweeney and other labor leaders hailed the measure using language almost identical to that enlisted by Hillary Rodham Clinton six years later to defend the administration's Health Security Act. The SEIU president said the measure fell squarely within "a long tradition of uniquely American solutions that rely on setting minimum standards for private enterprise rather than providing comprehensive coverage through government programs." U.S. Senate, Committee on Labor and Human Resources, "Minimum Health Benefits for All Workers Act of 1987," 100th Cong., 1st Sess. (June 24, 1987), pt. 1:75. See also "Push Health Insurance Plan," *UAW Washington Report* (May 29, 1987): 1; and David Jacobs, "Labor and the Strategy of Mandated Health Benefits," *Labor Studies Journal* 14, no. 3 (Fall 1989): 23–33.

⁶ David A. Weeks, *Rethinking Employee Benefit Assumptions* (New York: Conference Board, 1978).

⁷ Karen Swartz, *The Medically Uninsured: Special Focus on Workers* (Washington, D.C.: Urban Institute Press, July 1989).

⁸ Thomas A. Kochan, Harry C. Katz, and Robert B. McKersie, *The Transformation of American Industrial Relations* (New York: Basic Books, 1986), 9.

⁹ Though the work lives of contingent employees vary greatly, they share at least one common and agreed-upon characteristic—"a lack of attachment between the worker and employer." Anne E. Polivka and Thomas Nardone, "On the Definition of 'Contingent' Work," *Monthly Labor Review* (December 1989): 10. See also Kathleen Christensen and Mary Murphree, "Introduction to," in *Flexible Workstyles: A Look at Contingent Labor* (Washington, D.C.: Women's Bureau, U.S. Department of Labor, 1988); and U.S. House, Committee on Government Operations, *Rising Use of Part-Time and Temporary Workers: Who Benefits and Who Loses?* (Washington, D.C.: Government Printing Office, 1988).

It is difficult to get a precise fix on the number of contingent workers because nationally representative employment surveys have not measured the extent of contingent arrangements and because of differences in defining a "contingent" worker. Belous estimates that contingent workers comprise at least one-quarter of the labor force, while Gordon arrives at a lower figure of 10 percent. Richard S. Belous, "How Human Resource Systems Adjust to the Shift Toward Contingent Workers," *Monthly Labor Review* (March 1989): 10–11; and David M. Gordon, *Fat and Mean: The Corporate Squeeze of Working Americans and the Myth of Managerial "Downsizing"* (New York: Martin Kessler Books, The Free Press, 1996), 226–27.

¹⁰ Kochan et al., *The Transformation of American Industrial Relations*, 21. See also George Strauss, "Industrial Relations: Time of Change," *Industrial Relations* 23, no. 1 (Winter 1984): 3.

¹¹ For a development of this point, see Kochan et al., *The Transformation of American Industrial Relations*, 18. This two-track approach to labor-management relations has important parallels with the good cop, bad cop, approach of the National Civic Foundation and the NAM in the 1920s. See Larry J. Griffin, Michael E. Wallace, and Beth A. Rubin, "Capitalist Resistance to the Organization of Labor Before the New Deal: Why? How? Success?" *American Sociological Review* 51 (April 1986): 147–67.

¹² Richard S. Belous, *The Contingent Economy: The Growth of the Temporary, Part-Time, and Subcontracted Workforce* (Washington, D.C.: National Planning Association, 1989); "The Downsizing of America," seven-part series, *The New York Times* (March 3–9, 1996); Joel Bleifuss, "The Terminators," *In These Times* (March 4, 1996): 12; Kirk Johnson, "Evolution of the Workplace Alters Office Relationships," *The New York Times* (October 5, 1994): B-1; Louis Uchitelle, "More Downsized Workers Are Returning as Rentals," *The New York Times* (December 8, 1996): A-1; and Christopher D. Cook, "Workers for Rent," *In These Times* (July 22, 1996): 26–28.

¹³ On the ascendance of commercial Keynesianism, see Robert M. Collins, *The Business Response to Keynes, 1929–1964* (New York: Columbia University Press, 1981), esp. chs. 6 and 7. On the demise of the Keynesian consensus, see Margaret Weir, *Politics and Jobs: The Boundaries of Employment Policy in the United States* (Princeton, N.J.: Princeton University Press, 1992); Thomas Ferguson and Joel Rogers, *Right Turn: The Decline of the Democrats and the Future of American Politics* (New York: Hill and Wang, 1986); Isabel V. Sawhill, "Reaganomics in Retrospect," in *Perspectives on the Reagan Years*, ed. John L. Palmer (Washington, D.C.: Urban Institute Press, 1986); Aaron Wildavsky, *The Politics of the Budgetary Process* (Boston: Little Brown, 1984); and Paul E. Peterson, "The New Politics of Deficits," in *The New Direction in American Politics*, ed. John Chubb and Paul E. Peterson (Washington, D.C.: The Brookings Institution, 1985).

¹⁴ David Plotke, "The Political Mobilization of Business," in *The Politics of Interests: Interest Groups Transformed*, ed. Mark Petracca (Boulder, Colo.: Westview Press, 1992), 175–98; Wolfgang Streeck, "The Uncertainties of Management in the Management of Uncertainty: Employers, Labor Relations and Industrial Adjustment in the 1980s," *Work, Employment & Society* 1, no. 3 (September 1987): 281–308; and *Business Credibility: The Critical Factors*, ed. Phyllis S. McGrath (New York: The Conference Board, 1976).

¹⁵ By contrast, in the immediate postwar years, long-term employment relations and some semblance of job security and guarantee of benefits were valued because they demonstrated the rationality and trustworthiness of corporations to government officials, competitors, and potential employees. As such they were an important source of legitimacy for firms. John W. Meyer and Brian Rowan, "Institutionalized Organizations: Formal Structure as Myth and Ceremony," *American Journal of Sociology* 83, no. 2 (September 1977): 340–63.

¹⁶ The term "flexibility" has come to mean many different things in economic policymaking and firm strategies. The discussion here is concerned primarily with attempts to achieve "flexibility" by maximizing an employer's freedom to lay off and discharge workers, to shorten or lengthen the work week, and to vary other conditions of employment in response to the local or international economic situation.

For a good discussion of the various understandings of and policies associated with the search for "flexibility," see Robert Boyer, "Defensive or Offensive Flexibility?" in *The Search for Labor Market Flexibility: The European Economies in Transition*, ed. Robert Boyer (Oxford: Clarendon Press, 1988). See also Michael J. Piore, "Perspectives on Labor Market Flexibility," *Industrial Relations* 25, no. 2 (Spring 1986): 146–66; Michael J. Piore, "Adjustments in Organizational Structure and Their Implications for Social Standards in an Integrated Market," in *Industrial Restructuring and Industrial Relations in Canada and the United States*, ed. Elaine B. Willis (Kingston, Ontario: Industrial Relations Centre, Queen's University, 1989); Thierry J. Noyelle, *Beyond Industrial Dualism: Market and Job Segmentation in the New Economy* (Boulder, Colo.: Westview Press, 1987); Paul Osterman, *Employment Futures: Reorganization, Dislocation, and Public Policy* (New York: Oxford University Press, 1988); and *Grand Designs: The Impact of Corporate Strategies on Workers, Unions, and Communities*, ed. Charles Craypo and Bruce Nissen (Ithaca, N.Y.: ILR Press, 1993).

¹⁷ George Gonos, "The Contest Over 'Employer' Status in the Postwar United States: The Case of Temporary Help Firms," *Law & Society Review* 31, no. 1 (1997): 98.

¹⁸ Gonos, "The Contest Over 'Employer' Status," 98–99.

¹⁹ For more on the Carter administration and the employer mandate, see ch. 4.

²⁰ On the keen interest that business took in the White House's new labor market strategies and the growth of part-time employment in the private sector, see, "In Permanent Part-Time Work, You Can't Beat the Hours," *Nation's Business* 67, no. 1 (January 1979): 68.

²¹ Richard W. Hurd and Jill K. Kriesky, "The Rise and Demise of PATCO Reconstructed," *Labor and Industrial Relations Review* 40, no. 1 (October 1986): 115–22; and *Employee Rights in a Changing Economy: The Issue of Replacement Workers*, ed. William Spriggs (Washington, D.C.: Economic Policy Institute, 1991).

²² "Unions Blast Federal Move to Hire Temporaries," *AFL-CIO News* (January 5, 1985): 8.

²³ Gonos, "The Contest Over 'Employer' Status," 102.

²⁴ "Unions Score Defense Department on Contracting-Out Policy," *AFL-CIO News* (June 1, 1985): 5; and Paul C. Light, *The Tides of Reform: Making Government Work, 1945–1995* (New Haven, Conn.: Yale University Press, 1997), 85–86.

²⁵ Between 1982 and the onset of the recession in 1990, temporary jobs expanded at a rate 10 times as fast as overall employment. Eileen Appelbaum, "Structural Change and the Growth of Part-Time and Temporary Employment," in *New Policies for the Part-Time and Contingent Workforce*, ed. Virginia L. duRivage (Armonk, N.Y.: M.E. Sharpe, 1992), 2. See also Philip Mattera, "Temping Fate," *In These Times* (September 18, 1995): 14–17; John R. Oravec, "Part-time, Temp Jobs Fuel 'Joyless' Recovery," *AFL-CIO News* (September 20, 1993): 10; and Christopher Cook, "Temps—The Forgotten Workers," *The Nation* (January 31, 1994): 124–28.

²⁶ By the early 1990s, part-time employees comprised almost 20 percent of the nonagricultural workforce, up from 12 percent in the 1950s. Chris Tilly, "Reasons for the Continuing Growth of Part-Time Employment," *Monthly Labor Review* (March 1991): 10. From the early 1970s onward, the number of self-employed individuals as a percentage of the workforce grew, reversing a decline under way since the early part of the century. Louis Uchitelle, "Many Are Forced Into Ranks of Self-Employed at Low Pay," *The New York Times* (November 15, 1993): A-1.

²⁷ Only one-third of part-time workers, or fewer, receives health-insurance coverage through their employers, compared to nearly three-quarters of full-time, year-round workers. Sar A. Levitan and Elizabeth Conway, *Part-Time Employment: Living on Half-Rations* (Center for Social Policy Studies, George Washington University, 1988), working paper no. 101, as cited in Belous, "How Human Resource Systems Adjust," 11. Some part-timers who do not receive benefits directly from their employers are covered by another arrangement—such as a spouse's plan or a public program like Medicaid.

Fewer than one-quarter of those employed by temporary help agencies work for temp firms that offer health benefits. As for the self-employed, one out of four has no health insurance coverage. Harry B. Williams, "What Temporary Workers Earn; Findings from New BLS Survey," *Monthly Labor Review* (March 1989): 3–6, as cited in Polivka and Nardone, "On the Definition of 'Contingent' Work," 15, f.n. 10; *EBRI Databook on Employee Benefits*, 3rd ed., ed. Carolyn Pemberton and Deborah Holmes (Washington, D.C.: Employee Benefit Research Institute, 1995), 263.

²⁸ The legislation required employers to pay for a minimum package of health benefits for all employees working at least 17.5 hours per week, and their dependents. Employers would be required to pay at least 80 percent of the premium (100 percent for workers making less than 125 percent of the minimum wage). The Senate Labor Committee approved the controversial bill over the objections of the Republican minority, but the measure went no further in the 100th Congress. *Congress and the Nation, 1985–1988*, vol. 7 (Washington, D.C.: Congressional Quarterly Press, 1990), 599.

²⁹ See John J. Sweeney, U.S. Senate, Committee on Labor and Human Resources, "Minimum Health Benefits for All Workers Act of 1987," 100th Cong., 1st Sess. (June 24, 1987), pt. 1:91.

Ironically, conservative opponents of the legislation, notably Sen. Orin G. Hatch (R-Utah), the ranking minority member of the Senate Labor Committee, raised the issue of how the legislation did little or nothing for the contingent workforce. U.S. Senate, "Minimum Health Benefits for All Workers Act of 1988," 100th Cong., 2nd Sess. (May 25, 1988), 68–69.

³⁰ The recommendation, which was approved by a bare majority, would require all employers to provide health insurance to their workers or pay a tax to help fund a public program for the uninsured (the "play-or-pay" option). Judith Feder, "The Pepper Commission

Proposals," in *Social Insurance Issues for the Nineties, Proceedings of the Third Conference of the National Academy of Social Insurance,* ed. Paul N. Van Dewater (Dubuque, Iowa: Kendall/Hunt, 1992).

[31] See the remarks by Rep. Thomas J. Tauke (R-Iowa), Pepper Commission, U.S. Bipartisan Commission on Comprehensive Health Care, "A Call for Action" (Washington, D.C.: 1990), 247.

[32] Rep. Pete Stark (D-Calif.), "A Call for Action," 2 and 233.

[33] See the testimony of Princeton professor Paul Starr, U.S. Senate, Finance Committee, "Comprehensive Health Care Reform and Cost Containment," 102nd Cong., 2nd Sess. (May 6 and 7, 1992), pt. 1:37; Nolan W. Hancock of the OCAW, prepared statement, U.S. Senate, Finance Committee, "Comprehensive Health Care Reform and Cost Containment," 102nd Cong., 2nd Sess. (June 1992), pt. 2:497; and Karen Swartz, "Why Requiring Employers to Provide Health Insurance Is a Bad Idea," *Journal of Health Politics, Policy and Law* 15, no. 4 (1990): 779–92.

[34] This is not to say that legislators, other government officials, and organized labor were entirely sanguine or oblivious to the expanding contingent workforce. In 1988 the U.S. Labor Department released a lengthy and detailed study of contingent work. That same year the Government Operations Committee of the U.S. House held several days of hearings on the subject. In the early 1990s, organized labor took a keen interest in legislation that would clarify who should be considered a "leased employee" for pension purposes. U.S. Department of Labor, *Flexible Workstyles: A Look at Contingent Labor;* U.S. House, Committee on Government Operations, *Rising Use of Part-Time and Temporary Workers;* and James B. Parks, "Pension Reform Bills a Mixed Bag for Labor," *AFL-CIO News* (October 28, 1991): 6.

[35] Hillary Rodham Clinton testified before Congress in the fall of 1993 that business "bears the bulk of the responsibility, pays most of the bills," yet "until very recently had very little to say or very little control over the kinds of costs in the health care system that have increased their costs and, in many industries, lowered their competitiveness." The First Lady went on to say, "What I believe is the fair approach to what we are doing is to recognize that business has borne the burden for taking care of most Americans." U.S. Senate, Committee on Labor and Human Resources, "Health Security Act of 1993," 103rd Cong., 1st Sess. (September–October 1993), pt. 1:48.

Mrs. Clinton was not entirely uncritical of the corporate sector. For a brief period she cast around for "villains" in the health-care crisis and publicly castigated the insurance companies. Bob Woodward, *The Agenda: Inside the Clinton White House* (New York: Simon & Schuster, 1994), 147.

[36] The media helped perpetuate this view. For example, a lengthy article in *Fortune* magazine lauded how employers were the "prime movers behind medical care's re-engineering" because "in the working years" they "are responsible for paying much of the medical bill." Edmund Faltermayer, "Why Health Costs Can Keep Slowing," *Fortune* (January 24, 1994): 76.

[37] Families USA, "Health Spending: The Growing Threat to the Family Budget" (Washington, D.C.: Families USA Foundation, December 1991). Between 1980 and 1991, aggregate spending on health care by business increased 221 percent while aggregate spending by families rose almost 300 percent. Business spending includes health-insurance premiums (55 percent), general taxes (20 percent), Medicare (16 percent), and other miscellaneous items (8 percent).

[38] That year the average family paid nearly $4,300 to support the health-care system through out-of-pocket expenses (32 percent), insurance premiums (17 percent), Medicare payroll taxes (9 percent), Medicare premiums (3 percent), and general taxes (40 percent). That individuals and families pay the bulk of the nation's health-care tab often goes unrecognized because the U.S. public pays for health care through several disparate avenues while the business contribution is concentrated in health-insurance premiums. In 1991 business

footed the bill for 67 percent of all private insurance costs in the United States. Families USA, "Health Spending."

[39] Uwe E. Reinhardt, "Health Care Spending and American Competitiveness," *Health Affairs* (Winter 1989): 5–21; Mark Pauly, *Health Benefits at Work: An Economic and Political Analysis of Employment-Based Health Insurance* (Ann Arbor: University of Michigan Press, 1997); and Clay Chandler, "Health Reform's Competitiveness Case: Oversold? Most Economists Predict Little Impact on Trade and Investment," *The Washington Post* (November 7, 1993): H-1. For a challenge to this perspective, see Carl J. Schramm et al., "Perspectives: Responses to an Essay by Uwe Reinhardt on Health Care Spending and American Competitiveness," *Health Affairs* (Spring 1990): 162–77; and the testimony of Walter B. Maher of Chrysler and Paul H. O'Neill of Alcoa in Joint Economic Committee, "Rising Health Care Costs: Are They Really Making It Harder for U.S. Firms to Compete," 101st Cong., 2nd Sess. (May 23, 1990), 2–136.

[40] *EBRI Databook on Employee Benefits*, 3rd ed., 261. The term "employment-based plans," as used here, designates health insurance provided through workers' jobs. The insurance cost may be paid for by employers, unions, employees themselves, or a combination.

[41] John J. Motley III, vice-president for federal-governmental relations of the NFIB, estimated that only 42 to 45 percent of U.S. employers provide employment-based health benefits. See U.S. House, Subcommittee on Small Business, "The Small Business Community's Recommendations for National Health Care Reform," 103rd Cong., 1st Sess. (August 4, 1993), 17.

[42] Olveen Carrasquillo et al., "A Reappraisal of Private Employers' Role in Providing Health Insurance," *New England Journal of Medicine* 340, no. 2 (January 14, 1999): 109–14.

[43] Ida Hellander et al., "The Growing Epidemic of Uninsurance: New Data on the Health Insurance Coverage of Americans" (Washington, D.C.: Physicians for a National Health Program, December 15, 1994), 2 and 4.

[44] Angela M. O'Rand, "The Hidden Payroll: Employee Benefits and the Structure of Workplace Inequality," *Sociological Forum* 1 no. 4 (Fall 1986): 657. See also Lawrence B. Root, "Employee Benefits and Social Welfare: Complement and Conflict," *The Annals of the American Academy of Political and Social Science* 479 (1985): 101–18; and Sheila B. Kamerman and Alfred J. Kahn, *The Responsive Workplace: Employers and a Changing Labor Force*, (New York: Columbia University Press, 1987).

[45] Peter Passell, "Benefits Dwindle Along With Wages for the Unskilled," *The New York Times* (June 14, 1998): A-1.

[46] Laurie Perman and Beth Stevens, "Industrial Segregation and the Gender Distribution of Fringe Benefits," *Gender and Society* 3, no. 3 (September 1988): 388–404; and Nancy S. Jecker, "Can an Employer-Based Health Insurance System Be Just?," in *The Politics of Health Care Reform: Lessons From the Past, Prospects for the Future*, ed. James A. Morone and Gary S. Belkin (Durham, N.C.: Duke University Press, 1994). When wages are controlled for, differences in pension, health, and disability coverage for men and women disappear. Janet Currie, "Gender Gaps in Benefit Coverage," NBER working paper no. 4265 (Cambridge, Mass.: National Bureau of Economic Research, January 1983).

[47] "Health Inequities Put Hispanic Workers at Risk," *AFL-CIO News* (May 25, 1992): 6; and Peter T. Kilborn, "Denver's Hispanic Residents Point to Ills of the Uninsured," *The New York Times* (April 9, 1999): A-1.

[48] *EBRI Databook on Employee Benefits*, 3rd ed., 263.

[49] Rashid Bashshur and Cater Webb, "Nature and Dimensions of the Problem of Access," in *Improving Access to Health Care: What Can the States Do?*, ed. John H. Goddeeris and Andrew J. Hogan (Kalamazoo, Mich.: W.E. Upjohn Institute for Employment Research, 1992), 41–42. See also *EBRI Databook on Employee Benefits*, 3rd ed., 248–53. Analysts attribute these regional and state disparities in the number of uninsured to the absence of strong unions in the South and West, as well as more limited Medicaid programs in certain states. Swartz, *The Medically Uninsured*.

[50] Passell, "Benefits Dwindle"; and *EBRI Databook on Employee Benefits*, 3rd ed., 259–60. See also Richard Kronick, "Health Insurance, 1979–1989: The Frayed Connection Between Employment and Insurance," *Inquiry* 28, no. 4 (Winter 1991): 318; and Laura A. Scofea, "The Development and Growth of Employer-Provided Health Insurance," *Monthly Labor Review* (March 1994): 3–10.

[51] Joel C. Cantor, "Expanding Health Insurance Coverage: Who Will Pay?," *Journal of Health Politics, Policy and Law* 15, no. 4 (Winter 1990): 762.

[52] A 1983 study of the tax exclusion benefit found that three-quarters of households with incomes in the $50,000–$100,000 range benefited from the employer tax deduction, compared with only 31 percent in the $10,000–$15,000 range, and just 13 percent in the under $10,000 category. Furthermore, those in the higher income bracket get a proportionately higher break because they are in higher tax brackets to begin with. Rashi Fein, *Medical Care, Medical Costs: The Search for Health Insurance Policy* (Cambridge: Harvard University Press, 1986), 182.

[53] When executives were asked how they intended to control spending for health care, the overwhelming majority said they would shift more costs onto employees. "The 1990 National Executive Poll on Health Care Costs and Benefits," *Business and Health* (April 1990): 30.

[54] Kochan et al., *The Transformation of American Industrial Relations*, ch. 4. Between 1978 and 1983, the number of companies demanding tightened provisions for benefits or outright takebacks increased for all 12 items included on a Conference Board survey of several hundred firms. Conference Board report by Audrey Freeman cited in Andrew Remes, "The Attack on Benefits," *Economic Notes* 53, no. 9 (September 1985): 1–2.

[55] Asked to rank their top six negotiating priorities, management and labor put "employee cost sharing for health benefits" at the top of their lists in a 1989 survey by Metropolitan Life. Wages came in number two. Faith Lyman Ham, "Who Will Pay for Health Benefits? Management and Labor Face Off," *Business & Health* (August 1989): 29–39. See also Suzanne S. Taylor, *Negotiating Health Insurance in the Workplace: A Basic Guide* (Washington, D.C.: Bureau of National Affairs, 1992).

[56] Congressional Research Service, "Health Insurance and the Uninsured: Background Data and Analysis" (Washington, D.C.: Government Printing Office, May 1988), 3; and Ida Hellander et al., "The Growing Epidemic of Uninsurance: New Data on the Health Insurance Coverage of Americans," *International Journal of Health Services* 25, no. 3 (1995): 377–92.

[57] For full-time, year-round workers earning less than the poverty level, the decline was more pronounced—from 57 percent in 1979 to 34 percent in 1992. These figures are for direct employer coverage and do not include people covered as dependents in family plans. *EBRI Databook on Employee Benefits*, 3rd ed., 261. In 1992, working adults comprised over 55 percent of the uninsured in the United States, or nearly 23 million people. Children comprised 27.2 percent of the uninsured, or 11.1 million, and nonworkers comprised the remaining 17.3 percent, or 7.1 million people. These figures are based on the civilian nonelderly population. *EBRI Databook on Employee Benefits*, 3rd. ed., 247.

[58] EBRI *Databook on Employee Benefits*, 3rd ed., 305. For more on the extent of the cost shift, see J. Peter Nixon, "Health Care Reform: A Labor Perspective," *Healthcare Reform in The Nineties*, ed. Pauline Vaillancourt Rosenau (Thousand Oaks, Calif.: Sage, 1994); and Pseudonymous, "Unions Face the Crisis of Health Care Cost Containment," *Labor Notes* (July 1985): 7–10.

[59] Peter T. Kilborn, "Uninsured in U.S. Span Many Groups," *The New York Times* (February 26, 1999): A-1.

[60] According to the U.S. Department of Labor, in 1980 just over half of all employees received health insurance for their families entirely funded by employers. By 1986, the figure fell to 35 percent. U.S. Senate, Committee on Labor and Human Resources, "Minimum Health Benefits for All Workers Act of 1988," Report no. 360, 100th Cong., 2nd Sess. (May

25, 1988), 20–21. Between 1987 and 1989, payroll deductions for health-insurance premiums for family plans, adjusted for inflation, rose 56 percent. SEIU, department of public policy, "Employer-Paid Health Insurance is Disappearing" (SEIU: Washington, D.C., July 1989). See also Clifford Staples, "The Politics of Employment-Based Insurance in the United States," *International Journal of Health Services* 19, no. 3 (1989): 415–31; and Gail A. Jensen, Michael A. Morrisey, and John W. Marcus, "Cost Sharing and the Changing Pattern of Employer-Sponsored Health Benefits," *The Milbank Quarterly* 65, no. 4 (1987): 521–50.

⁶¹ Congressional Research Service, "Health Insurance and the Uninsured," xiv–xv, 3, and 112–13.

⁶² Mark J. Warshawsky, *The Uncertain Promise of Retiree Health Benefits: An Evaluation of Corporate Obligations* (Washington, D.C.: The AEI Press, 1992). One needs to be careful not to overstate the degree to which ERISA protects employee pensions. The 1980s saw the beginnings of a drastic restructuring of pension coverage due to the termination of a rash of healthy pension plans, radical changes in pension rules, and the widespread use of pension funds to relocate capital or restructure firms to the detriment of workers. Ellen E. Schultz, "The Pension Eraser: 'Integrating' Social Security Can Cut Benefits," *The Wall Street Journal* (March 12, 1997): C-1; and Teresa Ghilarducci, *Labor's Capital: The Economics and Politics of Pensions* (Cambridge, Mass.: MIT Press, 1992).

⁶³ The United Steel Workers responded by going on strike and appealing to Congress to compel LTV to reinstate the benefits. Congress approved a stopgap measure specifically for the LTV case as legislators continued to seek a more permanent solution to the problem of retiree health benefits in instances of bankruptcy.

⁶⁴ Warshawsky, *The Uncertain Promise; AFL-CIO News* (March 3, 1987): 5, and (March 28, 1987): 6; "USWA Retirees From Six States Tell Congress: 'Protect Our Health Benefits,' " *Steelabor* (March–April 1987): 10–11.

⁶⁵ "Mine Workers Hold Firm Against Pittston Tactics," *AFL-CIO News* (June 24, 1989): 9; "Mine Workers Battle Cutoff of Retiree Benefits," *AFL-CIO News* (February 3, 1992): 6; John Enagonio, "Health Care Issues Remain as Miners Go Back to Work," *Labor Notes* (April 1990): 3; Mike Hall, "Energy Bill Saves Miners' Benefits, Creates Jobs," *AFL-CIO News* (October 12, 1992); Jim Woodward, "Health Cuts May Spark Coal Strikes," *Labor Notes* (March 1992): 1; and Woodward, "United Mine Workers Union Wins Fight for Retiree Health Care," *Labor Notes* (September 1992): 7.

⁶⁶ Karen Ignagni, "Retiree Health: Bargaining for the 1990s," *AFL-CIO News* (August 5, 1989): 4.

⁶⁷ Phill Kwik, "Welcome to Class Warfare," *Labor Notes* (October 1989). The leadership's sit-in protest was even more surprising in light of a letter the federation had sent to its members discouraging them from participating in illegal activities. Kim Moody, "Despite Fines, Pittston Strikers Resume Civil Disobedience," *Labor Notes* (September 1989): 15.

⁶⁸ Erik Melander, "Coming Soon: An Assault on Retiree Health Care," *Labor Notes* (October 1988): 6; Warshawsky, *The Uncertain Promise;* M. R. Traska, "A Rule that Could Sink Your Company," *Business & Health* (January 1989): 31–33; Pamela Toulbee, "What's Ahead for Retiree Health," *Business & Health* (December 1990): 25–36; "New Accounting Rule Would Bring Retiree Health Cost to $2500 Per Employee," *Medical Benefits* (April 15, 1991): 9; and L. Kertesz, "Workers to Pay Now for Retiree Health Plan," *Medical Benefits* 7, no. 4 (April 15, 1990).

⁶⁹ Under the accounting convention that existed, companies were required to count only money actually spent on retiree benefits during a given year—and not future obligations—as a liability on corporate balance sheets. Under the new rule, each year companies would have to report a sufficient amount on their financial statements so that by the time their current employees retired, the full cost of the promised health benefits for the golden years would have been reported.

[70] Ignagni, "Retiree Health."

[71] A 1992 survey by William Mercer, Inc., the prominent benefit consulting firm, found that 83 percent of employers polled had tightened their retiree benefit programs because of the new FASB rule. Nixon, "Health Care Reform: A Labor Perspective," 207.

[72] Among firms offering benefits to early retirees, 38 percent paid the full cost of the premium in 1988, compared with just 32 percent in 1992. *EBRI Databook on Employee Benefits*, 3rd ed., 400–402.

[73] Richard Ostuw, "How Can Employers Cope With Soaring Retiree Health Care Costs?," *Pension World* (March 1987): 53–55; Deborah Lohse, "Early Retirees Get Healthy Dose of Reality," *The Wall Street Journal* (October 25, 1993): C-1; James B. Parks, "Public, Private Pensions Face Growing Threats," *AFL-CIO News* (March 20, 1995): 4; and Polly Callaghan, "1990 Contract Innovations Address Family Security," *AFL-CIO News* (April 15, 1991): 7.

[74] Nearly all U.S. citizens aged 65 and older qualify for Medicare, the federal health-care program for older Americans. Those who retire before age 65 are usually ineligible. Some employers provide health insurance to retired workers until Medicare kicks in and/or provide so-called Medigap coverage to retirees aged 65 and above to cover items or expenses not included in Medicare.

[75] The Internal Revenue Service facilitated this shift from defined benefits to defined contributions. The IRS in the 1970s began to relax its restrictions regarding the particular "benefits" that employers could consider tax-exempt. As employees subsequently began to pick and choose from a menu of tax-free benefits, employers felt less obligated to cover the full cost of any single benefit, including health insurance. Root, "Employee Benefits and Social Welfare," 111.

[76] P. Milligan, "Health Care Reform: A New Employer/Employee 'Deal'?" *Employment Relations Today* (Summer 1994): 117. Another commentator advised managers not to "underestimate the employee's savvy. He's aware of the erosion of entitlements in other areas of his life—in checking account requirements at the bank, for example—and has more or less accepted it as inevitable." Stanley Siegelman, "Communicating the Bad News," *Business and Health* (November 1990): 13.

[77] Conference Board, *Public Interest in a Private Economy* (New York: Conference Board, 1994), 15.

[78] See Alan Peres, benefits manager for Ameritech, prepared statement submitted on behalf of the Washington Business Group on Health, U.S. Senate, Subcommittee on Labor of the Committee on Labor and Human Resources, "Retiree Health Benefits: The Impact on Workers and Businesses," 103rd. Cong., 1st Sess. (1992), 65; and Regina Herlinger and Jeffrey Schwartz, "How Companies Tackle Health Care Costs, Part I," *Harvard Business Review* (July/August 1985): 78.

Some management prescriptions for reevaluating the deal and slashing medical costs bordered on the macabre. One commentator suggested legalizing physician-assisted suicide for the hopelessly ill as a way to broaden patient choice and conserve scarce resources. The dying person would "be given a choice on how to spend the money that would otherwise be spent ineffectively on postponing death." K.K. Fung, "Containing Health Care Cost Through Compensated Death," *Challenge* 37, no. 2 (1994): 1.

[79] The average unionized employer spent 12.7 percent of payroll to cover workers while nonunion employers (including those who provided no coverage) averaged 7.1 percent. "Unions Explore Options on Health Care Bargaining Strategies," *AFL-CIO News* (May 2, 1994): 2.

[80] See the exchange between David E. Scherb, vice-president, compensation, Pepsico, and Martin B. Zimmerman, chief economist, Ford, U.S. House, Committee on Ways and Means, "Effects of Health Care Reform on the National Economy and Jobs," 103rd Cong., 1st Sess. (December 15, 1993), 119–146; Bruce Atwater, chairman, General Mills, Inc., U.S.

House, Subcommittee on Health and the Environment of the Committee on Energy and Commerce, "Health Care Reform," 103rd Cong., 2nd Sess. (February 1994), pt. 9:69–71; and John J. Motley III, vice-president, federal-government relations, NFIB, U.S. House, Committee on Ways and Means, "Employer Mandate and Related Provisions of the Administration's Health Security Act," 103rd Cong., 2nd Sess. (February 3, 1994), 137.

[81] Alan Reuther, legislative director of the UAW, interview, Washington, D.C., June 7, 1996.

[82] See the exchange between Rep. Pete Stark (D-Calif.) and Martin B. Zimmerman, chief economist, Ford, "Effects of Health Care Reform on the National Economy and Jobs," 135–37. One noteworthy exception was Senator Kennedy. See U.S. Senate, Committee on Labor and Human Resources, "Health Security Act of 1993," 103rd Cong., 1st Sess. (September–October 1993), pt. 1:332–43.

[83] Mel Bass, director, health and benefit policy, American Automobile Manufacturers Association, U.S. Senate, Committee on Labor and Human Resources, "Health Security Act," 103rd Cong., 2nd Sess. (January–March 1994), pt. 4:498.

[84] Kochan et al., *The Transformation of American Industrial Relations*, 131–32.

[85] SEIU, "Out of Control, Into Decline" (Washington, D.C.: SEIU, 1992), 1–10. For other examples of the emphasis that union officials put on the competitiveness question in discussions of health care, see Nixon and Ignagni, "Health Care Reform: A Labor Perspective,"; and "Williams Pledges USWA Support for Clinton Plan," *Steelabor* (November–December 1993): 8–9.

[86] John J. Sweeney, U.S. House, Subcommittee on Health of the Committee on Ways and Means, "Health Care Reform," vol. 1, 103rd Cong., 1st Sess. (January–March 1993), 281. See also U.S. Senate, Committee on Labor and Human Resources, "Health Security Act of 1993," 103rd Cong., 1st Sess. (September–October 1993), pt. 1:320.

[87] This phrase comes from Paul Krugman, *Peddling Prosperity: Economic Sense and Nonsense in the Age of Diminished Expectations* (New York: W.W. Norton, 1994), 171.

[88] For example, an article on health-care costs in the *Harvard Business Review* began with a dire prediction: "Corporate expenses for health care are rising at such a fast rate that, if unchecked, they will eliminate all profits for the average Fortune '500' company and the largest 250 nonindustrials." Herlinger and Schwartz, "How Companies Tackle Health Care Costs, Part I," 69.

[89] D. Diblase, "Group Health Bills Equal A Third of Profits," *Business Insurance* (May 29, 1989): 37–38, cited in Martin, "Managing National Health Reform," 190. See also Katherine R. Levit and Cathy A. Cowan, "The Burden of Health Care Costs: Business, Households, and Governments," *Health Care Financing Review* 12, no. 2 (Winter 1990): 127–37; and Katherine R. Levit and Cathy A. Cowan, "Business, Households, and Governments: Health Care Costs, 1990," *Health Care Financing Review* 13, no. 2, (Winter 1991): 83–93.

[90] SEIU, "Out of Control, Into Decline," 7. See also the graph included in Ignagni, "Retiree Health: Bargaining for the 1990s." The Clinton administration also used profits as a yardstick to measure how much medical expenses purportedly hurt U.S. firms. See Robert Reich, U.S. House, Committee on Education and Labor, "Hearings on the President's Health Care Reform Proposal," vol. 1, 103rd Cong., 1st Sess. (October 7 and 14, 1993), 183.

[91] From 41 percent of after-tax profits in 1980 to 88 percent in 1985, by some estimates. During this same period, employer spending on health-insurance premiums as a percentage of after-tax profits increased from 31 percent to 65 percent. These figures are based on contributions by business to health-insurance premiums, Medicare, workers' compensation, temporary disability insurance, and industrial plant health services and are calculated from the *EBRI Databook on Employee Benefits*, 3rd ed., Table 10.14, 368.

[92] From $156 billion in 1980 to $129 billion in 1985, or a fall of 17 percent. Had corporate after-tax profits held steady between 1980 and 1985, employer spending on health care as a percentage of after-tax profits would have been 73 percent, not 88 percent, in 1985. Sim-

ilarly, employer spending on health-insurance premiums as a percentage of after-tax profits would have been 54 percent, not 65 percent, if profits had held steady between 1980 and 1985. Calculated from *EBRI Databook on Employee Benefits*, 3rd ed., Table 10.14, 368.

⁹³ Spending on wages and salaries as expressed as a percentage of after-tax profits dropped from a high point of 1255 percent in 1985 to 958 percent in 1992, a figure nearly identical to that of 1970 (986 percent). Employer spending on total compensation fell from a high of 1486 percent of after-tax profits in 1985 to 1143 percent in 1992, again a figure comparable to that of 1970 (1104 percent). Calculated from *EBRI Databook on Employee Benefits*, 3rd ed., Table 10.14, 368.

⁹⁴ Reuters, "The Transition: Excerpts from Clinton's Conference on the State of the Economy," *The New York Times* (December 15, 1992): B-10, as cited in Pauly, *Health Benefits at Work*, 28–29.

⁹⁵ Louis Uchitelle, "Insurance as a Job Benefit Shows Signs of Overwork," *The New York Times* (May 1, 1991): A-1.

⁹⁶ A 1984 Congressional report found that fringe benefits were equal to almost 83 percent of compensation for actual time worked in Italy; Japan came in at 75 percent; West Germany at 71 percent; the United Kingdom at 38 percent; and the United States at just 37 percent. Congressional Research Service, "An International Comparison of Fringe Benefits," cited in Remes, "The Attack on Benefits." See also Patricia Capdevielle, "International Comparisons of Hourly Compensation Costs," *Monthly Labor Review* (June 1989): 10–12; Martin Rein, "The Social Policy of the Firm," *Policy Sciences* 14 (1982): 126; and Richard Freeman, "How Labor Fares in Advanced Economies," in *Working Under Different Rules*, ed. Richard Freeman (New York: Russell Sage Foundation, 1994), 22–23.

⁹⁷ Robert Reich, "Who is Us?," *Harvard Business Review* (January/February 1990): 53–64. See also William J. Holstein et al., "The Stateless Corporation," *Business Week* (May 14, 1990): 98–105; and Gerald Epstein, "Mortgaging America: Debts, Lies, and Multinationals," *World Policy Journal* 8, no. 1 (Winter 1990–91): 27–59.

⁹⁸ See Paul Krugman, "Fantasy Economics," *The New York Times* (September 26, 1994): A-17; Krugman, *Peddling Prosperity;* David M. Gordon, "The Global Economy: New Edifice or Crumbling Foundations?," *New Left Review* no. 168 (March/April 1988): 37, 58–59, and 61; Linda Weiss, "Globalization and the Myth of the Powerless State," *New Left Review* no. 225 (September/October 1997): 3–27; Doug Henwood and Hector Figueroa, "Dialogue: Does Globalization Matter?" *In These Times* (March 31, 1997): 14–18; and Robert Wade, "Globalization and Its Limits: Reports of the Death of the National Economy are Greatly Exaggerated," in *National Diversity and Global Capitalism*, ed. Suzanne Berger and Ronald Dore (Ithaca, N.Y.: Cornell University Press, 1996), 60–88.

⁹⁹ Reinhardt, "Health Care Spending and American Competitiveness," 15; and Pauly as quoted in Uchitelle, "Insurance as a Job Benefit Shows Signs of Overwork."

¹⁰⁰ Although leading business executives stressed in public the need to cut labor and benefit costs to remain competitive, in more select audiences they took a position surprisingly similar to Gordon's. A 1994 report by the Conference Board suggested that "wage costs are of only secondary importance in the global expansion process." The Conference Board, "U.S. Manufacturers in the Global Marketplace: A Research Report" (New York: The Conference Board, 1994), 17.

¹⁰¹ Kim Moody, *Workers in a Lean World: Unions in the International Economy* (New York: Verso, 1997), 36.

Chapter 7: Adrift and on the Defensive

¹ Labor opposed proposals that mandated that employers pay only 50 percent of their employees' health premiums, fearing this would encourage employers who currently paid a larger portion to view the 50 percent figure as a new norm. David Rogers and Hilary Stout,

"Labor Turns Up Heat on Senate Health-Care Bill," *The Wall Street Journal* (August 5, 1994): A-3; see also the accounts in the *AFL-CIO News* (esp. May 16, 1994; May 30, 1994; June 27, 1994; July 25, 1994; August 9, 1994; and August 22, 1994).

[2] According to one survey, by the late 1980s, 22 of 26 unions polled favored a federally funded national health plan. Heather Kennedy, "The Attitudes and Perspectives of Organized Labor Toward Health Care Cost Management" (Washington, D.C.: Employee Benefit Research Institute, 1990).

[3] Robert Kearns, "Unions Set Drive to Overhaul Health Care," Reuter Business Report (November 15, 1989): electronic database.

[4] AFL-CIO, "The Case for Health Care Reform: The People Speak, Transcripts from Regional Hearings, September–October 1990" (Washington, D.C.: AFL-CIO, 1990).

[5] Jobs With Justice newsletter, "Report on Health Care Action Day—October 3, 1990," Sheinkman Papers, Amalgamated Clothing Workers of America Records, Labor-Management Documentation Center, Cornell University, Box 5, "Jobs With Justice"; and Laura McClure, "Does a 'Reformed' System Mean a Better System?," *Labor Notes* (July 1990): 9.

[6] Robert McGarrah to Gerald McEntee, November 6, 1990, "AFL-CIO Health Care Committee Meeting," McGarrah Papers; and Robert McGarrah to Gerald McEntee, May 21, 1990, "AFL-CIO Health Care Meetings," McGarrah Papers.

[7] Camille Colatosti, "What Are Unions Doing About Fixing the Health Care System?," *Labor Notes* (July 1990): 8–9. Sweeney reportedly was a widely acceptable choice to head the federation's health-care committee precisely because his union had extensive Taft-Hartley commitments. J. Peter Nixon, senior policy analyst, SEIU, interview, Washington, D.C., June 3, 1996. By one estimate, 350,000 of the SEIU's 1 million members receive health benefits through the union's own Taft-Hartley fund. "The Health Care Debate," *Economic Notes* (January–February 1991): 9–13.

[8] This account of the meeting is based on the handwritten notes of Robert McGarrah, AFSCME director of public policy, who was present. "Notes Re: 1/31/91 Meeting of the Health Care Committee," McGarrah Papers.

[9] Unions voting for the single-payer plan were: AFSCME, CWA, UAW, ACTWU, ILGWU, APWU, UMW, and IAM. Those voting for the "play-or-pay" proposal were: SEIU, AFT, USWA, UFCW, RWDSU, TCU, and the building and construction trades department of the AFL-CIO. Joyce Frieden, "Unions Rev Up Health Reform Engines," *Business and Health* 9, no. 8 (August 1991): 42–44.

[10] Statement of the executive council of the AFL-CIO on national health reform, February 1991, George Meany Memorial Archives, Silver Spring, Md., pamphlet collection. See also Frieden, "Unions Rev Up Health Reform Engines"; and Colleen M. O'Neill, "Health Care Campaign Reaches Hill," *AFL-CIO News* (February 4, 1991): 1.

[11] Suzanne Gordon, "AFL-CIO Steps Backwards on National Health Insurance," *Labor Notes* (April 1991): 1.

[12] Morton Bahr et al., letter to Lane Kirkland, August 9, 1991, McGarrah Papers; and Camille Colatosti, "AFL-CIO Takes Health Care Reform 'One Step at a Time'," *Labor Notes* (January 1992): 3.

[13] In the months leading up to the introduction of the measure, Sen. Edward Kennedy had convinced many of his Democratic colleagues on the Labor Committee that there was no viable alternative to the employer mandate. Individual supporters of national health insurance on the Labor Committee reportedly "kept silent and by their silence inadvertently persuaded other like-minded members that there was no support for alternatives to employment-based plans." Mark A. Peterson, "Report from Congress: Momentum Toward Health Care Reform in the U.S. Senate," *Journal of Health Politics, Policy and Law* 17, no. 3 (Fall 1992): 560–61.

[14] Colatosti, "AFL-CIO Takes Health Care Reform 'One Step at a Time'." Barry Gordon, president of the Screen Actors Guild, was one of the few who spoke up in defense of a single-payer system. He sparked rounds of applause as he urged the leadership to speak "loudly

and strongly for a single-payer solution." AFL-CIO, "Proceedings of the AFL-CIO 19th Constitutional Convention," Detroit, November 11–14, 1991 (Washington, D.C.: AFL-CIO, 1991), 119.

[15] AFL-CIO, "Proceedings of the AFL-CIO 19th Constitutional Convention."

[16] Colatosti, "AFL-CIO Takes Health Care Reform 'One Step at a Time'."

[17] A June 1991 study by the General Accounting Office buoyed the single-payer forces, concluding that a Canadian-style health-care system could save the United States as much as $67 billion a year in administrative and insurance overhead costs. The savings would be more than enough to provide adequate insurance for the uninsured and the underinsured. Testimony of Charles A. Bowsher, comptroller general of the General Accounting Office, U.S. House, Committee on Government Operations, "Efficiency and Cost Effectiveness of the U.S. Health Care System: A Comparison With Canada," 102nd Cong., 1st Sess. (June 4, 11, and 18, 1991), 24.

A poll of Democratic House members taken by the Democratic Study Group in early 1992, but not released until May, found that legislators decidedly favored the single-payer option over "play-or-pay" proposals. Some charge that this poll was suppressed because it defied the conventional wisdom of the Democratic leadership, which claimed that legislators overwhelmingly supported an employer-mandate solution over the single-payer option. "The Suppressed Democratic Study Group's 'Stealth' Survey Surfaces," *Health Letter* (Public Citizen Research Group) 8, no. 7 (July 1992): 10.

[18] Harry Bernstein, "The Hidden Player in Clinton's War," *Los Angeles Times* (November 10, 1992): D-3; Harry Bernstein, "How Unions Must Revive Under Clinton," *Los Angeles Times* (December 22, 1992): D-3; and Greg Tarpinian, *Trade Union Advisor* (November 24, 1992), reprinted in *OCAW Reporter* (January–February 1993).

[19] Alan Reuther, legislative director, UAW, interview, Washington, D.C., June 7, 1996.

[20] Sara Nichols, former staff attorney, Public Citizen, interview, Washington, D.C., June 13, 1996.

[21] "Whoa, It's Not Over Yet," *The Nation* (December 7, 1992): 1.

[22] Lynn Williams, former president of the USWA, personal correspondence with the author, July 5, 1999.

[23] Laura McClure, "Will Managed Competition Cure the Health Care System?," *Labor Notes* (February 1993): 8–9.

[24] Laura McClure, "Unions Desert Single-Payer Coalition for Clinton's Managed Competition," *Labor Notes* (February 1993): 10; and Evelyn Dubrow, former legislative director, ILGWU, interview, Washington, D.C., June 24, 1996.

[25] Glen Boatman, "AFSCME's Switch to 'Managed Competition' Upsets Single-Payer Movement in Ohio," *Labor Notes* (March 1993): 5.

[26] Statement adopted by the AFL-CIO Executive Council, February 1993, pamphlet collection, George Meany Memorial Archives, Silver Spring, Md.

Around this time, the AFL-CIO joined the Coalition to Preserve Health Benefits, a group comprised primarily of business organizations opposed to the taxation of employee benefits. Several labor leaders chafed at the coalition's conservative leanings, however, and three months later the federation dropped out of the group. Naftali Bendavid, "Shattering the Old Order in Health-Care Politics," *Legal Times* (October 11, 1993): 27.

[27] Kim Moody, "Is There a Future for Unions in the Clinton Administration's Plans?," *Labor Notes* (October 1993): 13; Moody, "Labor in the Clinton Era: New Opportunities, New Problems," *Labor Notes* (February 1993): 1; Keith Brooks, "Clinton's 'Economic Stimulus Package': Much Ado About Not Too Much," *Labor Notes* (June 1993): 12; and Christina Del Valle, "Labor Didn't Expect Much From Bill and Is Getting Even Less," *Business Week* (June 21, 1993): 51.

[28] James Ridgeway, "Who Spiked Single Pay," *The Texas Observer* (October 1, 1993): 13.

[29] AFL-CIO, "Proceedings of the AFL-CIO Twentieth Constitutional Convention," San Francisco, Calif., October 4–7, 1993 (Washington, D.C.: AFL-CIO, 1993), 9.

³⁰ Elizabeth Drew, *On the Edge: The Clinton Presidency* (New York: Simon and Schuster, 1994), 340.

³¹ David Moberg, "The Morning NAFTA," *In These Times* (December 13, 1993): 20–21; Louis S. Richman, "Why Labor Hates NAFTA," *Fortune* (November 15, 1993): 28; and Ken Jennings and Jeffrey W. Steagall, "Unions and NAFTA's Legislative Passage," *Labor Studies Journal* 21, no. 1 (Spring 1996): 61–79.

³² Even Labor Secretary Robert B. Reich, a defender of the treaty, conceded that NAFTA resonated with the U.S. public in ways that went well beyond any of the specific provisions in the trade treaty. "This debate has become so emotional," he declared, "because NAFTA is a symbol of the almost subliminal debate going on in the American psyche about whether our kids will live better than we are." Thomas L. Friedman, "Scholars' Advice and New Campaign Help the President Hit His Old Stride," *The New York Times* (November 17, 1993): A-20.

³³ The resolutions adopted by the UAW at its 1992 convention epitomized this mixed message. On the one hand, the autoworkers attacked NAFTA, charging that the "main beneficiaries of these policies are the multinational corporations who are searching out the lowest costs and the highest profits over the short term, all at the expense of workers." In the next breath, the union appeared acutely sensitive to corporations and to how the "skyrocketing costs of health care adversely affect the international competitiveness of many businesses and threaten the job security of millions of Americans." UAW, "Proceedings of the 30th Constitutional Convention," San Diego, Calif., June 14–18, 1992 (Detroit: UAW, 1992), 123 and 142.

³⁴ "Williams Pledges USWA Support for Clinton Plan," *Steelabor* (November–December 1993): 8–9.

³⁵ Ian Robinson, "NAFTA, Social Unionism, and Labour Movement Power in Canada and the United States," *Relations industrielles/Industrial Relations* 49, no. 4 (1994); and Rand Wilson, "Winning Lessons from the NAFTA Loss," *Labor Research Review* 13, no. 1 (Fall 1994): 29–37.

³⁶ Dana Priest and Michael Weisskopf, "Health Care Reform: The Collapse of a Quest," *The Washington Post* (October 11, 1994): A-6; and Friedman, "Scholars' Advice."

³⁷ Colleen M. O'Neill, "Health Care Reform Battle Lines Drawn," *AFL-CIO News* (September 20, 1993): 1.

³⁸ John R. Oravec, "Side Deals Fail; AFL-CIO Fights NAFTA," *AFL-CIO News* (August 23, 1993): 1.

³⁹ In a June 1993 memorandum, Al From, the president of the conservative Democratic Leadership Council, advised Clinton that he could use support for NAFTA to "gain real credibility as a new Democrat and an agent of fundamental change." Memorandum cited in James Ridgeway, "Bill to Losers: Drop Dead," *The Village Voice* (November 30, 1993): 19.

⁴⁰ Friedman, "Scholars' Advice."

⁴¹ For example, the UAW's toll-free hotline had a recorded message urging members to call their representatives regarding striker replacement legislation and NAFTA, but never mentioned health care. Kevin Salwen, "Dueling Initiatives: NAFTA vs. Health Care," *The Wall Street Journal* (September 3, 1993): A-10. See also Gordon L. Clark, "NAFTA: Clinton's Victory, Organized Labor's Loss," *Political Geography* 13, no. 4 (July 1994): 377–84.

⁴² Evoking distasteful stereotypes of labor thugs strong-arming opponents in a televised interview, Clinton denounced what he called the "roughshod, muscle-bound tactics" of unions in their campaign to block NAFTA. John R. Oravec, " 'No NAFTA' Drive Goes Down to Wire," *AFL-CIO News* (November 15, 1993): 4.

⁴³ Michael Byrne, "Clinton-Republican Coalition Passes NAFTA," *AFL-CIO News* (November 29, 1993): 6.

⁴⁴ This quotation comes from a *Labor Party Advocate* article by Bob Kasen that was reprinted in *OCAW Reporter* (January–February 1994).

⁴⁵ Asra Q. Nomani, "Empty Threats," *The Wall Street Journal* (October 28, 1994): special section, R-11; R. W. Apple, Jr., "Unions Faltering in Reprisals Against Trade Pact Backers,"

The New York Times (February 21, 1994): A-1; and Suzanne Gordon, "Let's Have Real Payback for Politicians Who Voted 'Yes' on NAFTA," *Labor Notes* (January 1994): 11.

⁴⁶ Haynes Bonner Johnson and David S. Broder, *The System: The American Way of Politics at the Breaking Point* (Boston: Little, Brown, 1996), 292.

⁴⁷ "There was this deep period of mourning within the AFL-CIO [after the NAFTA loss]," said Claudia Bradbury St. John of the AFL-CIO. "People were angry. People wouldn't be motivated." St. John, former senior health policy specialist, AFL-CIO, interview, Washington, D.C., June 7, 1996. Also, Willie L. Baker, Jr., director of civil rights and community relations of the UFCW, interview, Washington, D.C., June 24, 1996; and Reuther, interview.

⁴⁸ Colleen M. O'Neill, "Labor Teaching ABCs of Health Care Reform," *AFL-CIO News* (December 13, 1993): 2.

⁴⁹ And once in the field, the federation's staff scrupulously avoided referring to the Health Security Act as the "Clinton plan," for fear of further igniting the ire of union members. St. John, interview.

⁵⁰ Peter T. Kilborn, "Clinton and Unions, Burying Hatchets, Focus on Common Interests," *The New York Times* (February 21, 1994): A-12; and Thomas L. Friedman, "President Confers With Labor Leaders for Fence Mending," *The New York Times* (December 11, 1993): A-1. On labor's initial endorsement, see Colleen M. O'Neill, "Clinton Plan Meets Labor's Longtime Goals," *AFL-CIO News* (October 4, 1993): 1.

⁵¹ Colleen M. O'Neill, "Unions Plan Aggressive Drive," *AFL-CIO News* (January 17, 1994): 1–2.

⁵² Mary Kay Henry, health-care division director, SEIU, interview, Washington, D.C., June 3 and 4, 1996.

⁵³ Robert M. McGlotten, former legislative director of the AFL-CIO, interview, Washington, D.C., June 13, 1996.

⁵⁴ Nichols, interview.

⁵⁵ Max Fine, memorandum to Carol Galaty, n.d., Re: An attempt to appeal to Ralph Nader, Committee for National Health Insurance Collection, Walter P. Reuther Library, Wayne State University, Detroit, Box 40, Folder 25, "Nader Memo, n.d."

⁵⁶ These included differences in the constituencies served by organized labor and public-interest groups. See Michael W. McCann, *Taking Reform Seriously: Perspectives in Public Interest Liberalism* (Ithaca, N.Y.: Cornell University Press, 1986), chs. 2 and 3; Thomas Byrne Edsall, "The Changing Shape of Power: A Realignment in Public Policy," in *The Rise and Fall of the New Deal Order, 1930–1980*, ed. Steve Fraser and Gary Gerstle (Princeton, N.J.: Princeton University Press, 1989), esp. 277–78; and Graham K. Wilson, *Unions in American National Politics* (New York: St. Martin's Press, 1979), 40–41 and 83–84. On friction with consumer advocates over labor's lukewarm support for tougher health and safety standards for consumer products and tougher campaign finance laws, see Fraser Collection, Box 65, Folder 36, "Nader, Ralph"; Wilson, *Unions in American National Politics*, 83–84; and coverage of campaign finance issues in major labor publications, especially the *AFL-CIO News*. On the strident opposition of well-known public-interest groups and left-leaning think tanks to the unionization of their staffs, see "Don't Buy: National Boycotts Sanctioned by the AFL-CIO Executive Council," *UAW Washington Report* (June 10–17, 1988): 4; and T.R. Reid, "Liberal Think Tank Fights a Union," *The Washington Post* (January 23, 1977): A-4.

⁵⁷ *OCAW Reporter* (July–August 1988): 22.

⁵⁸ "Labor-Management Cooperation: Is There a Future?," *OCAW Reporter* (March–April 1988); and OCAW, "Proceedings of the 20th Constitutional Convention" (August 12–16, 1991), 6.

⁵⁹ Bill Hoyle, "Health Care Activism Bolsters LPA Organizing," *OCAW Reporter* (July–August 1993); Robert Wages, "Time to Take a Stand, Build a Movement," *OCAW Reporter* (May–June 1993): 4; Jane Slaughter, "We Were Never Meant to Be Business Unionists: Interview with Robert Wages," *Labor Notes* (September 1992): 5.

⁶⁰ See the *OCAW Reporter* cover story on health care (January–February 1990); and Hoyle, "Health-Care Activism Bolsters LPA Organizing."

⁶¹ See the remarks of OCAW president Joseph M. Misbrener in OCAW, "Proceedings of the 20th Constitutional Convention," 6; " 'Safe' Approach Won't Win National Health Care," OCAW *Reporter* (July–August 1992); and OCAW *Reporter* (September–October 1991): 3. Robert Wages of the OCAW directly attacked the federation's support of the employer-mandate approach. "Even George Meany, that flaming liberal leader, laughed it off Capitol Hill when Nixon threw it there," he charged. *OCAW Reporter* (November–December 1993): 3.

⁶² In late 1993, OCAW president Wages charged, "Clinton's plan will create an insurance business oligopoly that will own a full one-seventh of the economy." OCAW *Reporter* (November–December 1993): 3.

⁶³ Baker, interview.

⁶⁴ By late summer 1993, single-payer measures had the backing of 87 representatives in the House and five co-sponsors in the Senate. The CBO ended up awarding a very positive "scoring" to the McDermott-Wellstone single-payer legislation and agreed that this approach would save more than enough money to ensure universal health care. Theda Skocpol, *Boomerang: Clinton's Health Security Effort and the Turn Against Government in U.S. Politics* (New York: W.W. Norton & Co., 1996), 202, f.n. 47.

⁶⁵ Mike McNamee, "Snickers and Sniping at Clinton—From the Left," *Business Week* (August 30, 1993): 34–35.

⁶⁶ Johnson and Broder, *The System*, 44.

⁶⁷ Nichols, interview; and Barbara Markham Smith, former legislative aide to Rep. Jim McDermott (D-Wash.), interview Washington, D.C., June 24, 1996.

⁶⁸ "We were schizophrenic. We endorsed the McDermott bill, but also supported the Clinton plan in the meantime," explained Daniel J. Schulder, director, department of legislation, National Council of Senior Citizens (NCSC), interview, Washington, D.C., June 4, 1996.

⁶⁹ Tamar Lewin, "The Health Care Debate: Behind the Scenes," *The New York Times* (July 28, 1994): A-20. Although the leadership of Citizen Action drew closer to the White House on health care, much of its rank and file remained skeptical. For example, hundreds of members of Citizen Action booed Ira Magaziner, Clinton's health-care czar, when he addressed a gathering in July 1993. Ridgeway, "Who Spiked Single Pay."

⁷⁰ Ridgeway, "Who Spiked Single Pay"; and Nichols, interview.

⁷¹ Indeed, the ARRP did not officially endorse the Clinton plan, even though John Rother, its director of legislation and public policy, headed the Health Care Reform Project. Johnson and Broder, *The System*, 480–81.

⁷² John Rother, director of legislation and public policy, ARRP, interview, Washington, D.C., June 15, 1996; Schulder, interview; Fernando Trevino, executive director, APHA, interview, Washington, D.C., June 14, 1996; Jeff P. Jacobs, director of Congressional affairs, APHA, interview, Washington, D.C., June 21, 1996; Ronald Pollack and Phyllis Torda, "The Pragmatic Road Toward National Health Insurance," *The American Prospect*, no. 6 (Summer 1991): 92–100; Phyllis Torda, former director of health policy, Families USA, interview, Washington, D.C., June 4, 1996; and Gail Shearer, director of health policy analysis, Consumers Union, interview, Washington, D.C., June 7, 1996. For more on the internal divisions within the AARP over health-care reform, see coverage of this issue in *Health Letter* (Public Citizen's Health Research Group), especially September 1994: 1; February 1994: 10; April 1992: 7; and March 1992: 3.

⁷³ David Abernethy, former majority staff director, Subcommittee on Health of the Committee on Ways and Means, U.S. House of Representatives, interview, Washington, D.C., June 14, 1996.

⁷⁴ His remarks were not for attribution.

⁷⁵ The aim of the alliances was to pool the buying power of companies and individuals in a specified region or state to spur insurers to compete among themselves by improving qual-

ity and lowering costs. Under this arrangement, most health-care purchasers would be required to join an alliance, which would sponsor all health-insurance plans and would also evaluate available plans. Skocpol, *Boomerang*, 43–44. See also James R. Tallon and Lawrence D. Brown, "Health Alliances: Functions, Forms, and Federalism," in *Making Health Reform Work: The View From the States*, ed. John J. DiIulio and Richard Nathan (Washington, D.C.: The Brookings Institution, 1994).

[76] Ray, interview; and SEIU, *Industrial and Allied Update* (Fall/Winter 1993): 9.

[77] Georgine even went so far as to characterize these multiemployer plans as "prototype health alliances." See U.S. House, Subcommittee on Health and the Environment of the Committee on Energy and Commerce, "Health Care Reform Act," 103rd Cong., 1st Sess. (November 1993), pt. 5:103.

[78] They pursued their interests primarily through the Corporate Health Care Coalition, a group of large, self-insured, multistate employers, which counted McDonnell Douglas, Dow Chemical, Hershey Foods, General Electric, and other leading corporations among its membership.

[79] James B. Parks, "Kirkland: Undaunted Unionists 'Agents of Change'," *AFL-CIO News* (October 18, 1993): 5.

[80] For more on experience rating, see ch. 3.

[81] AFSCME, whose membership is comprised primarily of government employees, was particularly upset because the Health Security Act, as originally proposed, permitted large employers in the private sector and private-sector unions with big Taft-Hartley funds to keep their employees and members out of the alliances. However, it required all public employees to participate in the new system. McGarrah, interview; and Robert McGarrah, memorandum to Gerald McEntee, April 22, 1994, Re: Meeting with Magaziner, McGarrah Papers, Box 4, "National Health Care Reform" folder.

[82] Testimony of Jerry J. Jasinowski, president of the NAM, U.S. House, Subcommittee on Health of the Committee on Ways and Means, "Health Care Reform Proposals," vol. 7, 103rd Cong., 1st Sess. (October 28, November 2, and November 4, 1993), 403; and Skocpol, *Boomerang*, 66.

[83] Consumers Union, "The Clinton Health Care Act," rev. (Washington, D.C.: Consumers Union, 1994), 26; and Shearer, interview.

[84] Abernethy, interview.

[85] G. Lawrence Atkins, coordinator, Corporate Health Care Coalition, interview, Washington, D.C., June 6, 1996. See also the testimony of Bruce Karrh, vice-president of DuPont Co., who appeared on behalf of the Corporate Health Care Coalition, U.S. House, Subcommittee on Health and the Environment of the Committee on Energy and Commerce, "Health Care Reform Act," 103rd Cong., 1st Sess. (November–December 1993): pt. 6:667–69 and 707. For more on self-insurance and the ERISA preemption, see ch. 3.

[86] Ray, interview; and Georgine, "Health Care Reform Act," (November–December 1993), pt 5:103–105.

[87] D. Wise, "What Happens to ERISA Under Health Care Reform," *Business & Health* 11, no. 12 (1993): 53–56.

[88] In the words of James Ray of the NCCMP, unions with Taft-Hartley funds "went berserk" over the Mitchell proposal and were proud to have brought it down. James S. Ray, legislative representative, NCCMP, interview, Washington, D.C., June 13, 1996.

[89] Reuther, interview.

[90] See John J. Sweeney, editorial, *Industrial and Allied Update* (Spring/Summer 1991). In 1991, Sweeney tried to get the Ohio AFL-CIO to rescind its support of legislation that would create a single-player system in Ohio. Glen Boatman, "AFL-CIO Leadership Is Failing in Its National Health Care Campaign," *Labor Notes* (February 1991): 11.

[91] Gerald M. Shea, assistant to the president for governmental affairs, AFL-CIO, interview, Washington, D.C., June 13, 1996.

⁹² Glen Boatman, "AFSCME's Switch to 'Managed Competition' Upsets Single-Payer Movement in Ohio," *Labor Notes* (March 1993): 5; and "Healthy States?," *Health Letter* (Public Citizen's Health Research Group) 8, no. 7 (July 1992): 8–9.

⁹³ Nichols, interview.

⁹⁴ Smith, interview.

⁹⁵ The commercials and all the free media attention they garnered helped create the impression that the HIAA was a "major player" in health-care issues, giving the organization "influence in the legislative process that it otherwise lacked." The Annenberg Public Policy Center of the University of Pennsylvania, "Media in the Middle: Fairness and Accuracy in the 1994 Health Care Reform Debate" (Philadelphia, Pa.: Annenberg Center, February 1995), 17.

Between mid-January and late July of 1994, the HIAA received four times more broadcast coverage than the AFL-CIO in connection with the health-care issue. The Annenberg Public Policy Center of the University of Pennsylvania, "Newspaper and Television Coverage of the Health Care Reform Debate, January 16–July 25, 1994" (Philadelphia, Pa.: Annenberg Center, August 12, 1994), 7–9.

⁹⁶ See Nancy Donaldson and Ned McCulloch, memorandum to Bob Welsh and Gerry Shea, October 2, 1993, Nixon Papers, "The Clinton Plan-SEIU Materials" folder.

⁹⁷ Johanna Schneider, director of communications, Business Roundtable, interview, Washington, D.C., June 5, 1996; Hilary Stout and Rick Wartzman, "White House Lobbies Strongly to Block Business Support of Rival Health Plan," *The Wall Street Journal* (February 2, 1994): 37; Gwen Ifill, "Clintons Campaigning to Scuttle Endorsement of Rival Health Plan," *The New York Times* (February 2, 1994): A-1; and Priest and Weisskopf, "Health Care Reform: The Collapse of a Quest."

⁹⁸ U.S. House, Committee on Ways and Means, "Employer Mandate and Related Provisions of the Administration's Health Security Act," 103rd Cong., 2nd Sess. (February 3, 1994), 16–17 and 54; and Lisa M. Sprague, former manager of employee benefits, U.S. Chamber of Commerce, interview, Washington, D.C., June 24, 1996.

⁹⁹ National Association of Manufacturers, "Health Care Reform Recommendations," mimeo, March 23, 1994; and Johnson and Broder, *The System*, 316–18.

¹⁰⁰ Henry, interview. By contrast, nine months earlier the heads of the Big Three and the president of the UAW were willing to sign a joint letter to Hillary Rodham Clinton stating their support for the "administration's commitment to reform our country's health care system." Robert J. Eaton (Chrysler), Harold A. Poling (Ford), John F. Smith, Jr. (GM), and Owen Bieber (UAW), letter to Hillary Rodham Clinton, May 5, 1993, McGarrah Papers, Box 1, "National Health Care Reform" folder.

¹⁰¹ In private, drafters of the Health Security Act were uneasy about how the Congressional Budget Office would ultimately choose to categorize the employer mandate for budgeting purposes. Skocpol, *Boomerang*, 67–8; and Jacob S. Hacker, *The Road to Nowhere: The Genesis of President Clinton's Plan for Health Security* (Princeton, N.J.: Princeton University Press, 1997), 124.

¹⁰² Theodore R. Marmor and Jerry L. Mashaw, "A Tortured Fiction Is Swept From the Table," *Los Angeles Times* (February 18, 1994): B-7; and Joseph White, "Budgeting and Health Policymaking," in *Intensive Care: How Congress Shapes Health Policy*, ed. Thomas E. Mann and Norman J. Ornstein (Washington, D.C.: American Enterprise Institute and The Brookings Institution, 1995).

¹⁰³ Rex Hardesty, "Labor Pledges to Keep Fighting for Health Care," *AFL-CIO News* (October 3, 1994): 1.

¹⁰⁴ AFSCME, "National Health Care: The Battle Begins," *Public Employee* (January 1994): 7.

¹⁰⁵ "Carey Calls on Clinton to Change Strategy on Health Care Reform," PR Newswire (February 7, 1994): electronic database.

¹⁰⁶ Nichols, interview; and McGarrah, memorandum to Gerald McEntee, February 17, 1994, McGarrah Papers, Box 4, "National Health Care Reform" folder.

107   David Corn, "Left Out of The Party? The Left and the Democratic Party," *The Nation* (February 7, 1994): 156; Peter Kilborn, "Unions Plan to Spend $10 Million to Promote Clinton Health Plan," *The New York Times* (February 22, 1994): A-1. See also McGarrah memorandum to McEntee, March 21, 1994, McGarrah Papers, Box 4, "National Health Care Reform" folder.

108   Lawrence A. Weil, "Organized Labor and Health Reform: Union Interests and the Clinton Plan," *Journal of Public Health Policy* 18, no. 1 (1997): 30–48; Johnson and Broder, *The System*, 287–91; and Kevin Salwen, "Labor Unions Consider How to Spend Funds in Drive for Health Reform," *The Wall Street Journal* (February 22, 1994): A-2.

109   Canadian-style reform had few maverick and outspoken advocates in the Senate. Even Sen. Paul Wellstone (D-Minn.), ostensibly its main Senate champion, came under criticism because he was ambivalent about his own bill and refused to hand off sponsorship of the single-payer legislation to a more committed and forceful advocate like Sen. Russell D. Finegold (D-Wis.). Smith, interview. Numerous requests to interview key members of Sen. Wellstone's staff who were involved in health-care reform were ignored.

110   U.S. House, Subcommittee on Health of the Committee on Ways and Means, "Health Care Reform," vol. 8, 103rd Cong., 2nd Sess. (February 9, 1994), 210; U.S. House, Committee on Education and Labor, "Hearings on Health Care Reform," vol. 2, 103rd Cong., 2nd Sess. (January 31, 1994, and February 7, 1994), 205, 212, and 219.

111   U.S. House, Committee on Ways and Means, "Employer Mandate and Related Provisions of the Administration's Health Security Act," 103rd Cong., 2nd Sess. (February 3, 1994), 25.

112   U.S. House, Committee on Ways and Means, "Financing Provisions of the Administration's Health Security Act and Other Health Reform Proposals," 103rd Cong., 1st Sess. (November 16, 18, and 19, 1993), 119.

113   See U.S. House, Subcommittee on Labor-Management Relations of the Committee on Education and Labor, "Hearings on Health Care Reform," 103rd Cong., 2nd. Sess. (February 1994), 7–75.

114   U.S. House, Committee on Education and Labor, "Hearings on Health Care Reform," vol. 2, 103rd Cong., 2nd Sess. (February 7, 1994), 255 and 294.

115   Theda Skocpol, "The Aftermath of Defeat," *Journal of Health Politics, Policy and Law* 20, no. 2 (Summer 1995): 485–89; Lawrence R. Jacobs and Robert Y. Shapiro, "Don't Blame the Public for Failed Health Care Reform," *Journal of Health Politics, Policy and Law* 20, no. 2 (Summer 1995): 411–23; and Shea, interview.

116   For more on the Canadian case, see ch. 2.

117   Gwen Ifill, "Clinton's Standard Campaign Speech: A Call for Responsibility," *The New York Times* (April 26, 1992): sec. 1, pt. 1:24.

118   See Bill Clinton, "September 1993 Health Security Speech," in *Solving America's Health-Care Crisis*, ed. Erik Eckholm (New York: Times Books, Random House, 1993), 301–14.

119   For instance, Secretary of Labor Robert B. Reich told legislators in the fall of 1993, "In the absence of reform, health care costs will continue to strangle public investment, business competitiveness, job creation, and wage growth." He assured legislators that "Clinton's health care reform plan offers the bold medicine necessary to release this chokehold." Robert B. Reich, U.S. House, Committee on Education and Labor, "Hearings on the President's Health Care Reform Proposal," vol. 1, 103rd Cong., 1st Sess. (October 7 and 14, 1993), 183–84.

120   For more on the polarized political environment, see Alberto Alesina and Howard Rosenthal, *Partisan Politics, Divided Government, and the Economy* (Cambridge and New York: Cambridge University Press, 1995); and David W. Rohde, *Parties and Leaders in the Postreform House* (Chicago and London: The University of Chicago Press, 1991). On the determination of labor's opponents to kill any health-care reform bill, see Skocpol, *Boomerang;* and Johnson and Broder, *The System*.

[121] "Health-Care Debate Spawns Flood of Lobbyists' Cash," *The Philadelphia Inquirer* (July 22, 1994), cited in "Health Care Reform: Biggest Lobbying Campaign Ever," *Health Letter* (Public Citizen's Health Research Group) (November 1994): 11–12; Thomas Scarlett, "Killing Health Care Reform: How Clinton's Opponents Used a Political Media Campaign to Lobby Congress and Sway Public Opinion," *Campaigns and Elections* (October–November 1994): 34–37; and Center for Public Integrity, "Well-Healed: Inside Lobbying for Health Care Reform" (Washington, D.C.: Center for Public Integrity, 1994), 593–632.

[122] Mark A. Peterson, "The Health Care Debate: All Heat and No Light," *Journal of Health Politics, Policy and Law* 20, no. 2 (Summer 1995): 425–30; and Theodore R. Marmor, "A Summer of Discontent: Press Coverage of Murder and Medical Care Reform," *Journal of Health Politics, Policy and Law* 20, no. 2 (Summer 1995): 485–89.

[123] The broadcast media, for example, devoted twice as much time to the health-care activities of the Christian Coalition, with its 1 million members, as to the activities of the AFL-CIO, with its 13 million members. Annenberg Center, "Newspaper and Television Coverage of the Health Care Reform Debate," 7. See also Hacker, *The Road to Nowhere*, 63–67; Trudy Lieberman, "Covering Health Care Reform: Round One," *Columbia Journalism Review* (September–October 1993): 33; Annenberg Center, "Newspaper and Television Coverage of the Health Care Reform Debate," Table 2, 11; and J. Brundin, "How the U.S. Press Covers the Canadian Health Care System," *International Journal of Health Services* 23, no. 2: 275–77, cited in Sven Steinmo and Jon Watts, "It's the Institutions, Stupid! Why Comprehensive National Health Insurance Always Fails in America," *Journal of Health Politics, Policy and Law* 20, no. 2 (Summer 1995): 461.

[124] For more on crises and cross-class coalitions, see Peter Swenson, "Arranged Alliance: Business Interests in the New Deal," *Politics & Society* 25, no. 1 (March 1997): 66–116. For a detailed critique of Skocpol's *Boomerang* that stresses the importance of "popular activism and mass protests in compelling elites to accept political change," see Jennifer Klein, "Bringing Politics Back In: Health Security and Social Politics in America," *Radical History Review* 69 (1997): 271.

[125] For more on the difficulties of coalition building today, see *The Social Divide: Political Parties and the Future of Activist Government*, ed. Margaret Weir (Washington, D.C.: Brookings Institution, 1998).

Chapter 8: Conclusion

[1] Sven Steinmo and Kathleen Thelen, "Historical Institutionalism in Comparative Politics," in *Structuring Politics: Historical Institutionalism in Comparative Analysis*, ed. Sven Steinmo, Kathleen Thelen, and Frank Longstreth (Cambridge: Cambridge University Press, 1992), 3. Or as David B. Truman reminds us, institutions do not "prescribe all the meanderings of politics." Rather, they "mark some of its limits" and "designate certain points through which it must flow." Truman, *The Governmental Process* (New York: Knopf, 1953), 322.

[2] For a good discussion of the intersection between political economy and historical institutionalism, see Jonas Pontusson, "From Comparative Public Policy to Political Economy: Putting Political Institutions in Their Place and Taking Interests Seriously," *Comparative Political Studies* 28, no. 1 (April 1995): 117–47.

[3] For a good overview of the three main waves—rational choice institutionalism, sociological institutionalism, and historical institutionalism—and their relationship to one another, see Peter A. Hall and Rosemary C. R. Taylor, "Political Science and the Three Institutionalisms," *Political Studies* 44 (1996): 936–57.

[4] For a development of this point, see Stephen Skowronek, *Building a New American State: The Expansion of National Administrative Capacities, 1877–1920* (Cambridge: Cambridge University Press, 1982), esp. 8–9 and 13; *The Politics of Social Policy in the United States*, ed. Mar-

garet Weir, Ann Shola Orloff, and Theda Skocpol (Princeton, N.J.: Princeton University Press, 1988); and Margaret Weir and Theda Skocpol, "State Structures and Social Keynesianism," *International Journal of Comparative Sociology* 24 (1983): 4–29.

⁵ Frank R. Dobbin, "The Origins of Private Social Insurance: Public Policy and Fringe Benefits in America, 1920–1950," *American Journal of Sociology* 97, no. 5 (1992): 1420. See also, Margaret Weir, *Politics and Jobs: The Boundaries of Employment Policy in the United States* (Princeton, N.J.: Princeton University Press, 1992), esp. 16.

⁶ Karen Orren and Stephen Skowronek, "Beyond the Iconography of Order: Notes for a New Institutionalism," in *The Dynamics of American Politics: Approaches and Interpretations*, ed. Larry C. Dodd and Calvin Jillson (Boulder, Colo.: Westview, 1993); and Rogers M. Smith, "Beyond Tocqueville, Myrdal, and Hartz: The Multiple Traditions in America," *American Political Science Review* 87, no. 3 (September 1993): 549–66.

⁷ E. E. Schattschneider, *The Semi-Sovereign People: A Realist's View of Democracy in America* (New York: Holt, Rinehart, and Winston, 1960), 68.

⁸ On path dependency, see Paul Pierson, "The Path to European Integration: A Historical Institutionalist Analysis," *Comparative Political Studies* 29, no. 2 (April 1996): 123–63; *The Politics of Social Policy in the United States*, ed. Weir, Orloff, and Skocpol; and Weir, *Politics and Jobs*, esp. 18.

⁹ The well known "switchmen" metaphor comes, of course, from Max Weber, "The Social Psychology of the World Religions" (1913), in *From Max Weber: Essays in Sociology*, ed. H. H. Gerth and C. Wright Mills (New York: Oxford University Press, 1958), 280.

¹⁰ See the contributions to Judith Goldstein and Robert O. Keohane, *Ideas and Foreign Policy: Beliefs, Institutions, and Political Change*, ed. Judith Goldstein and Robert O. Keohane (Ithaca, N.Y.: Cornell University Press, 1993); and *The Political Power of Economic Ideas: Keynesianism Across Nations*, ed. Peter A. Hall (Princeton, N.J.: Princeton University Press, 1989).

¹¹ For the alternative definitions or understandings of ideas, see, respectively, Sheri Berman, *The Social Democratic Moment: Ideas and Politics in the Making of Interwar Europe* (Cambridge: Harvard University Press, 1998), 33; Goldstein and Keohane, "Ideas and Foreign Policy," in *Ideas and Foreign Policy*, ed. Goldstein and Keohane, 8–11; and Peter Hall, "Policy Paradigms, Social Learning, and the State," *Comparative Politics* 25, no. 3 (April 1993): 275–96.

¹² For a development of this point, see Theodore R. Marmor, "Introduction," *Political Analysis and American Medical Care: Essays* (Cambridge: Cambridge University Press, 1983).

¹³ Julius Getman, *The Betrayal of Local 14* (Ithaca, N.Y., and London: ILR and Cornell University Press, 1998).

¹⁴ James A. Morone, "The Bureaucracy Empowered," in *The Politics of Health Care Reform: Lessons From the Past, Prospects for the Future*, ed. James A. Morone and Gary S. Belkin (Durham, N.C.: Duke University Press, 1994), 149.

¹⁵ Colin Gordon, *New Deals: Business, Labor, and Politics in America, 1920–1935* (Cambridge: Cambridge University Press, 1994).

¹⁶ Peter Swenson, "Arranged Alliance: Business Interests in the New Deal," *Politics & Society* 25, no. 1 (March 1997): 100.

¹⁷ Arthur Neef and James Thomas, "International Comparisons of Productivity and Unit Labor Cost Trends in Manufacturing," *Monthly Labor Review* (December 1988): 28. Judged in terms of output growth, the economic expansion of the 1980s was comparable to the expansion of the 1960s. Rebecca M. Blank and David Card, "Poverty, Income Distribution, and Growth: Are They Still Connected?," in *Brookings Papers on Economic Activity* 2 (Washington, D.C.: The Brookings Institution, 1993), 287. Blank and Card contend that the two expansions were distinct in some other important respects. The economic expansion of the 1980s had far weaker redistributive effects and failed to substantially reduce poverty or narrow income inequality, unlike other postwar expansions.

¹⁸ Edwin Amenta and Yvonne Zylan, "It Happened Here; Political Opportunity, the New Institutionalism, and the Townsend Movement," *American Sociological Review* 56 (April

1991): 250–65; Arthur M. Schlesinger, Jr., *The Politics of Upheaval: The Age of Roosevelt* (Boston: Houghton Mifflin, 1960), 33–37 and 551; Martha Derthick, *Policymaking for Social Security* (Washington, D.C.: The Brookings Institution, 1979), 194–205; Sheryl R. Tynes, *Turning Points in Social Security: From 'Cruel Hoax' to Sacred Entitlement* (Stanford, Calif.: Stanford University Press, 1996), 33–34; and Alan Brinkley, *The End of Reform* (New York: Vintage, 1996), 12.

For a more general discussion of how the bargaining position of moderates can be strengthened by the presence of more radical groups or alternatives, see Herbert Haines, "Black Radicalization and the Funding of Civil Rights: 1957–1970," *Social Problems* 32, no. 1 (October 1984): 31–43.

[19] John R. Commons, *Institutional Economics: Its Place in Political Economy* (Madison: University of Wisconsin, 1959 [1934]), 854, in Peter Swenson, "Arranged Alliance," 103.

[20] Mike Davis, *Prisoners of the American Dream: Politics and Economy in the History of the US Working Class* (London: Verso, 1986), 52; and Joel Rogers, "The Folks Who Brought You the Weekend: Labor and Independent Politics," in *Audacious Democracy: Labor, Intellectuals, and the Social Reconstruction of America*, ed. Steven Fraser and Joshua B. Freeman (Boston: Mariner, 1997), 255.

[21] Dan Balz and Ronald Brownstein, *Storming the Gates: Protest Politics and the Republican Revival* (Boston: Little, Brown, 1996), 116–17 and 142–43; and "Mr. Speaker: The Rise of Newt Gingrich," four-part series, *The Washington Post* (December 18–21, 1994): A-1.

[22] David Brody, *Workers in Industrial America*, 2nd ed. (New York: Oxford University Press, 1993), esp. 249–53; Brody, "Labor's Crisis in Historical Perspective," in *The State of the Unions*, ed. George Strauss, Daniel G. Gallagher, and Jack Fiorito (Madison, Wis.: Industrial Relations Research Association, 1991); and Charles C. Heckscher, *The New Unionism: Employee Involvement in the Changing Corporation* (New York: Basic Books, 1987), 237.

[23] Moreover, the founders of the CIO hailed from the AFL, and some of them even served on its executive council. Solomon Barkin, "Pure and Simple Unionism: An Adequate Base for Union Growth?" in Strauss et al., *The State of the Unions*.

[24] Edward Ian Robinson, "Organizing Labour: Explaining Canada–U.S. Union Diversity in the Post-War Period" (Ph.D. dissertation, Yale University, 1992).

[25] Between the early 1960s and the early 1980s, Canadian unions more than doubled their membership. By the early 1980s, the unionized sector of the Canadian workforce approached 40 percent, more than double the figure for the United States. Brody, *Workers in Industrial America*, 245–46.

For a more pessimistic view of the recent political prospects for organized labor in Canada, see Leo Panitch and Donald Swartz, *The Assault on Trade Union Freedom: From Wage Controls to Social Contract* (Toronto: Garamond Press, 1993); and Miriam Catherine Smith, "Labour Without Allies: The Canadian Labour Congress in Politics, 1956–1988" (Ph.D. dissertation, Yale University, 1990).

[26] Rex Hardesty, "Labor Pledges to Keep Fighting for Health Care," *AFL-CIO News* (October 3, 1994): 1.

[27] David Moberg, "Heeding the Call," *In These Times* (November 13, 1995): 20–22. For more on the AFL-CIO electoral contest, see Laura McClure, "AFL-CIO: A New Era?," *Labor Notes* (December 1995): 1; and David Moberg, "State of the Unions; interview with Richard Trumka," *In These Times* (April 1, 1996): 22–23.

[28] He opposed both the direct election of international officers by the membership and a prohibition on dual salaries for the SEIU's top officers. Furthermore, Sweeney has supported on occasion the hounding of SEIU dissident reformers. Kay Eisenhower, "First-Ever Contested Election Gives Service Employees a Taste of Democracy," *Labor Notes* (June 1992): 5; Martha Gruelle, "Service Employees Open Debate on Their Union's Future," *Labor Notes* (March 1996): 8–9; and Kim Moody, "American Labor: A Movement Again?" *Monthly Review* 49, no. 3 (July–August 1997): 63–79.

[29] John J. Sweeney, "How Much?" *Service Employees Union* (March/April 1995).

[30] Shortly after he became the federation's new president, Sweeney commended Clinton for doing "a lot of pro-worker business" and assured the rank and file that the president of the United States "would not take us for granted." Harry Bernstein, "John J. Sweeney: Can the Vigor Be Restored to America's Labor Movement?" *Los Angeles Times* (October 29, 1995): H-3.

[31] John J. Sweeney, with David Kusnet, *America Needs a Raise: Fighting for Economic Security and Social Justice* (Boston: Houghton Mifflin, 1996), 5–6 and 32; Steven Greenhouse, "Labor Chief Asks Business for a New 'Social Compact'," *The New York Times* (December 7, 1995): A-20; and Jane Slaughter, "AFL-CIO Seeks Partnership With GE's 'Neutron Jack'," *Labor Notes* (October 1998): 1.

[32] "Sweeney's Wake-Up Call to Business," *Economic Notes* (January 1996): 3.

[33] Gerald M. Shea, assistant to the president for governmental affairs, AFL-CIO, interview, Washington, D.C., June 13, 1996. See also, Sweeney, *America Needs a Raise.*

[34] "AFL-CIO Is Planning to Focus Anew On Social Issues," *The Wall Street Journal* (February 18, 1997): 1; David Moberg, "Union Pension Power," *The Nation* (June 1, 1998): 16–20; and *Not Your Father's Union Movement: Inside the AFL-CIO*, ed. Jo-Ann Mort (London and New York: Verso, 1998).

[35] One needs to be careful not to overstate the significance of this victory. Republicans tacked onto the minimum wage legislation billions of dollars in tax breaks and subsidies that were on the wish lists of the Fortune 500 and the small business sector for years. Elizabeth Lee, "The Minimum Wage Increase Act of 1996: Minimum Wage Increase, Maximum Benefits for Business" (senior essay, Yale University, April 1997).

[36] Estimates vary enormously on just how much organized labor spent. The oft-cited figure of $35 million actually was a supplement to other spending for political purposes that did not have to be reported to the Federal Election Commission because it was not spent on advertisements that specifically advocated the election of a Democratic candidate. Morton M. Kondracke, "Payback Time: GOP Plots Attack on Labor Unions," *Roll Call* (November 21, 1996): 6.

[37] "The unions fired and missed," gloated an aide to Rep. Bill Paxon (R-N.Y.), a leading House Republican, soon after the election. "The best retribution is that we have 218 votes and they don't." Kondracke, "Payback Time."

[38] Twelve of the 44 freshmen who were targeted were defeated, while every one of the 27 who were not targeted retained their seats. Other things being equal, "the vote for Republican freshmen who were targets of the AFL-CIO video campaigns was typically about eight percentage points lower than the vote for freshmen who were not targeted." Gary C. Jacobson, "The 105th Congress: Unprecedented and Unsurprising," in *The Elections of 1996*, ed. Michael Nelson (Washington, D.C.: Congressional Quarterly Press, 1997), 156–57.

[39] Paul A. Gigot, "Terminator II: Why Big Labor Keeps on Coming," *The Wall Street Journal* (April 11, 1997): A-14.

[40] Jill Abramson and Steven Greenhouse, "Labor Victory on Trade Bill Reveals Power," *The New York Times* (November 12, 1997): A-1.

[41] William Safire, "The Demo-Labor Party," *The New York Times* (November 12, 1997): A-31.

[42] Frank Swoboda, "AFL-CIO Fights Proposed Union Spending Curbs," *The Washington Post* (March 20, 1998): A-8.

[43] "A Few Good Victories," *The Nation* (November 23, 1998): 3–4; and Steven Greenhouse, "Republicans Credit Labor for Success by Democrats," *The New York Times* (November 6, 1998): A-28.

[44] Sarah Luthens, "Labor to Join the 'Protest of the Century' Against World Trade Organization," *Labor Notes* (October 1999): 16.

[45] Kim Moody, "On Eve of Seattle Trade Protests, Sweeney Endorses Clinton's Agenda," *Labor Notes* (December 1999): 1.

⁴⁶ For example, in June 1998, in a controversial move, Sweeney dismissed Richard Bensinger, the widely respected organizing director of the AFL-CIO. Sweeney reportedly fired Bensinger because he had alienated labor's old guard with his strident emphasis on the need to organize new members. Leah Samuel, "AFL's Top Organizer Ousted," *Labor Notes* (August 1998): 2; and David Moberg, "Organizing to Win?," *In These Times* (August 9, 1998): 11–13.

⁴⁷ In defense of efforts to explore the possibility of launching a third party, Stern declared, "As the Democrats continue to support Republican anti-worker policies, the need for an independent labor-based strategy is clearer than ever." Andy Stern, letter to the editor, *The Nation* (June 23, 1997): 2.

⁴⁸ J. Peter Nixon, senior policy analyst, SEIU, interview, Washington, D.C., June 3, 1996.

⁴⁹ The one exception here is the OCAW and other unionists associated with the fledgling Labor Party, which kicked off a national campaign for a single-payer health-care system at the party's constitutional convention in late 1998. Kim Moody, "Labor Party's Convention Clears the Way to Run Candidates, Sets Health Care Campaign," *Labor Notes* (December 1998): 3.

⁵⁰ Lisa Belkin, "The Ellwoods; But What About Quality?," *The New York Times Magazine* (December 8, 1996): 68; SEIU, "Demanding Quality: SEIU Principles for Quality Care" (Washington, D.C.: SEIU 1996); and the home page for FACCT at http://www.facct.org. See also David Bacon, "Whose Side Are You On?," *In These Times* (August 11, 1997): 28–29; and Marc Cooper, "Labor's Hardest Drive: Organizing a New Politics," *The Nation* (November 24, 1997): 18.

⁵¹ For more on the origins of the Jackson Hole Group, see Jacob S. Hacker, *The Road to Nowhere: The Genesis of President Clinton's Plan for Health Security* (Princeton, N.J.: Princeton University Press, 1997), 52–60.

⁵² Milt Freudenheim, "Employees Face Steep Increases in Health Costs," *The New York Times* (November 27, 1998): A-1; Jennifer Steinhauer, "Health Insurance Costs Rise, Hitting Small Business Hard," *The New York Times* (January 19, 1999): A-1; and Robert Pear, "Government Lags in Steps to Widen Coverage," *The New York Times* (August 9, 1998): sec. 1, 1.

⁵³ "Medicare Recommendations Delayed," *St. Petersburg Times* (February 27, 1999): A-2; William M. Welch, "Medicare Reform Plan Raises Age Threshold," *USA Today* (January 27, 1999): A-2; and Michael M. Weinstein, "The Nation: Fixing Medicare; Light at a Tunnel's End," *The New York Times* (January 10, 1999): sec. 4, 3.

⁵⁴ Elisabeth Rosenthal, "Union Plans to Market Own HMO," *The New York Times* (December 17, 1996): B-1.

⁵⁵ Ian Fisher, "Empire Blue Cross Rejects Takeover Plan," *The New York Times* (February 26, 1998): B-6.

⁵⁶ David Lefer, "Rivera's Star Rising: Local 1199 Chief Is Emerging as Rights Leader," *The Daily News* (April 18, 1999): 39.

⁵⁷ James S. Ray, legislative representative, NCCMP, interview, Washington, D.C., June 13, 1996, and U.S. House, Subcommittee on Health of the Committee on Ways and Means, "Prepared Testimony of James S. Ray," Federal News Service (May 25, 1995): electronic database. Ray concedes that some of his comrades-in-arms in organized labor, as well as key legislators like Rep. Pete Stark (D-Calif.), view such measures with alarm and predict that they would hasten the demise of Medicare as yet another piece of the public welfare state is returned to the private sector.

⁵⁸ Steven Greenhouse, "The Most Innovative Figure in Silicon Valley? Maybe This Labor Organizer," *The New York Times* (November 14, 1999): sec. 1, 32.

⁵⁹ The same is true for public-interest groups. For instance, the AARP cannot be counted on to champion national health insurance or even ardently defend Medicare. Because it is a major provider of supplemental health insurance to the aged, the AARP is unlikely to lead the

charge for eliminating private insurance in the United States. Furthermore, because of the AARP's extensive role in insurance provision and its other revenue-producing activities, its tax-exempt status remains the soft underbelly of its political activism. Adriel Bettelheim, "Its Clout Often Makes AARP a Target," *The Denver Post* (May 20, 1996): A-1; and John Rother, AARP director of legislation and public policy, interview, June 5, 1996, Washington, D.C.

⁶⁰ Robert Pear, "Health Care Proposals Help Define Democrats," *The New York Times* (December 20, 1999): A-32; "A Health Care Proposal by Bill Bradley" (September 28, 1999), http://www.billbradley.com; and James Dao, "Bradley Presents Health Plan for Almost All the Uninsured," *The New York Times* (September 29, 1999): A-1.

⁶¹ Robert Pear, "Insurers Ask Government to Extend Health Plans," *The New York Times* (May 23, 1999): sec. 1, 16.

⁶² See Andrew Richards, "Down But Not Out: Labour Movements in Late Industrial Societies," working paper (Madrid: Instituto Juan March de Estudios e Investigaciones, May 1995), esp. 45; and *Building Bridges: The Emerging Grassroots Coalition of Labor and Community*, ed. Jeremy Brecher and Tim Costello (New York: Monthly Review Press, 1990). For a critical view of this perspective, see Kim Scipes, "Labor-Community Coalitions: Not All They're Cracked Up to Be," *Monthly Review Press* 43, no. 7 (December 1991): 34–46; and the response by Brecher and Costello, 47–51.

⁶³ For a moving account of the P-9 strike, see *American Dream*, the Oscar-winning documentary directed by Barbara Kopple. See also Kim Moody, "Review: Austin Nightmare," *Labor Notes* (May 1992): 10; and Nicolaus Mills, "The Hormel Strike: Why Local P-9 Is Going It Alone," *The Nation* (April 26, 1986): 578–81.

⁶⁴ Jonathan D. Rosenblum, *Copper Crucible: How the Arizona Miners' Strike of 1983 Recast Labor-Management Relations in America* (Ithaca, N.Y.: ILR Press, 1995).

⁶⁵ Adolph Reed, "Toward a More Perfect Union," *The Village Voice* (October 3, 1995): 24.

⁶⁶ Brody, *Workers in Industrial America*, 2nd ed., 238.

⁶⁷ Weir, "American Politics and the Future of Social Policy," in *The Social Divide: Political Parties and the Future of Activist Government*, ed. Weir (Washington, D.C.: Brookings Institution, 1998), 525. See also, Rogers, "The Folks Who Brought You the Weekend"; and Richard Oestreicher, "The Rules of the Game: Class Politics in Twentieth Century America," in *Organized Labor and American Politics, 1894–1994: The Labor-Liberal Alliance*, ed. Kevin Boyle (Albany: SUNY Press, 1998), 44.

Abbreviations

AARP	American Association of Retired Persons
ACTWU	Amalgamated Clothing and Textile Workers Union
AFL-CIO	American Federation of Labor–Congress of Industrial Organizations
AFSCME	American Federation of State, County and Municipal Employees
AFT	American Federation of Teachers
AMA	American Medical Association
APHA	American Public Health Association
APWU	American Postal Workers Union
BAC	International Union of Bricklayers and Allied Craftsmen
CCF	Cooperative Commonwealth Federation
CNHI	Committee for National Health Insurance
COPE	Committee on Political Education
CWA	Communications Workers of America
ERIC	ERISA Industry Committee
ERISA	Employee Retirement Income Security Act
HMO	Health maintenance organization
IAM	International Association of Machinists
ILGWU	International Ladies Garment Workers Union
NAFTA	North American Free-Trade Agreement
NAM	National Association of Manufacturers
NCCMP	National Coordinating Committee of Multiemployer Plans
NCSC	National Council of Senior Citizens
NDP	New Democratic Party
NFIB	National Federation of Independent Business
NLCHCR	National Leadership Coalition for Health Care Reform
OCAW	Oil, Chemical, and Atomic Workers
PNHP	Physicians for a National Health Program
RWDSU	Retail, Wholesale and Department Store Union
SEIU	Service Employees International Union

TCU	Transportation and Communications International Union
UAW	United Automobile, Aerospace and Agricultural Implement Workers
UFCW	United Food and Commercial Workers
UMW	United Mine Workers
UNITE	Union of Needletrades, Industrial and Textile Employees
USWA	United Steelworkers of America
WBGH	Washington Business Group on Health

Interviewees

DAVID ABERNETHY, former majority staff director, Subcommittee on Health of the Committee on Ways and Means, U.S. House of Representatives. At the time of the interview, Abernethy was an executive with the Health Insurance Plan of Greater New York.

G. LAWRENCE ATKINS, coordinator, Corporate Health Care Coalition and senior vice president, government relations, The Jefferson Group.

WILLIE L. BAKER, JR., director of civil rights and community relations, United Food and Commercial Workers (UFCW).

DAVID BUCHANAN, senior legislative assistant for Rep. John Conyers (D-Mich.).

JULIE CANTOR-WEINBERG, associate director, employee benefits, National Association of Manufacturers (NAM).

JANE DELGADO, executive director, National Coalition of Hispanic Health and Human Services Organizations (COSSMHO).

EVELYN DUBROW, former legislative director, International Ladies Garment Workers Union (ILGWU). At the time of the interview, Dubrow was the legislative director of the Union of Needletrades, Industrial and Textile Employees (UNITE), which was formed by the merger of the ILGWU and the Amalgamated Clothing and Textile Workers Union (ACTWU) in 1995.

MARY KAY HENRY, director, health-care division, Service Employees International Union (SEIU).

JEFF P. JACOBS, director of Congressional affairs, American Public Health Association (APHA).

JAMES JOHNSTON, former vice president of industry-government relations, General Motors. At the time of the interview, Johnston was a resident fellow at the American Enterprise Institute.

KAREN KERRIGAN, director, Small Business Survival Committee.

WILLIAM F. LITTLE, health and benefits manager, Ford.

WALTER B. MAHER, director of public policy, Chrysler Corporation.

ROBERT MCGARRAH, director of public policy, American Federation of State, County and Municipal Employees (AFSCME).

ROBERT M. MCGLOTTEN, legislative director of the AFL-CIO from 1986 to 1995. At the time of the interview, McGlotten was employed with McGlotten & Jarvis.

SARA NICHOLS, former staff attorney, Public Citizen. At the time of the interview, Nichols was Washington director of the Physicians for a National Health Program (PNHP).

J. PETER NIXON, senior policy analyst, Service Employees International Union (SEIU).

JAMES S. RAY, legislative representative for the National Coordinating Committee for Multiemployer Plans (NCCMP). At the time of the interview, Ray was also an attorney with Connerton, Ray & Simon.

ALAN REUTHER, legislative director, United Automobile, Aerospace and Agricultural Implement Workers (UAW).

MARGARET M. RHOADES, executive director, National Leadership Coalition on Health Care.

JOHN ROTHER, director of legislation and public policy, American Association of Retired Persons (AARP). Rother also headed the Health Care Reform Project, a broad coalition of labor, consumer, and health groups.

MICHAEL O. ROUSH, director of federal governmental relations, Senate, National Federation of Independent Business (NFIB).

CLAUDIA BRADBURY ST. JOHN, former senior health policy specialist, AFL-CIO. At the time of the interview, she was director of the Consumer Healthcare Center of the National Consumers League.

ANDREAS "ANDY" SCHNEIDER, former counsel, Subcommittee on Health of the Committee on Energy and Commerce, U.S. House of Representatives. At the time of the interview, Schneider was a member of the professional staff of the House Democratic Leadership Policy Committee.

JOHANNA SCHNEIDER, director of communications, Business Roundtable.

DANIEL J. SCHULDER, director, department of legislation, National Council of Senior Citizens (NCSC).

BERT SEIDMAN, director of the department of social security of the AFL-CIO from 1966 until his retirement in 1990. At the time of the interview, Seidman was a consultant for the National Council of Senior Citizens (NCSC).

GERALD M. SHEA, director of the health-care division of the Service Employees International Union (SEIU) until September 1993, when he moved to the AFL-CIO to direct its employee benefits department. At the time of the interview, Shea was assistant to the president for governmental affairs, AFL-CIO.

GAIL SHEARER, director, health policy analysis, Consumers Union.

KATHLEEN M. SKRABUT, senior legislative representative, Service Employees International Union (SEIU).

BARBARA MARKHAM SMITH, former legislative aide for health policy for Rep. James McDermott (D-Wash.). At the time of the interview, Smith was a senior research staff scientist with the Center for Health Policy Research, Washington, D.C.

LISA M. SPRAGUE, former manager of employee benefits, U.S. Chamber of Commerce. At the time of the interview, Sprague was director of legislative affairs for the Association of Managed Healthcare Organizations.

PHYLLIS TORDA, former director of health policy, Families USA. At the time of the interview, Torda was an assistant vice president of the National Committee for Quality Assurance.

FERNANDO TREVINO, executive director, American Public Health Association (APHA).

DR. YVONNECRIS VEAL, president, National Medical Association.

LYNN WILLIAMS, former president, United Steelworkers of America (USWA).

STEVE WILSON, chief of staff for Rep. Marge Roukema (R-N.J.).

Bibliography

Archives

AFL, AFL-CIO Department of Legislation, 1906–78 Legislation, George Meany Memorial Archives, Silver Spring, Md.
AFSME Office of the President: Jerry Wurf Papers, Walter P. Reuther Library, Wayne State University, Detroit, Mich.
Amalgamated Clothing Workers of America Records: Jack Sheinkman Papers, Labor-Management Documentation Center, Cornell University, Ithaca, N.Y.
Committee for National Health Insurance (CNHI) Collection, Walter P. Reuther Library, Wayne State University, Detroit.
Chamber of Commerce of the United States Records: Statements, Speeches, Etc., Arch N. Booth, Accession 1960, Hagley Library, Wilmington, Del.
UAW President's Office: Douglas A. Fraser Collection, Wayne State University, Walter P. Reuther Library, Detroit.
UAW Washington Office: Stephen Schlossberg Collection, Walter P. Reuther Library, Wayne State University, Detroit.

Periodicals

AFL-CIO, *AFL-CIO News*
AFSCME, *Public Employee*
Business and Health
California AFL-CIO News
Economic Notes
Labor Notes
Monthly Labor Review
National Journal
OCAW, *OCAW Reporter*
Public Citizen Research Group, *Health Letter*
SEIU, *Service Employees Union*
———, *Leadership Newsletter*
———, *Political and Legislative Newsletter*
———, *SEIU Leadership News Update*
———, *Service Employee*
UAW, *Solidarity*
———, *UAW Washington Report*

249

U.S. Chamber of Commerce, *Nation's Business*
USWA, *Steelabor*

Books and Articles

Abramson, Paul R., John H. Aldrich, and David W. Rohde, *Change and Continuity in the 1988 Elections*. Washington, D.C.: Congressional Quarterly Press, 1990.
————, *Change and Continuity in the 1992 Elections*. Washington, D.C.: Congressional Quarterly Press, 1994.
————. *Change and Continuity in the 1996 Elections*. Washington, D.C.: Congressional Quarterly Press, 1998.
AFL-CIO. "The Case for Health Care Reform: The People Speak, Transcripts from Regional Hearings, September–October 1990." Washington, D.C.: AFL-CIO, 1990.
Akard, Patrick J. "Corporate Mobilization and Political Power: The Transformation of U.S. Economic Power in the 1970s." *American Sociological Review* 57 (1992): 597–615.
Alesina, Alberto, and Howard Rosenthal. *Partisan Politics, Divided Government, and the Economy*. Cambridge: Cambridge University Press, 1995.
Alford, Robert R. *Health Care Politics: Ideological and Interest Group Barriers to Reform*. Chicago: University of Chicago Press, 1975.
Allen, Donna. *Fringe Benefits: Wages or Social Obligation?* Ithaca, N.Y.: Cornell University Press, 1964.
Amberg, Stephen. *Union Inspiration in American Politics: The Autoworkers and the Making of a Liberal Industrial Order*. Philadelphia: Temple University Press, 1994.
————. "The CIO Political Strategy in Historical Perspective: Creating a High-Road Economy in the Post-War Era." *Organized Labor and American Politics, 1894–1994: The Liberal-Labor Alliance*. Kevin Boyle, ed. Albany: SUNY Press, 1998: 159–94.
Amenta, Edwin, et al. "The Political Origins of Unemployment Insurance in Five American States." *Studies in American Political Development* 2 (1987): 137–82.
Amenta, Edwin, and Theda Skocpol. "States and Social Policies." *Annual Review of Sociology* 12 (1986): 131–57.
Amenta, Edwin, and Yvonne Zylan. "It Happened Here: Political Opportunity, the New Institutionalism, and the Townsend Movement." *American Sociological Review* 56 (April 1991): 250–65.
Annenberg Public Policy Center of the University of Pennsylvania. "Media in the Middle: Fairness and Accuracy in the 1994 Health Care Reform Debate." Philadelphia: February 1995.
————. "Newspaper and Television Coverage of the Health Care Reform Debate: January 16–July 25, 1994." Philadelphia: August 12, 1994.
Aronowitz, Stanley. "The Labor Movement and the Left in the United States." *Socialist Review* 9.2 (1979): 9–61.
————. *Working Class Hero: A New Strategy for Labor*. New York: The Pilgrim Press, 1983.
Atkins, G. Lawrence, and Kristin Bass. *ERISA Preemption: The Key to Market Innovation in Health Care*. Washington, D.C.: Corporate Health Care Coalition, 1995.
Axelrod, Robert. "Presidential Election Coalitions in 1984." *American Political Science Review* 80 (March 1986): 281–84.
Barkin, Solomon. "Pure and Simple Unionism: An Adequate Base for Union Growth?" *The State of the Unions*. George Strauss, Daniel G. Gallagher, and Jack Fiorito, eds. Madison, Wis.: Industrial Relations Research Association, 1991.
Barlett, Donald L., and James B. Steele. *America: What Went Wrong?* Kansas City: Andrews and McMeel, 1992.

Bashshur, Rashid, and Cater Webb. "Nature and Dimensions of the Problem of Access." *Improving Access to Health Care: What Can the States Do?* John H. Goddeeris and Andrew J. Hogan, eds. Kalamazoo, Mich.: W.E. Upjohn Institute for Employment Research, 1992.

Battista, Andrew. "Political Divisions in Organized Labor." *Polity* 24.2 (Winter 1991): 173–97.

Baumgartner, Frank R., and Bryan D. Jones. *Agendas and Instability in American Politics.* Chicago: Chicago University Press, 1993.

Bean, Jonathan J. *Beyond the Broker State: Federal Policies Toward Small Business, 1936–1961.* Chapel Hill: The University of North Carolina Press, 1996.

Bell, Deborah E. "Unionized Women in State and Local Government." *Women, Work and Protest: A Century of U.S. Women's Labor History.* Ruth Milkman, ed. Boston: Routledge & Kegan Paul, 1985.

Belous, Richard S. *The Contingent Economy: The Growth of the Temporary, Part-Time, and Subcontracted Workforce.* Washington, D.C.: National Planning Association, 1989.

Bendix, Reinhard. *Work and Authority in Industry: Ideologies of Management in the Course of Industrialization.* Berkeley: University of California Press, 1974.

Bennett, James T. "Private Sector Unions: The Myth of Decline." *Journal of Labor Research* 12.1 (Winter 1991): 1–12.

Bennett, James T., and John T. Delaney. "Research on Unions: Some Subjects in Need of Scholars." *Journal of Labor Research* 14.2 (Spring 1993): 95–110.

Bergthold, Linda. "American Business and Health Care Reform." *American Behavioral Scientist* 36.6 (July 1993): 802–12.

———. *Purchasing Power in Health: Business, the State, and Health Care Politics.* New Brunswick, N.J.: Rutgers University Press, 1990.

———. "American Business and Health Reform." *Health Care Reform in the Nineties.* Pauline Vaillancourt Rosenau, ed. Thousand Oaks, Calif.: Sage, 1994.

———. "The Frayed Alliance: Business and Health Care in Massachusetts." *Journal of Health Politics, Policy and Law* 15.4 (Winter 1990): 915–28.

Berkowitz, Edward, and Kim McQuaid. *Creating the Welfare State: The Political Economy of Twentieth-Century Reform.* New York: Praeger, 1988.

Berman, Sheri. *The Social Democratic Moment: Ideas and Politics in the Making of Interwar Europe.* Cambridge: Harvard University Press, 1998.

Bernstein, Anya. "Inside or Outside? The Politics of Family and Medical Leave." *Policy Studies Journal* 25.1 (Spring 1997): 87–99.

Bernstein, Irving. *The Lean Years.* Boston: Houghton, Mifflin, 1960.

Blank, Rebecca M., and David Card. "Poverty, Income Distribution, and Growth: Are They Still Connected?" *Brookings Papers on Economic Activity* 2. Washington, D.C.: The Brookings Institution, 1993.

Blendon, Robert J., and Tracey Stelzer Hyams, eds. *Reforming the System: Containing Health Care Costs in an Era of Universal Coverage.* New York: Faulkner and Grey, 1992.

Bluestone, Barry, and Bennett Harrison. *The Deindustrialization of America: Plant Closings, Community Abandonment, and the Dismantling of Basic Industry.* New York: Basic Books, 1982.

Blum, Linda M. *Between Feminism and Labor: The Significance of the Comparative Worth Movement.* Berkeley: University of California Press, 1991.

Bok, Derek C., and John T. Dunlop. *Labor and the American Community.* New York: Simon & Schuster, 1970.

Boyer, Robert. "Defensive or Offensive Flexibility?" *The Search for Labor Market Flexibility: The European Economies in Transition.* Robert Boyer, ed. Oxford: Clarendon Press, 1988.

Boyle, Kevin. *The UAW and the Heyday of American Liberalism.* Ithaca, N.Y.: Cornell University Press, 1995.

————, ed. *Organized Labor and American Politics, 1894–1994: The Labor-Liberal Alliance.* Albany: SUNY Press, 1998.

————. "Little More Than Ashes: The UAW and American Reform in the 1960s." *Organized Labor and American Politics, 1894–1994: The Labor-Liberal Alliance.* Kevin Boyle, ed. Albany: SUNY Press, 1998.

Bradford, David F., and Derrick A. Max. *Intergenerational Transfers Under Community Rating.* Washington, D.C.: The AEI Press, 1996.

Brady, David W., and Kara M. Buckley. "Health Care Reform in the 103rd Congress: A Predictable Failure." *Journal of Health Politics, Policy and Law* 20.2 (Summer 1995): 447–54.

Brandes, Stuart D. *American Welfare Capitalism, 1880–1940.* Chicago: University of Chicago Press, 1976.

Braverman, Harry. *Labor and Monopoly Capital: The Degradation of Work in the Twentieth Century.* New York: Monthly Review Press, 1975.

Brecher, Jeremy, and Tim Costello, eds. *Building Bridges: The Emerging Grassroots Coalition of Labor and Community.* New York: Monthly Review Press, 1990.

Brinkley, Alan. *The End of Reform: New Deal Liberalism in Recession and War* (New York: Vintage, 1996).

Brodie, Janine. *Politics on the Margins: Restructuring and the Canadian Women's Movement.* Halifax, Nova Scotia: Fernwood Publishing, 1995.

Brodie, Mollyann, and Robert J. Blendon. "The Public's Contribution to Congressional Gridlock on Health Care Reform." *Journal of Health Politics, Policy and Law* 20.2 (Summer 1995): 403–10.

Brody, David. "Labor Movement." *Encyclopedia of American Political History.* Jack P. Greene, ed. New York: Charles Scribner's Sons, 1984.

————. "Labor's Crisis in Historical Perspective." *The State of the Unions.* George Strauss, Daniel G. Gallagher, and Jack Fiorito, eds. Madison, Wis.: Industrial Relations Research Association, 1991.

————. "On the Failure of U.S. Radical Politics: A Farmer-Labor Analysis." *Industrial Relations* 22.2 (1983): 141–163.

————. *Workers in Industrial America.* 2nd ed. New York: Oxford University Press, 1993.

Brown, Charles, James Hamilton, and James Medoff. *Employers Large and Small.* Cambridge: Harvard University Press, 1990.

Brown, Lawrence D. "Dogmatic Slumbers: American Business and Health Policy." *The Politics of Health Care Reform: Lessons From the Past, Prospects for the Future.* James A. Morone and Gary S. Belkin, eds. Durham, N.C.: Duke University Press, 1994.

————, ed. *Health Policy in Transition: A Decade of Health Politics, Policy and Law.* Durham, N.C.: Duke University Press, 1987.

————. "The Medically Uninsured: Problems, Policies, and Politics." *Journal of Health Politics, Policy and Law* 15.2 (Summer 1990).

————. *Politics and Health Care Organization: HMOs as Federal Policy.* Washington, D.C.: The Brookings Institution, 1983.

Brown, Michael K. "Bargaining for Social Rights: Unions and the Reemergence of Welfare Capitalism." *Political Science Quarterly* 112.4 (1997–98): 645–74.

Buchmueller, Thomas C. "Health Risk and Access to Employer-Provided Health Insurance." *Inquiry* 32.1 (1995): 75–86.

Budrys, Grace. *When Doctors Join Unions.* Ithaca, N.Y.: ILR Press/Cornell University Press, 1996.

Buffa, Dudley W. *Union Power and American Democracy: The U.A.W. and the Democratic Party, 1935–72.* Ann Arbor: The University of Michigan Press, 1984.

Burch, Philip H., Jr. "The NAM as an Interest Group." *Politics and Society* 4.1 (Fall 1973): 97–130.

Butler, Patricia A. "Roadblock to Reform: ERISA Implications for State Health Care Initiatives." Washington, D.C.: National Governors' Association, 1994.

Cameron, David R. "Social Democracy, Corporatism, Labour Quiescence, and the Representation of Economic Interests in Advanced Capitalist Society." *Order and Conflict in Contemporary Capitalism: Studies in the Political Economy of Western European Nations.* John H. Goldthorpe, ed. New York: Oxford University Press, 1984.

———. "The Politics and Economics of the Business Cycle." *The Political Economy: Readings in the Politics and Economics of American Public Policy.* Thomas Ferguson and Joel Rogers, eds. Armonk, N.Y.: M.E. Sharpe, 1984.

Cantor, Daniel, and Juliet Schor. *Tunnel Vision: Labor, the World Economy, and Central America.* Boston: South End Press, 1987.

Cantor, Joel C. "Expanding Health Insurance Coverage: Who Will Pay?" *Journal of Health Politics, Policy and Law* 15.4 (Winter 1990): 755–78.

Carrasquillo, Olveen, et al. "A Reappraisal of Private Employers' Role in Providing Health Insurance." *New England Journal of Medicine* 340.2 (January 14, 1999): 109–14.

Cates, Jerry R. *Insuring Inequality: Administrative Leadership in Social Security, 1935–54.* Ann Arbor: University of Michigan Press, 1983.

Chandler, William M. "Canadian Socialism and Policy Impact: Contagion From the Left?" *Canadian Journal of Political Science* 10.4 (December 1977): 755–80.

Christensen, Kathleen, and Mary Murphree. "Introduction." *Flexible Workstyles: A Look at Contingent Labor.* Washington, D.C.: Women's Bureau, U.S. Department of Labor, 1988.

Citizens Fund. "Premiums Without Benefits: The Decade-Long Growth in Commercial Health Insurance Industry Waste and Inefficiency." Citizens Fund, April 1992.

Clark, Gordon L. *Unions and Communities Under Siege: American Communities and the Crisis of Organized Labor.* Cambridge: Cambridge University Press, 1989.

———. "NAFTA: Clinton's Victory, Organized Labor's Loss." *Political Geography* 13.4 (July 1994): 377–84.

Clawson, Dan. *Bureaucracy and the Labor Process: The Transformation of U.S. Industry, 1860–1920.* New York: Monthly Review Press, 1980.

Clinton, Bill, and Al Gore. *Putting People First: How We Can All Change America.* New York: Times Books, 1992.

Coburn, David, et al. "Medical Dominance in Canada in Historical Perspective: The Rise and Fall of Medicine?" *International Journal of Health Services* 13.3 (1983): 407–32.

Cohen, Isaac. "Political Climate and Two Airline Strikes: Century Air in 1932 and Continental Airlines in 1983–85." *Industrial and Labor Relations Review* 43.2 (1990): 308–23.

Cohen, Lizabeth. *Making a New Deal: Industrial Workers in Chicago, 1919–1939.* Cambridge: Cambridge University Press, 1990.

Cohen, Richard E. *Changing Course in Washington: Clinton and the New Congress* (New York: Macmillan College Publishing Company, 1994).

Coleman, Vernon. "Labor Power and Social Equality: Union Politics in a Changing Economy." *Political Science Quarterly* 103.4 (1988): 687–705.

Collins, Robert M. *The Business Response to Keynes, 1929–1964.* New York: Columbia University Press, 1981.

Colon, Dominique M. "Labor's Dilemma in Providing Health Care Benefits and Services to American Workers: A Study of a Union's Approach to Health Planning in the 1980s." M.A. thesis, Yale University, 1983.

Conference Board. "U.S. Manufacturers in the Global Marketplace: A Research Report." New York: The Conference Board, 1994.

Cook, Timothy I. *Governing With the News: The News as a Political Institution.* Chicago: Chicago University Press, 1998.

Cornfield, Daniel B. "Labor Unions, Corporations, and Families: Institutional Competition in the Provision of Social Welfare." *Marriage and Family Review* 15.3/4 (1990): 37–57.

———. "The U.S. Labor Movement: Its Development and Impact on Social Inequality." *Annual Review of Sociology* 17 (1991): 27–49.

———. "Union Decline and the Political Demands of Organized Labor." *Work and Occupations* 16.3 (August 1989): 292–322.

Cotton, Paul. "Pre-Existing Conditions 'Hold Americans Hostage' to Employers and Insurers." *Journal of the American Medical Association* 265 (1991): 2451–53.

Craypo, Charles, and Bruce Nissen, eds. *Grand Designs: The Impact of Corporate Strategies on Workers, Unions, and Communities.* Ithaca: ILR Press, 1993.

Croteau, David. *Politics and the Class Divide: Working People and the Middle-Class Left.* Philadelphia: Temple University Press, 1995.

Currie, Janet. "Gender Gaps in Benefit Coverage." NBER working paper no. 4265. Cambridge, Mass.: National Bureau of Economic Research, January 1983.

Daley, Anthony. "The Steel Crisis and Labor Politics in France and the United States." *Bargaining for Change: Union Politics in North America and Europe.* Miriam Golden and Jonas Pontusson, eds. Ithaca, N.Y.: Cornell University Press, 1992.

Dark, Taylor E. "Organized Labor and the Congressional Democrats: Reconsidering the 1980s." *Political Science Quarterly* 111.1 (1996): 83–104.

———. "Organized Labor and the Presidential Nominating Process: Reconsidering the 1980s." *Presidential Studies Quarterly* 26.2 (Spring 1996): 391–401.

———. *The Unions and the Democrats: An Enduring Alliance.* Ithaca, N.Y.: Cornell University Press, 1999.

Davis, Mike. *Prisoners of the American Dream: Politics and Economy in the History of the U.S. Working Class.* London: Verso, 1986.

Delaney, John, Jack Fiorito, and Marick F. Masters. "The Effects of Union Organizational and Environmental Characteristics on Union Political Action." *American Journal of Political Science* 32.3 (August 1988): 616–42.

Delaney, John Thomas. "The Future of Unions as Political Organizations." *Journal of Labor Research* 12.4 (1991): 373–87.

Delaney, John T., and Marick F. Masters, "Unions and Political Action." *The State of the Unions.* George Strauss, Daniel G. Gallagher, and Jack Fiorito, eds. Madison, Wis.: Industrial Relations Research Association, 1991.

Derickson, Alan. "Health Security for All? Social Unionism and Universal Health Insurance, 1935–1958." *The Journal of American History* 80.4 (March 1994): 1333–56.

———. *Workers' Health, Workers' Democracy: The Western Miners' Struggle, 1891–1925.* Ithaca, N.Y.: Cornell University Press, 1988.

Derthick, Martha. *Policymaking for Social Security.* Washington, D.C.: The Brookings Institution, 1979.

Dickinson, Harley D. "The Struggle for State Health Insurance: Reconsidering the Role of Saskatchewan Farmers." *Studies in Political Economy* 41 (Summer 1993): 133–56.

Dobbin, Frank R. "The Origins of Private Social Insurance: Public Policy and Fringe Benefits in America, 1920–1950." *American Journal of Sociology* 97.5 (1992): 1416–50.

Dobbin, Frank, and Terry Boychuk. "Public Policy and the Rise of Private Pensions: The US Experience Since 1930." *The Privatization of Social Policy? Occupational Welfare and the Welfare State in America, Scandinavia and Japan.* Michael Shalev, ed. Great Britain: St. Martin's Press, 1996.

Domhoff, G. William. *The Higher Circles: The Governing Class in America.* New York: Vintage Books, 1971.

Draper, Alan. *A Rope of Sand : The AFL-CIO Committee on Political Education, 1955–1967.* New York: Praeger, 1989.

Dubofsky, Melvyn. "Jimmy Carter and the End of the Politics of Productivity." *The Carter Presidency: Policy Choices in the Post-New Deal Era.* Gary M. Fink and Hugh D. Graham, eds. Lawrence: University Press of Kansas, 1998.

———. *The State and Labor in Modern America.* Chapel Hill: The University of North Carolina Press, 1994.

Dunlop, John T., ed. *Business and Public Policy.* Cambridge: Harvard University Press, 1980.
———. *Dispute Resolution: Negotiation and Consensus Building.* Dover, Mass.: Auburn House, 1984.
———. "Health Care Coalitions." *Private Sector Coalitions: A Fourth Party in Health Care.* B. Jon Jaeger, ed. Durham, N.C.: Department of Health Administration, 1983.
———. *Industrial Relations Systems.* New York: Holt, 1958.
Eckholm, Erik, ed. *Solving America's Health-Care Crisis.* New York: Times Books, Random House, 1993.
Edsall, Thomas Byrne. "The Changing Shape of Power: A Realignment in Public Policy." *The Rise and Fall of the New Deal Order, 1930–1980.* Steve Fraser and Gary Gerstle, eds. Princeton, N.J.: Princeton University Press, 1989.
———. *The New Politics of Inequality.* New York: W.W. Norton & Co., 1984.
Edwards, Jennifer, et al. "Will Small Business Reform Improve Access in the 1990s." *Reforming the System: Containing Health Care Costs in an Era of Universal Coverage.* Robert J. Blendon and Tracey Stelzer Hyams, eds. New York: Faulkner and Grey, 1992.
Edwards, Richard. *Contested Terrain: The Transformation of the Workplace in the Twentieth Century.* New York: Basic Books, 1979.
Edwards, Richard, and Michael Podgursky. "The Unraveling Accord: American Unions in Crisis." *Unions in Crisis and Beyond: Perspectives from Six Countries.* Richard Edwards, ed. Dover, Mass.: Auburn House Publishing Co., 1986.
Eisinger, Peter K. *The Rise of the Entrepreneurial State: State and Local Economic Development in the United States.* Madison: The University of Wisconsin Press, 1988.
Elving, Ronald D. *Conflict and Compromise: How Congress Makes the Law.* New York: Simon & Schuster, 1995.
Enthoven, Alain. "The History and Principles of Managed Competition." *Health Affairs* 13 (Supplement 1993): 24–48.
Enthoven, Alain, and Richard Kronick. "A Consumer-Choice Plan for the 1990s." *New England Journal of Medicine* 320.1 (January 5, 1989): 29–37 and 320.2 (January 12, 1989): 94–110.
Epstein, Gerald. "Mortgaging America: Debts, Lies, and Multinationals." *World Policy Journal* 8.1 (Winter 1990–91): 27–59.
Erlich, Mark. *Labor at the Ballot Box: The Massachusetts Prevailing Wage Campaign of 1988.* Philadelphia: Temple University Press, 1990.
Esping-Andersen, Gosta. *Politics Against Markets: The Social Democratic Road to Power.* Princeton, N.J.: Princeton University Press, 1985.
———. "Power and Distributional Regimes." *Politics and Society* 14.2 (1985): 223–56.
———. *The Three Worlds of Welfare Capitalism.* London: Polity, 1990.
Esping-Andersen, Gosta, and Walter Korpi. "Social Policy as Class Politics in Post-War Capitalism: Scandinavia, Austria, and Germany." *Order and Conflict in Contemporary Capitalism.* John H. Goldthorpe, ed. Oxford: Clarendon Press, 1984.
Esping-Andersen, Gosta, Martin Rein, and Lee Rainwater, eds. *Stagnation and Renewal in Social Policy: The Rise and Fall of Policy Regimes.* Armonk, N.Y.: M.E. Sharpe, 1987.
Evans, C. Lawrence. "Committees and Health Jurisdiction in Congress." *Intensive Care: How Congress Shapes Health Policy.* Thomas E. Mann and Norman J. Ornstein, eds. Washington, D.C.: American Enterprise Institute and The Brookings Institution, 1995.
Evans, Peter B., Dietrich Rueschemeyer, and Theda Skocpol, eds. *Bringing the State Back In.* Cambridge: Cambridge University Press, 1985.
Fallows, James. *Breaking the News: How the Media Undermines American Democracy.* New York: Pantheon, 1996.
Families, USA. "Health Spending: The Growing Threat to the Family Budget." Washington, D.C.: Families USA Foundation, December 1991.

Feder, Judith. "The Pepper Commission Proposals." *Social Insurance Issues for the Nineties, Proceedings of the Third Conference of the National Academy of Social Insurance.* Paul N. Van Dewater, ed. Dubuque, Iowa: Kendall/Hunt, 1992.

Fein, Rashi. *Medical Care, Medical Costs: The Search for Health Insurance Policy.* Cambridge: Harvard University Press, 1986.

———. "The Politics of Health Reform." *Dissent* 41.4 (Winter 1994): 43–56.

Ferguson, Thomas, and Joel Rogers, eds. *The Political Economy: Readings in the Politics and Economics of American Public Policy.* Armonk, N.Y.: M.E. Sharpe, 1984.

———. *Right Turn: The Decline of the Democrats and the Future of American Politics.* New York: Hill and Wang, 1986.

Fink, Gary M., ed. *AFL-CIO Executive Council Statements and Reports, 1956–1975.* Westport, Conn.: Greenwood Press, 1977.

Fink, Leon, and Brian Greenberg. *Upheaval in the Quiet Zone: A History of Hospital Workers' Union 1199.* Urbana: University of Illinois Press, 1989.

Fiorito, Jack, and Charles R. Greer. "Determinants of U.S. Unionism: Past Research and Future Needs." *Industrial Relations* 21.1 (1982): 1–32.

Flood, Lawrence, ed. *Unions and Public Policy: The New Economy, Law, and Democratic Politics.* Westport, Conn.: Greenwood Press, 1995.

Foley, Michael, and John E. Owens. *Congress and the Presidency: Institutional Politics in a Separated System.* Manchester: Manchester University Press, 1996.

Foner, Eric. "Why Is There No Socialism in the United States?" *History Workshop* 17 (Spring 1984): 57–80.

Foner, Philip S. *Organized Labor and the Black Worker, 1619–1973.* New York: Praeger Publishers, 1974.

———. *Women and the American Labor Movement: From World War I to the Present.* New York: The Free Press, 1980.

Fones-Wolf, Elizabeth A. *Selling Free Enterprise: The Business Assault on Labor and Liberalism, 1945–60.* Urbana: University of Illinois Press, 1994.

Forbath, William E. *Law and the Shaping of the American Labor Movement.* Cambridge: Harvard University Press, 1991.

Form, William. *Segmented Labor, Fractured Politics: Labor Politics in American Life.* New York: Plenum Press, 1995.

Foster, James Caldwell. *The Union Politic: The CIO Political Action Committee.* Columbia: University of Missouri, 1975.

Fox, Daniel M. *Health Politics: The British and American Experience, 1911–1965.* Princeton, N.J.: Princeton University Press, 1986.

Fox, Daniel M., and Daniel C. Schaffer. "Health Policy and ERISA: Interest Groups and Semipreemption." *Journal of Health Politics, Policy and Law* 14.2 (Summer 1989): 239–60.

Fox, Peter D., Willis B. Goldbeck, and Jacob J. Spies. *Health Care Cost Management: Private Sector Initiatives.* Ann Arbor, Mich.: Health Administration Press, 1984.

Fraser, Douglas. "Inside the 'Monolith'." *The State of the Unions.* George Strauss, Daniel G. Gallagher, and Jack Fiorito, eds. Madison, Wis.: Industrial Relations Research Association, 1991.

Freeman, Richard B., ed. *Working Under Different Rules.* New York: Russell Sage Foundation, 1994.

Freeman, Richard B., and Casey Ichniowski, eds. *When Public Sector Workers Unionize.* Chicago: Chicago University Press, 1988.

Freeman, Richard B., and Morris M. Kleiner. "Employer Behavior in the Face of Union Organizing Drives." *Industrial and Labor Relations Review* 43.4 (April 1990): 351–65.

Freeman, Richard B., and James L. Medoff. *What Do Unions Do?* New York: Basic Books, 1984.

Friedman, Emily. "The Threat of Time." *Frontiers of Health Services Management* 12.2 (Winter 1995): 35–39.

Friedman, Sheldon, et al., eds. *Restoring the Promise of American Labor Law.* Ithaca, N.Y.: ILR Press, 1994.

Gabin, Nancy. *Feminism in the Labor Movement: Women and the United Auto Workers, 1935–75.* Ithaca, N.Y.: Cornell University Press, 1990.

Gall, Gilbert J. *The Politics of the Right to Work: The Labor Federation as Special Interests, 1943–1979.* New York: Greenwood Press, 1982.

Gamble, Andrew. *The Free Economy and the Strong State: The Politics of Thatcherism.* 2nd ed. London: Macmillan, 1994.

Garbarino, Joseph W. *Health Plans and Collective Bargaining.* Berkeley: University of California Press, 1960.

Garrett, Geoffrey, and Barry R. Weingast. "Ideas, Interests, and Institutions: Constructing the European Community's Internal Market." *Ideas and Foreign Policy: Beliefs, Institutions, and Political Change.* Judith Goldstein and Robert O. Keohane, eds. Ithaca, N.Y.: Cornell University Press, 1993.

Geoghegan, Thomas. *Which Side Are You On? Trying to Be for Labor When It's Flat on Its Back.* New York: Farrer, Straus & Giroux, 1991.

Ghilarducci, Teresa. *Labor's Capital: The Economics and Politics of Pensions.* Cambridge, Mass.: MIT Press, 1992.

Gifford, Courtney D., ed. *Directory of U.S. Labor Organizations.* Washington, D.C.: Bureau of National Affairs, 1988.

Gillon, Steven M. *Politics and Vision: The A.D.A. and American Liberalism, 1947–1985.* New York: Oxford University Press, 1987.

Gitterman, Daniel P. "Redistributing Earnings? The American System of Shared Powers and the Fair Labor Standards Act, 1938–1998." Ph.D. dissertation, Brown University, 1999.

Goldberger, Susan A. "The Politics of Universal Access: The Massachusetts Health Security Act of 1988." *Journal of Health Politics, Policy and Law* 15.4 (Winter 1990): 857–85.

Goldberg-Hiller, Jonathan. "The Limits to Union: Labor, Gays and Lesbians, and Marriage in Hawai'i." Paper presented at the annual meetings of the American Political Science Association, Boston, September 3–6,1998.

Golden, Miriam. "Conclusion: Current Trends in Trade Union Politics." *Bargaining for Change: Union Politics in North America and Europe.* Golden and Jonas Pontusson, eds. Ithaca, N.Y.: Cornell University Press, 1992.

———. *Heroic Defeats: The Politics of Job Loss.* Cambridge: Cambridge University Press, 1997.

Golden, Miriam, and Jonas Pontusson, eds. *Bargaining for Change: Union Politics in North America and Europe.* Ithaca, N.Y.: Cornell University Press, 1992.

Golden, Miriam A., Michael Wallerstein, and Peter Lange. "Postwar Trade-Union Organization and Industrial Relations." *Continuity and Change in Contemporary Capitalism.* Herbert Kitschelt, et al., eds. Cambridge: Cambridge University Press, 1999.

Goldfield, Michael. *The Decline of Organized Labor in the United States.* Chicago: The University of Chicago Press, 1987.

———. "Explaining New Deal Labor Policy." *American Political Science Review* 84.4 (1990): 1304–15.

———. "Labor in American Politics—Its Current Weakness." *Journal of Politics* 48 (1986): 2–29.

———. "Worker Insurgency, Radical Organization, and New Deal Labor Legislation." *American Political Science Review* 83.4 (1989): 1257–82.

Gonos, George. "The Contest Over 'Employer' Status in the Postwar United States: The Case of Temporary Help Firms." *Law & Society Review* 31.1 (1997): 81–110.

Gordon, Colin. "Dead on Arrival: Health Care Reform in the United States." *Studies in Political Economy* 39 (Fall 1992): 141–59.

———. "New Deal, Old Deck: Business and the Origins of Social Security." *Politics & Society* 19.2 (1991): 165–207.

———. *New Deals: Business, Labor, and Politics in America, 1920–1935.* Cambridge: Cambridge University Press, 1994.

———. "Why No National Health Insurance in the U.S.? The Limits of Social Provision in War and Peace, 1941–1948," *Journal of Policy History* 9.3 (1997): 277–310.

Gordon, David M. *Fat and Mean: The Corporate Squeeze of Working Americans and the Myth of Managerial "Downsizing.* New York: Martin Kessler Books, The Free Press, 1996.

———. "The Global Economy: New Edifice or Crumbling Foundations?" *New Left Review* 168 (March/April 1988): 24–64.

Gordon, David M., Richard Edwards, and Michael Reich. *Segmented Work, Divided Workers: The Historical Transformation of Labor in the United States.* Cambridge: Cambridge University Press, 1982.

Goulden, Joseph C. *Jerry Wurf: Labor's Last Angry Man.* New York: Atheneum, 1982.

Gourevitch, Peter, Peter Lange, and Andrew Martin. "Industrial Relations and Politics: Some Reflections." *Industrial Relations in International Perspective: Essays in Research and Policy.* Peter B. Doeringer, ed. New York: Holmes & Meier, 1981.

Green, Mark, and Andrew Buchsbaum. *The Corporate Lobbies: Political Profiles of the Business Roundtable & the Chamber of Commerce.* Washington, D.C.: Public Citizen, 1980.

Green, William C., and Ernest J. Yanarella, eds. *North American Auto Unions in Crisis: Lean Production as Contested Terrain.* Albany: SUNY Press, 1996.

Greene, Julie. *Pure and Simple Politics : The American Federation of Labor and Political Activism, 1881–1917.* Cambridge and New York: Cambridge University Press, 1998.

Greenstone, J. David. *Labor in American Politics.* Chicago: Chicago University Press, 1977.

Greider, William. *Who Will Tell the People? The Betrayal of American Democracy.* New York: Simon & Schuster, 1992.

Grenier, Guillermo J. *Inhuman Relations: Quality Circles and Anti-Unionism in American Industry.* Philadelphia: Temple University Press, 1988.

Griffin, Larry J., Holly J. McCammon, and Christopher Botsko. "The 'Unmaking' of a Movement? The Crisis of U.S. Trade Unions in Comparative Perspective." *Change in Societal Institutions.* Maureen T. Hallinan, David M. Klein, and Jennifer Glass, eds. New York: Plenum Press, 1990.

Griffin, Michael E. Wallace, and Beth A. Rubin. "Capitalist Resistance to the Organization of Labor Before the New Deal: Why? How? Success?" *American Sociological Review* 51 (April 1986): 147–67.

Griffith, Robert. "Forging America's Postwar Order: Domestic Politics and Political Economy in the Age of Truman." *The Truman Presidency.* Michael J. Lacey. ed. Cambridge: Cambridge University Press, 1989.

Grogan, Colleen M. "Federalism and Health Care Reform." *Health Care Reform in the Nineties.* Pauline Vaillancourt Rosenau, ed. Thousand Oaks, Calif.: Sage, 1994.

———. "Hope in Federalism? What Can the States Do and What Are They Likely To Do?" *Journal of Health Politics, Policy and Law* 20.2 (Summer 1995): 477–84.

Gross, James. *Broken Promises: The Subversion of U.S. Labor Relations Policy, 1947–1994.* Philadelphia: Temple University Press, 1995.

Guest, Dennis. *The Emergence of Social Security in Canada.* 2nd ed. Vancouver: University of British Columbia Press, 1985.

Hacker, Jacob S. *The Road to Nowhere: The Genesis of President Clinton's Plan for Health Security.* Princeton, N.J.: Princeton University Press, 1997.

Haines, Herbert. "Black Radicalization and the Funding of Civil Rights: 1957–1970." *Social Problems* 32.1 (October 1984): 31–43.

Hall, Peter A., and Rosemary C.R. Taylor. "Political Science and the Three Institutionalisms." *Political Studies* 44 (1996): 936–57.

Halpern, Martin. "Jimmy Carter and the UAW: Failure of an Alliance." *Presidential Studies Quarterly* 26.3 (Summer 1996): 755–77.

———. *UAW: Politics in the Cold War Era.* Albany: SUNY Press, 1988.

Hancke, Bob. "The Crisis of National Unions: Belgian Labor in Decline." *Politics and Society* 19.4 (1991): 463–87.

Harris, Howell John. *The Right to Manage: Industrial Relations Policies of American Business in the 1940s.* Madison: The University of Wisconsin Press, 1982.

Harrison, Bennett, and Barry Bluestone. *The Great U-Turn: Corporate Restructuring and the Polarizing of America.* New York: Basic Books, 1988.

Hartley, Fred A., Jr., *Our New National Labor Policy.* New York: Funk & Wagnalls, 1948.

Hartmann, Susan M. *Truman and the 80th Congress.* Columbia: University of Missouri Press, 1971.

Hattam, Victoria C. *Labor Visions and State Power: The Origins of Business Unionism in the United States.* Princeton, N.J.: Princeton University Press, 1993.

Heckscher, Charles C. *The New Unionism: Employee Involvement in the Changing Corporation.* New York: Basic Books, 1987.

Hellander, Ida, et al., "The Growing Epidemic of Uninsurance: New Data on the Health Insurance Coverage of Americans." *International Journal of Health Services* 25.3 (1995): 377–92.

Hendricks, Rickey Lynn. "A Necessary Revolution: The Origins of the Kaiser Permanente Medical Care Program." Ph.D. dissertation, University of Denver, 1987.

Herzenberg, Stephen. "Whither Social Unionism? Labor and Restructuring in the U.S. Auto Industry." *The Challenge of Restructuring: North American Labor Movements Respond.* Jane Jenson and Rianne Mahon, eds. Philadelphia: Temple University Press, 1993.

Hicks, Alex, Roger Friedlander, and Edwin Johnson. "Class Power and State Policy: The Case of Large Business Corporations, Labor Unions, and Governmental Redistribution in the American States." *American Sociological Review* 43 (June 1978): 302–15.

Hirschfield, Daniel S. *The Lost Reform: The Campaign for Compulsory Health Insurance in the United States from 1932 to 1943.* Cambridge: Harvard University Press, 1970.

Hollingsworth, J. Rogers. *A Political Economy of Medicine: Great Britain and the United States.* Baltimore: The Johns Hopkins University Press, 1986.

Horowitz, Ruth L. *Political Ideologies of Organized Labor.* New Brunswick, N.J.: Transaction Books, 1978.

Hout, Michael, Clem Brooks, and Jeff Manza. "The Democratic Class Struggle in the United States, 1948–1992." *American Sociological Review* 60 (December 1995): 805–28.

Howard, Christopher. *The Hidden Welfare State: Tax Expenditures and Social Policy in the United States.* Princeton, N.J.: Princeton University Press, 1997.

———. "The Hidden Side of the American Welfare State." *Political Science Quarterly* 108.3 (1993): 403–36.

Howard, Robert. *Brave New Workplace.* New York: Viking, 1985.

Huntington, Samuel P., and Jorge I. Dominguez. "Political Development." *Handbook of Political Science* 3. Fred I. Greenstein and Nelson W. Polsby, eds. Reading, Mass.: Addison-Wesley, 1975.

Hurd, Richard W., and Jill K. Kriesky. "The Rise and Demise of PATCO Reconstructed." *Labor and Industrial Relations Review* 40.1 (October 1986): 115–22.

Immergut, Ellen M. "Institutions, Veto Points, and Policy Results: A Comparative Analysis of Health Care." *Journal of Public Policy* 10.4 (1990): 391–416.

Inglehart, John. "Health Care and American Business." *New England Journal of Medicine* 306.2 (1982): 120–24.

Jacobs, David C. *Collective Bargaining as an Instrument of Social Change.* Westport, Conn.: Quorum Books, 1994.
———. "Labor and the Strategy of Mandated Health Benefits." *Labor Studies Journal* 14.3 (Fall 1989): 23–33.
———. "The UAW and the Committee for National Health Insurance: The Contours of Social Unionism." *Advances in Industrial and Labor Relations* 4. David Lewin, David B. Lipsky, and Donna Sockell, eds. Greenwich, Conn.: JAI Press, 1987.
———. "The United Auto Workers and the Campaign for National Health Insurance." Ph.D. dissertation, Cornell University, 1983.
Jacobs, Lawrence R. "Politics of America's Supply State: Health Reform and Technology." *Health Affairs* 14.2 (Summer 1995): 143–57.
Jacobs, Lawrence R., and Robert Y. Shapiro. "Don't Blame the Public for Failed Health Care Reform." *Journal of Health Politics, Policy and Law* 20.2 (Summer 1995): 411–23.
Jacobson, Gary C. "The 105th Congress: Unprecedented and Unsurprising." *The Elections of 1996.* Michael Nelson, ed. Washington, D.C.: Congressional Quarterly Press, 1997.
Jacoby, Sanford M. "American Exceptionalism Revisited: The Importance of Management." *Masters to Managers: Historical and Comparative Perspectives on American Employers.* Sanford M. Jacoby, ed. New York: Columbia University Press, 1991.
———, ed. *Masters to Managers: Historical and Comparative Perspectives on American Employers.* New York: Columbia University Press, 1991.
Jaeger, B. Jon, ed. *Private Sector Coalitions: A Fourth Party in Health Care.* Durham, N.C.: Department of Health Administration, 1983.
Jecker, Nancy S. "Can an Employer-Based Health Insurance System Be Just?" *The Politics of Health Care Reform: Lessons From the Past, Prospects for the Future.* James A. Morone and Gary S. Belkin, eds. Durham, N.C.: Duke University Press, 1994.
Jensen, Gail A., Michael A. Morrisey, and John W. Marcus. "Cost Sharing and the Changing Pattern of Employer-Sponsored Health Benefits." *The Milbank Quarterly* 65.4 (1987): 537–41.
Jenson, Jane, and Rianne Mahon, eds. *The Challenge of Restructuring: North American Labor Movements Respond.* Philadelphia: Temple University Press, 1993.
———. "Legacies for Canadian Labour of Two Decades of Crisis." *The Challenge of Restructuring: North American Labor Movements Respond.* Jenson and Mahon, eds. Philadelphia: Temple University Press, 1993.
Johnson, Haynes Bonner, and David S. Broder. *The System: The American Way of Politics at the Breaking Point.* Boston: Little, Brown, 1996.
Johnston, Paul. *Success Where Others Fail: Social Movement Unionism and the Public Workplace.* Ithaca, N.Y.: ILR Press, 1994.
Juravich, Tom, and Peter R. Shergold. "The Impact of Unions on the Voting Behavior of Their Members." *Industrial and Labor Relations Review* 41.3 (April 1988): 374–85.
Kamerman, Sheila B., and Alfred J. Kahn. *The Responsive Workplace: Employers and a Changing Labor Force.* New York: Columbia University Press, 1987.
Karson, Marc. *American Labor Unions and Politics; 1900–1918.* Carbondale: Southern Illinois University Press, 1958.
Katz, Harry. "Policy Debates Over Work Reorganization in North American Unions." *New Technology and Industrial Relations.* Richard Hyman and Wolfgang Streeck, eds. Oxford: Basil Blackwell, 1988.
Katznelson, Ira. "The State to the Rescue? Political Science and History Reconnect." *Social Research* 59.4 (Winter 1992): 719–37.
Kaufman, Burton I. *The Presidency of James Earl Carter, Jr.* Lawrence: University Press of Kansas, 1993.
Keeran, Roger, and Greg Tarpinian. "Public Policy and the Recent Decline of Strikes." *Policy Studies Journal* 18.2 (Winter 1989–90): 461–70.

Kennedy, Heather. "The Attitudes and Perspectives of Organized Labor Toward Health Care Cost Management." Washington, D.C.: Employee Benefit Research Institute, 1990.

Klein, Jennifer. "Bringing Politics Back In: Health Security and Social Politics in America." *Radical History Review* 69 (1997): 261–72.

Kochan, Thomas A., Harry C. Katz, and Robert B. McKersie. *The Transformation of American Industrial Relations.* New York: Basic Books, 1986.

Korpi, Walter. "Social Policy and Distributional Conflict in the Capitalist Democracies." *West European Politics* 3 (1980): 296–316.

———. *The Working Class in Welfare Capitalism.* London: Routledge & Kegan Paul, 1978.

Krajcinovic, Ivana. *From Company Doctors to Managed Care: The United Mine Workers' Noble Experiment.* Ithaca, N.Y.: Cornell University Press, 1997.

Kronick, Richard. "The Slippery Slope of Health Care Finance; Business Interests and Hospital Reimbursement in Massachusetts." *Journal of Health Politics, Policy and Law* 15.4 (Winter 1990): 887–913.

Krooss, Herman E. *Executive Opinion: What Business Leaders Said and Thought on Economic Issues, 1920s–1960s.* Garden City, N.Y.: Doubleday, 1970.

Krugman, Paul. *Peddling Prosperity: Economic Sense and Nonsense in the Age of Diminished Expectations.* New York: W.W. Norton, 1994.

LaBotz, Dan. *Rank-and-File Rebellion: Teamsters for a Democratic Union.* London: Verso, 1990.

Lankevich, George J. *Gerald R. Ford, 1913–: Chronology, Documents, Biographical Aids.* Dobbs Ferry, N.Y.: Oceana Publications, Inc., 1977.

Laycock, David. "Reforming Canadian Democracy? Institutions and Ideology in the Reform Party Project." *Canadian Journal of Political Science* 27.2 (June 1994): 213–47.

Lee, Elizabeth. "The Minimum Wage Increase Act of 1996: Minimum Wage Increase, Maximum Benefits for Business." Senior essay, Yale University, April 1997.

Lee, R. Alton. *Truman and Taft-Hartley: A Question of Mandate.* Lexington: University of Kentucky Press, 1966.

———. *Eisenhower and Landrum-Griffin: A Study in Labor-Management Politics* (Lexington: University Press of Kentucky, 1990).

Lemco, Jonathan, ed. *National Health Care: Lessons for the United States and Canada.* Ann Arbor: The University of Michigan Press, 1994.

Leuchtenburg, William E. *In the Shadow of FDR: From Harry Truman to Bill Clinton.* Ithaca, N.Y.: Cornell University Press, 1983.

Levine, Rhonda. *Class Struggle and the New Deal.* Lawrence: University Press of Kansas, 1988.

Levitan, Sar A. "Union Lobbyists' Contributions to Tough Labor Legislation." *Labor Law Journal* 10.10 (October 1959): 675–82.

Levitan, Sar A., and Martha R. Cooper. *Business Lobbies: The Public Good and the Bottom Line.* Baltimore: Johns Hopkins University Press, 1984.

Levy, Peter. *The New Left and Labor in the 1960s* (Urbana: University of Illinois Press, 1994).

Lewin, John C. "The Implementation of Health Care Reform: Lessons From Hawaii." *Implementation Issues and National Health Care Reform.* Charles Brecher, ed. Washington, D.C.: Josiah Macy, Jr. Foundation, 1992.

Lichtenstein, Nelson. "From Corporatism to Collective Bargaining: Organized Labor and the Eclipse of Social Democracy in the Postwar Era." *The Rise and Fall of the New Deal Order, 1930–1980.* Steve Fraser and Gary Gerstle, eds. Princeton, N.J.: Princeton University Press, 1989.

———. "Labor in the Truman Era: Origins of the 'Private Welfare State'." *The Truman Presidency.* Michael J. Lacey, ed. Cambridge: Cambridge University Press, 1989.

———. *Labor's War at Home: The CIO in World War II.* Cambridge: Cambridge University Press, 1982.

————. *The Most Dangerous Man in Detroit: Walter Reuther and the Fate of American Labor.* New York: Basic Books, 1995.

Light, Paul C. *The Tides of Reform: Making Government Work, 1945–1995.* New Haven, Conn.: Yale University Press, 1997.

Lindblom, Charles E. *Politics and Markets: The World's Political-Economic Systems.* New York: Basic Books, 1977.

Lipset, Seymour Martin. "Labor Unions in the Public Mind." *Unions in Transition: Entering the Second Century.* Seymour Martin Lipset, ed. San Francisco: ILR Press, 1986.

————, ed. *Unions in Transition: Entering the Second Century.* San Francisco: ILR Press, 1986.

MacIntyre, Duncan M. *Voluntary Health Insurance and Rate Making.* Ithaca: Cornell University Press, 1962.

Maier, Mark H. *City Unions: Managing Discontent in New York City.* New Brunswick, N.J.: Rutgers University Press, 1987.

Maioni, Antonia. *Parting at the Crossroads: The Emergence of Health Insurance in the United States and Canada.* Princeton, N.J.: Princeton University Press, 1998.

————. "Parting at the Crossroads: The Development of Health Insurance in Canada and the United States, 1940–65." *Comparative Politics* 29.4 (July 1997): 411–31.

Makinson, Larry, and Joshua Goldstein. *Open Secrets: The Encyclopedia of Congressional Money and Politics.* 4th ed. Washington, D.C.: Congressional Quarterly Press, 1996.

Mann, Thomas E., and Norman J. Ornstein, eds. *Intensive Care: How Congress Shapes Health Policy.* Washington, D.C.: American Enterprise Institute and The Brookings Institution, 1995.

March, J.G. "The Business Firm as a Political Coalition." *Journal of Politics* 24 (1962): 662–78.

Markovits, Andrei S. *The Politics of the West German Trade Unions: Strategies of Class and Interest Representation in Growth and Crisis.* Cambridge: Cambridge University Press, 1986.

Markowitz, Gerald, and David Rosner. "Seeking Common Ground: A History of Labor and Blue Cross." *Journal of Health Politics, Policy and Law* 16.4 (Winter 1991): 695–718.

Marks, Gary. *Unions in Politics: Britain, Germany, and the United States in the Nineteenth and Early Twentieth Centuries.* Princeton, N.J.: Princeton University Press, 1989.

Marmor, Theodore, Wayne L. Hoffman, and Thomas C. Heagy. "National Health Insurance: Lessons from the Canadian Experience." *Political Analysis and American Medical Care: Essays.* Theodore Marmor, ed. Cambridge: Cambridge University Press, 1983.

————. *Political Analysis and American Medical Care: Essays.* Cambridge: Cambridge University Press, 1983.

————. "A Summer of Discontent: Press Coverage of Murder and Medical Care Reform." *Journal of Health Politics, Policy and Law* 20.2 (Summer 1995): 485–89.

————. *Understanding Health Care Reform.* New Haven, Conn.: Yale University Press, 1994.

————. *The Politics of Medicare.* Chicago: Aldine Publishing Co., 1973.

Martin, Cathie Jo. "The Least Common Denominator Society: Business and Social Policy in the United States." Paper delivered at the annual meetings of the American Political Science Association, San Francisco, Calif., August 28–September 1, 1996.

————. "Inviting Business to the Party: The Corporate Response to Social Policy." *The Social Divide: Political Parties and the Future of Activist Government.* Margaret Weir, ed. Washington, D.C. and New York: Brookings Institution Press and Russell Sage Foundation, 1998.

————. "Managing National Health Reform: Business and the Politics of Policy Innovation." *Health Care Reform in the Nineties.* Pauline Vaillancourt Rosenau, ed. Thousand Oaks, Calif.: Sage, 1994.

————. "Mandating Social Change: The Business Struggle Over National Health Reform" (typescript, 1995).

———. "Nature or Nurture? Sources of Firm Preference for National Health Reform." *American Political Science Review* 89.4 (December 1995): 898–913.

———. "Stuck in Neutral: Big Business and the Politics of National Health Reform." *Journal of Health Politics, Policy and Law* 20.2 (Summer 1995): 430–36.

———. "Together Again: Business, Government, and the Quest for Cost Control." *Journal of Health Politics, Policy and Law* 18.2 (Summer 1993): 359–93.

Masters, Marick F. "Federal Employee Unions and Political Action." *Industrial and Labor Relations Review* 38.4 (July 1985): 612–28.

———. *Unions at the Crossroads: Strategic Membership, Financial, and Political Perspectives* (Westport, Conn.: Quorum Books, 1997).

Masters, Marick F., and John Thomas Delaney. "The Causes of Union Political Involvement: A Longitudinal Analysis." *Journal of Labor Research* 6 (1985): 341–62.

———. "Union Legislative Records During President Reagan's First Term." *Journal of Labor Research* 8.1 (Winter 1987): 1–18.

———. "Union Political Activities: A Review of the Empirical Literature." *Industrial and Labor Relations Review* 40.3 (April 1987): 336–53.

Masters, Marick F., Robert S. Atkin, and John Thomas Delaney. "Unions, Political Action, and Public Policies: A Review of the Past Decade." *Policy Studies Journal* 18.2 (Winter 1989–90): 471–80.

May, Martha. "Bread Before Roses: American Workingmen, Labor Unions, and the Family Wage." *Women, Work and Protest: A Century of U.S. Women's Labor History*. Ruth Milkman, ed. Boston: Routledge & Kegan Paul, 1985.

Mayfield, Jacqueline Rowley, Trevor Bain, and Milton Ray Mayfield. "Learning About Health Care Cost Containment: The CWA-Bell South Case." *Labor Studies Journal* 18.3 (Fall 1993): 50–61.

Mayhew, David R. *Placing Parties in American Parties: Organization, Electoral Settings, and Government Activity in the Twentieth Century*. Princeton, N.J.: Princeton University Press, 1986.

McAdams, Alan K. *Power and Politics in Labor Legislation*. New York: Columbia University Press, 1959.

McCann, Michael W. *Taking Reform Seriously: Perspectives in Public Interest Liberalism*. Ithaca, N.Y.: Cornell University Press, 1986.

McCartin, Joseph A. *Labor's Great War: The Struggle for Industrial Democracy and the Origins of Modern American Labor Relations, 1912–1921*. Chapel Hill: University of North Carolina Press, 1997.

McClure, Arthur F. *The Truman Administration and the Problems of Postwar Labor, 1945–48*. Rutherford, N.J.: Fairleigh Dickinson University Press, 1969.

McGrath, Phyllis S., ed. *Business Credibility: The Critical Factors*. New York: The Conference Board, 1976.

McQuaid, Kim. *Big Business and Presidential Power: From FDR to Reagan*. New York: William Morrow & Co., 1982.

Mehring, John. "AIDS at Work: The SEIU AIDS Project." *Labor Research Review* 14, no. 2 (1990): 83–89.

Meier, August, and Elliott Rudwick. *Black Detroit and the Rise of the UAW*. Oxford: Oxford University Press, 1979.

Melhado, Evan M. "Competition versus Regulation in American Health Policy." *Money, Power, and Health Care*. Evan M. Melhado, Walter Feinberg, and Harold M. Swartz, eds. Ann Arbor, Mich.: Health Administration Press, 1988.

Meyer, John W., and Brian Rowan. "Institutionalized Organizations: Formal Structure as Myth and Ceremony." *American Journal of Sociology* 83.2 (September 1977): 340–63.

Miliband, Ralph. *The State in Capitalist Society*. New York: Basic Books, 1969.

Milkman, Ruth. "The Anti-Concessions Movement in the UAW: Interview With Douglas Stevens." *Socialist Review* 12.5 (1982): 19–42.

———, ed. *Women, Work and Protest: A Century of U.S. Women's Labor History.* Boston: Routledge & Kegan Paul, 1985.

Millis, Harry A., and Emily Clark Brown. *From the Wagner Act to Taft-Hartley; A Study of National Labor Policy and Labor Relations.* Chicago: Chicago University Press, 1950.

Mills, D. Quinn. "Management Performance." *U.S. Industrial Relations, 1950–1980: A Critical Assessment.* Jack Stieber, Robert B. McKersie, and D. Q. Mills, eds. Madison, Wis.: Industrial Relations Research Association, 1981.

Milton, David. *The Politics of U.S. Labor: From the Great Depression to the New Deal.* New York: Monthly Review Press, 1982.

Mizruchi, Mark S. *The Structure of Corporate Political Action: Interfirm Relations and Their Consequences.* Cambridge: Harvard University Press, 1992.

Montgomery, David. *The Fall of the House of Labor: The Workplace, the State, and American Labor Activism, 1865–1925.* Cambridge: Cambridge University Press, 1987.

———. *Workers' Control in America: Studies in the History of Work, Technology, and Labor Struggles.* Cambridge: Cambridge University Press, 1979.

Moody, Kim. "American Labor: A Movement Again?" *Monthly Review* 49.3 (July–August 1997): 63–79.

———. *Workers in a Lean World: Unions in the International Economy* (New York: Verso, 1997).

Morone, James A. "The Bureaucracy Empowered." *The Politics of Health Care Reform: Lessons From the Past, Prospects for the Future.* James A. Morone and Gary S. Belkin, eds. Durham: Duke University Press, 1994.

———. *The Democratic Wish: Popular Participation and the Limits of American Government.* New York: Basic Books, 1990.

———. "Elusive Community: Democracy, Deliberation, and the Reconstruction of Health Policy." *The New Politics of Public Policy.* Marc K. Landy and Martin A. Levin, eds. Baltimore: The Johns Hopkins University Press, 1995.

———. "Nativism, Hollow Corporations, and Managed Competition: Why the Clinton Health Care Reform Failed." *Journal of Health Politics, Policy and Law* 20.2 (Summer 1995): 391–98.

Morone, James A., and Gary S. Belkin, eds. *The Politics of Health Care Reform: Lessons From the Past, Prospects for the Future.* Durham, N.C.: Duke University Press, 1994.

Morone, James A., and Theodore R. Marmor. "Representing Consumer Interests: The Case of American Health Planning." *Political Analysis and American Medical Care: Essays.* Theodore R. Marmor, ed. Cambridge: Cambridge University Press, 1983.

Morrison, Ellen M., and Gregory Schmid. "State Initiatives in Health Care." *Reforming the System: Containing Health Care Costs in an Era of Universal Coverage.* Robert J. Blendon and Tracey Stelzer Hyams, eds. New York: Faulkner and Grey, 1992.

Mort, Jo-Ann, ed. *Not Your Father's Union Movement: Inside the AFL-CIO.* London: Verso, 1998.

Mucciaroni, Gary. *Reversals of Fortune: Public Policy and Private Interests.* Washington, D.C.: The Brookings Institution, 1995.

Mulcahy, Richard Patrick. "Serving the Union: The United Mine Workers of America Welfare and Retirement Fund, 1946–1978." Ph.D. dissertation, West Virginia University, 1988.

Munts, Raymond. *Bargaining for Health: Labor Unions, Health Insurance, and Medical Care.* Madison: University of Wisconsin Press, 1967.

National Leadership Commission on Health Care. *For the Health of a Nation: A Shared Responsibility.* Ann Arbor, Mich.: Health Administration Press Perspectives, 1989.

Navarro, Vicente. *The Politics of Health Policy: The U.S. Reforms.* Cambridge: Blackwell, 1994.

———. "Why Congress Did Not Enact Health Reform." *Journal of Health Politics, Policy and Law* 20.2 (Summer 1995): 455–61.

————. "Why Some Countries Have National Health Insurance, Others Have National Health Services, and the U.S. Has Neither." *Social Science and Medicine* 28.9 (1989): 887–98.

Neubauer, Deane. "Hawaii: The Health State." *Health Policy Reform in America: Innovations from the States.* Howard M. Leichter, ed. Armonk, N.Y.: M.E. Sharpe, 1992.

North, Douglass C. *Institutions, Institutional Change and Economic Performance.* Cambridge: Cambridge University Press, 1990.

Noyelle, Thierry J. *Beyond Industrial Dualism: Market and Job Segmentation in the New Economy.* Boulder, Colo.: Westview Press, 1987.

Oestreicher, Richard. "The Rules of the Game: Class Politics in Twentieth Century America." *Organized Labor and American Politics, 1894–1994: The Labor-Liberal Alliance,* Kevin Boyle, ed. Albany: SUNY Press, 1998.

Oopay, Anne Ghislaine. "Welfare Organization: The Case of Worksite Health Promotion." Ph.D. dissertation, University of Illinois at Urbana–Champaign, 1991.

O'Rand, Angela M. "The Hidden Payroll: Employee Benefits and the Structure of Workplace Inequality." *Sociological Forum* 1.4 (Fall 1986): 657–83.

Orren, Karen. "Organized Labor and the Invention of Modern Liberalism in the United States." *Studies in American Political Development* 2 (1987): 317–36.

————. "Union Politics and Postwar Liberalism in the United States." *Studies in American Political Development* 1 (1986): 215–52.

Orren, Karen, and Stephen Skowronek. "Beyond the Iconography of Order: Notes for a New Institutionalism." *The Dynamics of American Politics: Approaches and Interpretations.* Larry C. Dodd and Calvin Jillson, eds. Boulder, Colo.: Westview, 1993.

Osterman, Paul. *Employment Futures: Reorganization, Dislocation, and Public Policy.* New York: Oxford University Press, 1988.

Parker, Mike, and Jane Slaughter. *Choosing Sides: Unions and the Team Concept.* Boston: South End Press, 1988.

Parmet, Wendy. "Regulation and Federalism: Legal Impediments to State Health Care Reform." *American Journal of Law and Medicine* 19.1 and 19.2 (1993): 131–40.

Patashnik, Eric. "A New Look in Welfare State Research." *Policy Currents* 7.3 (September 1997): 1–6.

Pauly, Mark. *Health Benefits at Work: An Economic and Political Analysis of Employment-Based Health Insurance.* Ann Arbor: University of Michigan Press, 1997.

Pemberton, Carolyn, and Deborah Holmes, eds. *EBRI Databook on Employee Benefits.* 3rd ed. Washington, D.C.: Employee Benefit Research Institute, 1995.

Pepper Commission, U.S. Bipartisan Commission on Comprehensive Health Care. "A Call for Action." Washington, D.C., 1990.

Perman, Laurie, and Beth Stevens. "Industrial Segregation and the Gender Distribution of Fringe Benefits." *Gender and Society* 3.3 (September 1988): 388–404.

Peterson, Mark A. "The Health Care Debate: All Heat and No Light." *Journal of Health Politics, Policy and Law* 20.2 (Summer 1995): 425–30.

————. "Political Influence in the 1990s: From Iron Triangles to Policy Networks." *Journal of Health Politics, Policy and Law* 18.2 (Summer 1993): 395–438.

————. "Congress in the 1990s: From Iron Triangles to Policy Networks." *The Politics of Health Care Reform: Lessons From the Past, Prospects for the Future.* James A. Morone and Gary S. Belkin, eds. (Durham, N.C.: Duke University Press, 1994).

————. "Institutional Change and the New Politics of Health Care in the 1990s." *Health Care Reform in the Nineties.* Pauline Vaillancourt Rosenau, ed. Thousand Oaks, Calif.: Sage, 1994.

————. "Report from Congress: Momentum Toward Health Care Reform in the U.S. Senate." *Journal of Health Politics, Policy and Law* 17.3 (Fall 1992): 553–73.

Peterson, Paul E. "The New Politics of Deficits." *The New Direction in American Politics.* John Chubb and Paul E. Peterson, eds. Washington, D.C.: The Brookings Institution, 1985.

Phillips, Kevin. *The Politics of Rich and Poor: Wealth and the American Electorate in the Reagan Aftermath.* New York: Random House, 1990.

Pierson, Paul. "The New Politics of the Welfare State." *World Politics* 48.2 (January 1996): 143–79.

———. "The Path to European Integration: A Historical Institutionalist Analysis." *Comparative Political Studies* 29.2 (April 1996): 123–63.

———. *Dismantling the Welfare State? Reagan, Thatcher, and the Politics of Retrenchment.* New York: Cambridge University Press, 1994.

Piore, Michael J. "Adjustments in Organizational Structure and Their Implications for Social Standards in an Integrated Market." *Industrial Restructuring and Industrial Relations in Canada and the United States.* Elaine B. Willis, ed. Kingston, Ontario: Industrial Relations Centre, Queen's University, 1989.

———. "The Future of Unions." *The State of the Unions.* George Strauss, Daniel G. Gallagher, and Jack Fiorito, eds. Madison, Wis.: Industrial Relations Research Association, 1991.

———. "Perspectives on Labor Market Flexibility." *Industrial Relations* 25.2 (Spring 1986): 146–66.

———. "Unions and Politics." *The Shrinking Perimeter: Unionism and Labor Relations in the Manufacturing Sector.* Hervey A. Jurvis and Myron Roomkin, eds. Lexington, Mass.: Lexington Books, 1980.

Piven, Frances Fox, ed. *Labor Parties in Postindustrial Societies.* Cambridge: Polity Press, 1991.

———. "Structural Constraints and Political Development." *Labor Parties in Postindustrial Societies.* Frances Fox Piven, ed. Cambridge: Polity Press, 1991.

Plotke, David. "The Political Mobilization of Business." *The Politics of Interests: Interest Groups Transformed.* Mark Petracca, ed. Boulder, Colo.: Westview Press, 1992.

———. *Building a Democratic Political Order: Reshaping American Liberalism in the 1930s and 1940s.* Cambridge: Cambridge University Press, 1996.

———. "The Wagner Act, Again: Politics and Labor, 1935–37." *Studies in American Political Development* 3 (1989): 105–56.

Poen, Monte M. *Harry S. Truman Versus the Medical Lobby: The Genesis of Medicare.* Columbia: University of Missouri Press, 1979.

Polsby, Nelson. *Consequences of Party Reform.* Oxford: Oxford University Press, 1983.

Polsby, Nelson W., and Aaron Wildavsky. *Presidential Elections: Strategies and Structures in American Politics.* 9th ed. Chatham, N.J.: Chatham House Publishers, 1996.

Pontusson, Jonas. "From Comparative Public Policy to Political Economy: Putting Political Institutions in Their Place and Taking Interests Seriously." *Comparative Political Studies* 28.1 (April 1995): 117–47.

Przeworski, Adam. *Capitalism and Social Democracy.* Cambridge: Cambridge University Press, 1985.

Public Papers of the Presidents of the United States: Harry S. Truman, 1950. Washington, D.C.: U.S. Government Printing Office, 1965.

Quadagno, Jill. *The Transformation of Old Age Security: Class and Politics in the American Welfare State.* Chicago: University of Chicago Press, 1988.

———. "Theories of the Welfare State." *Annual Review of Sociology* 13 (1987): 109–28.

———. "Two Models of Welfare State Development: Reply to Skocpol and Amenta." *American Sociological Review* 50.4 (1985): 575–78.

———. "Welfare Capitalism and the Social Security Act of 1935." *American Sociological Review* 49 (1984): 632–47.

Quadagno, Jill, and Madonna Meyer. "Organized Labor, State Structures, and Social Policy Development: A Case Study of Old Age Assistance in Ohio, 1916–1940." *Social Problems* 36.2 (1989): 181–96.

Quirk, Paul J. "Deregulation and the Politics of Ideas in Congress." *Beyond Self-Interest.* Jane J. Mansbridge, ed. Chicago: The University of Chicago Press, 1990.

Raffel, M.W., ed. *Comparative Health Systems: Descriptive Analyses of Fourteen National Health Systems.* University Park: Pennsylvania State University Press, 1984.

Ramsay, Craig, ed. *U.S. Health Policy Groups: Institutional Profiles.* Westport, Conn.: Greenwood Press, 1995.

Regini, Marino, ed. *The Future of Labour Movements.* London: Sage, 1992.

———. "Introduction: The Past and Future of Social Studies of Labour Movements." *The Future of Labour Movements.* Marino Regini, ed. London: Sage, 1992.

Rein, Martin. "The Social Policy of the Firm." *Policy Sciences* 14 (1982): 117–35.

———. "Is America Exceptional? The Role of Occupational Welfare in the United States and the European Community." *The Privatization of Social Policy? Occupational Welfare and the Welfare State in America, Scandinavia and Japan.* Michael Shalev, ed. (London: MacMillan Press, 1996).

Rein, Martin, and Lee Rainwater. "From Welfare State to Welfare Society." *Stagnation and Renewal in Social Policy: The Rise and Fall of Policy Regimes.* Gosta Esping-Andersen, Martin Rein, and Lee Rainwater, eds. Armonk, N.Y.: M.E. Sharpe, 1987.

———. "The Public/Private Mix." *Public/Private Interplay in Social Protection: A Comparative Study.* Rein and Rainwater, eds. Armonk, N.Y.: M.E. Sharpe, 1986.

Renner, Craig, and Vicente Navarro. "Why is Our Population of Uninsured and Underinsured Persons Growing? The Consequences of 'Deindustrialization' of the United States." *International Journal of Health Services* 19.3 (1989): 433–42.

Reynolds, Lloyd G. *Labor Economics and Labor Relations.* 8th ed. Englewood Cliffs, N.J.: Prentice Hall, 1982.

Riccucci, Norma H. *Women, Minorities, and Unions in the Public Sector.* New York: Greenwood Press, 1990.

Richards, Andrew. "Down But Not Out: Labour Movements in Late Industrial Societies." Working Paper, Instituto Juan March de Estudios e Investigaciones, Madrid, May 1995.

Riley, Charles A., II. *Small Business, Big Politics: What Entrepreneurs Need to Know to Use Their Growing Political Power.* Princeton, N.J.: Pacesetter Books, 1995.

Rimlinger, Gaston V. *Welfare Policy and Industrialization in Europe, America, and Russia.* New York: John Wiley & Sons, 1971.

Rixner, Brian. "Japanese Automobile Transplants: Redefining Relationships in the American Auto Industry." Senior essay, Yale University, 1995.

Robertson, David Brian. "The Bias of American Federalism: The Limits of Welfare-State Development in the Progressive Era." *Journal of Policy History* 1.3 (1989): 261–91.

Robinson, Ian. "NAFTA, Social Unionism, and Labour Movement Power in Canada and the United States." *Relations industrielles/Industrial Relations* 49.4 (1994): 657–95.

———. "Organizing Labour: Explaining Canada-U.S. Union Diversity in the Post-War Period." Ph.D. dissertation, Yale University, 1992.

Rochefort, David A., and Roger W. Cobb. "Problem Definition, Agenda Access, and Policy Choice." *Policy Studies Journal* 21.1 (1993): 56–71.

Roemer, Milton I. *National Health Systems of the World: Vol. 1, The Countries.* New York: Oxford University Press, 1991.

———. "National Health Systems Throughout the World." *Health Care Reform in the Nineties.* Pauline Vaillancourt Rosenau, ed. Thousand Oaks, Calif.: Sage, 1994.

Rogers, Joel. "Don't Worry, Be Happy: The Postwar Decline of Private-Sector Unionism in the United States." *The Challenge of Restructuring: North American Labor Movements Respond.* Jane Jenson and Rianne Mahon, eds. Philadelphia: Temple University Press, 1993.

———. "The Folks Who Brought You the Weekend: Labor and Independent Politics." *Audacious Democracy: Labor, Intellectuals, and the Social Reconstruction of America.* Steven Fraser and Joshua B. Freeman, eds. Boston: Mariner, 1997.

Rogin, Michael. "Voluntarism: The Political Functions of an Antipolitical Doctrine." *Labor and American Politics.* Charles M. Rehmus and Doris B. McLaughlin, eds. Ann Arbor: The University of Michigan, 1967.

Rohde, David W. *Parties and Leaders in the Postreform House.* Chicago: The University of Chicago Press, 1991.

Root, Lawrence S. "Employee Benefits and Social Welfare: Complement and Conflict." *The Annals of the American Academy of Political and Social Science* 479 (1985): 101–18.

——. *Fringe Benefits: Social Insurance in the Steel Industry.* Beverly Hills, Calif.: Sage, 1982.

Rosenau, Pauline Vaillancourt, ed. *Health Care Reform in the Nineties.* Thousand Oaks, Calif.: Sage, 1994.

Rosenblum, Jonathan D. *Copper Crucible: How the Arizona Miners' Strike of 1983 Recast Labor-Management Relations in America.* Ithaca, N.Y.: ILR Press, 1995.

Rosner, David, and Gerald Markowitz. "Hospitals, Insurance, and the American Labor Movement: The Case of New York in the Postwar Decades." *Journal of Policy History* 9.1 (1997): 74–95.

Rossiter, Louis F., and Amy K. Taylor. "Union Effects on the Provision of Health Insurance." *Industrial Relations* 21.2 (Spring 1982): 167–77.

Rosswurm, Steve, ed. *The CIO's Left-Led Unions.* New Brunswick, N.J.: Rutgers University Press, 1992.

Rothman, David J. "A Century of Failure: Health Care Reform in America." *Journal of Health Politics, Policy and Law* 18.2 (Summer 1993): 271–86.

Rothstein, Bo. "Labor-Market Institutions and Working-Class Strength." *Structuring Politics: Historical Institutionalism in Comparative Analysis.* Sven Steinmo, Kathleen Thelen, and Frank Longstreth, eds. Cambridge: Cambridge University Press, 1992.

Rovner, Julie. "Congress and Health Care Reform 1993–94." *Intensive Care: How Congress Shapes Health Policy.* Thomas E. Mann and Norman J. Ornstein, eds. Washington, D.C.: American Enterprise Institute and The Brookings Institution, 1995.

Ruggie, Mary. *Realignments in the Welfare State: Health Policy in the United States, Britain and Canada.* New York: Columbia University Press, 1996.

Sakala, Carol. "The Development of National Medical Care Programs in the United Kingdom and Canada: Applicability to Current Conditions in the United States." *Journal of Health Politics, Policy and Law* 15.4 (Winter 1990): 709–53.

Salmon, Jack Warren. "Corporate Attempts to Reorganize the American Health System." Ph.D. dissertation, Cornell University, 1978.

Sapolsky, H. M., et al. "Corporate Attitudes Toward Health Care Costs." *Milbank Memorial Fund Quarterly* 59.4 (1981): 561–85.

Sass, Steven A. *The Promise of Private Pensions: The First Hundred Years.* Cambridge: Harvard University Press, 1997.

Sawhill, Isabel V. "Reaganomics in Retrospect." *Perspectives on the Reagan Years.* John L. Palmer, ed. Washington, D.C.: Urban Institute Press, 1986.

Schattschneider, E.E. *The Semi-Sovereign People: A Realist's View of Democracy in America.* New York: Holt, Rinehart, and Winston, 1960.

Schatz, Ronald W. *The Electrical Workers: A History of Labor at General Electric and Westinghouse, 1923–60.* Urbana: University of Illinois Press, 1983.

Schenk, Christopher, and Elaine Bernard. "Social Unionism: Labor as a Political Force." *Social Policy* 23.1 (Summer 1992): 38–46.

Schick, Allen. "How a Bill Did Not Become a Law." *Intensive Care: How Congress Shapes Health Policy.* Thomas E. Mann and Norman J. Ornstein, eds. Washington, D.C.: American Enterprise Institute and The Brookings Institution, 1995.

Schlesinger, Arthur M., Jr. *The Politics of Upheaval: The Age of Roosevelt.* Boston: Houghton Mifflin, 1960.

Schramm, Carl J., et al. "Perspectives: Responses to an Essay by Uwe Reinhardt on Health Care Spending and American Competitiveness." *Health Affairs*, Spring 1990: 162–77.

Schrecker, Ellen W. "McCarthyism and the Labor Movement: The Role of the State." *The CIO's Left-Led Unions.* Steve Rosswurm, ed. New Brunswick, N.J.: Rutgers University Press, 1992.

SEIU. "Demanding Quality: SEIU Principles for Quality Care." Washington, D.C.: SEIU, 1996.

———. "Hammering the Middle Class: The Economic Impact of Taxing Benefits." Washington, D.C.: SEIU, April 1994.

———. "Out of Control, Into Decline." Washington, D.C.: SEIU, 1992.

———, Department of Public Policy. "Employer-Paid Health Insurance is Disappearing." SEIU: Washington, D.C., July 1989.

Shafer, Byron E. *Quiet Revolution: The Struggle for the Democratic Party and the Shaping of Post-Reform Politics.* New York: Russell Sage Foundation, 1983.

Shaiken, Harley. *Work Transformed: Automation and Labor in the Computer Age.* New York: Holt, Rinehart and Winston, 1984.

Shalev, Michael. "The Resurgence of Labor Quiescence." *The Future of Labour Movements.* Marino Regini, ed. London: Sage, 1992.

———, ed. *The Privatization of Social Policy? Occupational Welfare and the Welfare State in America, Scandinavia and Japan.* Great Britain: St. Martin's Press, 1996.

Shostak, Arthur B. *Robust Unionism: Innovations in the Labor Movement.* Ithaca, N.Y.: ILR Press, 1991.

Skocpol, Theda. "The Aftermath of Defeat." *Journal of Health Politics, Policy and Law* 20.2 (Summer 1995): 485–89.

———. *Boomerang: Clinton's Health Security Effort and the Turn Against Government in U.S. Politics.* New York: W.W. Norton & Co., 1996.

———. "Is the Time Finally Ripe? Health Insurance Reforms in the 1990s." *The Politics of Health Care Reform: Lessons From the Past, Prospects for the Future.* James Morone and Gary S. Belkin, eds. Durham, N.C.: Duke University Press, 1991.

Skocpol, Theda, and Edwin Amenta. "Did Capitalists Shape Social Security? Comment on Quadagno." *American Sociological Review* 50.4 (1985): 572–75.

Skowronek, Stephen. *Building a New American State: The Expansion of National Administrative Capacities, 1877–1920.* Cambridge: Cambridge University Press, 1982.

Smith, Miriam Catherine. "Labour Without Allies: The Canadian Labour Congress in Politics, 1956–1988." Ph.D. dissertation, Yale University, 1990.

Smith, Rogers M. "Beyond Tocqueville, Myrdal, and Hartz: The Multiple Traditions in America." *American Political Science Review* 87.3 (September 1993): 549–66.

———. "Political Jurisprudence, the 'New Institutionalism,' and the Future of Public Law." *American Political Science Review* 82.1 (March 1988): 89–108.

Sousa, David J. "Organized Labor in the Electorate, 1960–1988." *Political Research Quarterly* 46.4 (1993): 741 58.

Spriggs, William, ed. *Employee Rights in a Changing Economy: The Issue of Replacement Workers.* Washington, D.C.: Economic Policy Institute, 1991.

Staples, Clifford. "The Politics of Employment-Based Insurance in the United States." *International Journal of Health Services* 19.3 (1989): 415–31.

Starr, Paul. *The Logic of Health-Care Reform.* 1st ed. Knoxville, Tenn.: Grand Rounds Press, Whittle Direct Books, 1991.

———. *The Social Transformation of American Medicine.* New York: Basic Books, 1982.

Stebenne, David L. *Arthur J. Goldberg: New Deal Liberal.* New York: Oxford University Press, 1996.

Steinmo, Sven, and Kathleen Thelen. "Historical Institutionalism in Comparative Politics." *Structuring Politics: Historical Institutionalism in Comparative Analysis.* Sven

Steinmo, Kathleen Thelen, and Frank Longstreth, eds. Cambridge: Cambridge University Press, 1992.

Steinmo, Sven, Kathleen Thelen, and Frank Longstreth, eds. *Structuring Politics: Historical Institutionalism in Comparative Analysis.* Cambridge: Cambridge University Press, 1992.

Steinmo, Sven, and Jon Watts. "It's the Institutions, Stupid! Why Comprehensive National Health Insurance Always Fails in America." *Journal of Health Politics, Policy and Law* 20.2 (Summer 1995): 329–72.

Stepan-Norris, Judith, and Maurice Zeitlin. "Insurgency, Radicalism, and Democracy in America's Industrial Unions." *Social Forces* 75.1 (September 1996): 1–32.

Stephens, John D. *The Transition from Capitalism to Socialism.* New Jersey: Humanities Press, 1980.

Stevens, Beth. "Blurring the Boundaries: How the Federal Government Has Influenced Welfare Benefits in the Private Sector." *The Politics of Social Policy in the United States.* Margaret Weir, Ann Shola Orloff and Theda Skocpol, eds. Princeton, N.J.: Princeton University Press, 1988.

———. *Complementing the Welfare State: The Development of Private Pension, Health Insurance and Other Employee Benefits in the United States.* Geneva: International Labour Office, 1986.

———. "In the Shadow of the Welfare State: Corporate and Union Development of Employee Benefits." Ph.D. dissertation, Harvard University, 1984.

———. "Labor Unions, Employee Benefits, and the Privatization of the American Welfare State." *Journal of Policy History* 2.3 (1990): 233–60.

Stevens, Robert, and Rosemary Stevens. *Welfare Medicine in America: A Case Study of Medicaid.* New York: The Free Press, 1974.

Stevens, Rosemary. *American Medicine and the Public Interest.* New Haven: Yale University Press, 1971.

Stewart, John. *The Battle for Health: A Political History of the Socialist Medical Association, 1930–51.* Abingdon, England: Ashgate, 1999.

Stieber, Jack. *Governing the UAW.* New York: John Wiley and Sons, 1962.

Stone, Deborah. "Causal Stories and the Formulation of Agendas." *Political Science Quarterly* 104.2 (1989): 281–300.

———. "Drawing Lessons From Comparative Health Research." *Critical Issues in Health Policy.* Ralph A. Straetz, Marvin Lieberman, and Alice Sardell, eds. Lexington, Mass.: Lexington Books, 1981.

———. "The Resistible Rise of Preventive Medicine." *Health Policy in Transition: A Decade of Health Politics, Policy and Law.* Lawrence D. Brown, ed. Durham, N.C.: Duke University Press, 1987.

———. "The Struggle for the Soul of Health Insurance." *Journal of Health Politics, Policy, and Law* 18.2 (Summer 1993): 287–317.

Strauss, George. "Industrial Relations: Time of Change." *Industrial Relations* 23.1 (Winter 1984): 1–15.

Strauss, George, Daniel G. Gallagher, and Jack Fiorito, eds. *The State of the Unions.* Madison, Wis.: Industrial Relations Research Association, 1991.

Streeck, Wolfgang. "The Uncertainties of Management in the Management of Uncertainty: Employers, Labor Relations and Industrial Adjustment in the 1980s." *Work, Employment & Society* 1.3 (September 1987): 281–308.

Swartz, Karen. *The Medically Uninsured: Special Focus on Workers.* Washington, D.C.: Urban Institute Press, July 1989.

Swatz, D. "The Politics of Reform: Conflict and Accommodation in Canadian Health Policy." *The Canadian State: Political Economy and Political Power.* Leo Panitch, ed. Toronto: University of Toronto Press, 1977.

Sweeney, John J., with David Kusnet. *America Needs a Raise: Fighting for Economic Security and Social Justice.* Boston: Houghton Mifflin, 1996.

Swenson, Peter. "Arranged Alliance: Business Interests in the New Deal." *Politics & Society* 25.1 (March 1997): 66–116.

———. "Bringing Capital Back In; or Social Democracy Reconsidered: Employer Power, Cross-Class Alliances, and Centralization of Industrial Relations in Denmark and Sweden." *World Politics* 43 (July 1991): 513–44.

———. *Fair Shares: Unions, Pay and Politics in Sweden and West Germany.* Ithaca, N.Y.: Cornell University Press, 1989.

Tallon, James R., and Lawrence D. Brown. "Health Alliances: Functions, Forms, and Federalism." *Making Health Reform Work: The View From the States.* John J. DiIulio and Richard Nathan, eds. Washington, D.C.: The Brookings Institution, 1994.

Tasini, Jonathan. *The Edifice Complex: Rebuilding the American Labor Movement to Face the Global Economy.* New York: Labor Research Association, 1995.

Taylor, Andrew J. *Trade Unions and Politics: A Comparative Introduction.* Houndmills, England: Macmillan, 1989.

Taylor, Humphrey, Robert Leitman, and Robert Blendon. "Large Employers and Managed Care." *Reforming the System: Containing Health Care Costs in an Era of Universal Coverage.* Robert Blendon and Tracey Stelzer Hyams, eds. New York: Faulkner & Gray, 1992.

Taylor, Malcolm G. *Health Insurance and Canadian Public Policy: The Seven Decisions that Created the Canadian Health Insurance System.* Montreal: McGill-Queen's University Press, 1978.

———. *Insuring National Health Care: The Canadian Experience.* Chapel Hill: University of North Carolina Press, 1990.

Taylor, Suzanne S. *Negotiating Health Insurance in the Workplace: A Basic Guide.* Washington, D.C.: Bureau of National Affairs, 1992.

Thelen, Kathleen. "Beyond Corporatism: Toward a New Framework for the Study of Labor in Advanced Capitalism." *Comparative Politics* 27.1 (October 1994): 107–24.

Therborn, Goran, and Joop Roebroek. "The Irreversible Welfare State: Its Recent Maturation, Its Encounter with the Economic Crisis, and Its Future Prospects." *International Journal of Health Services* 16.3 (1986): 319–38.

Thompson, Frank J. "New Federalism and Health Care Policy: States and the Old Questions." *Health Policy in Transition: A Decade of Health Politics, Policy and Law.* Lawrence D. Brown, ed. Durham, N.C.: Duke University Press, 1987.

Tolliday, Steven, and Jonathan Zeitlin. "Employers and Industrial Relations Between Theory and History." *The Power to Manage? Employers and Industrial Relations in Comparative-Historical Perspective.* Steven Tolliday and Jonathan Zeitlin, eds. London: Routledge, 1991.

Tomlins, Christopher L. *The State and the Unions: Labor Relations, Law, and the Organized Labor Movement in America, 1880–1960.* Cambridge: Cambridge University Press, 1985.

Tone, Andrea. *The Business of Benevolence: Industrial Paternalism in Progressive America.* Ithaca, N.Y.: Cornell University Press, 1997.

Troy, Leo. *The New Unionism in the New Society: Public Sector Unions in the Redistributive State.* Fairfax, Va.: George Mason University Press, 1994.

Turner, Lowell. *Democracy at Work: Changing World Markets and the Future of Labor Unions.* Ithaca, N.Y.: Cornell University Press, 1992.

Tynes, Sheryl R. *Turning Points in Social Security: From 'Cruel Hoax' to Sacred Entitlement.* Stanford, Calif.: Stanford University Press, 1996.

U.S. House Committee on Government Operations. *Rising Use of Part-Time and Temporary Workers: Who Benefits and Who Loses?* Washington, D.C.: U.S. Government Printing Office, 1988.

Useem, Michael. *The Inner Circle: Large Corporations and the Rise of Business Political Activity in the U.S. and U.K.* New York: Oxford University Press, 1984.

Vielba, Carol. "Government and Industry: The Local Dimension." *Policy and Politics* 14.4 (1986): 507–18.

Visser, Jelle. "The Strength of Union Movements in Advanced Capitalist Democracies: Social and Organizational Variations." *The Future of Labour Movements.* Marino Regini, ed. London: Sage, 1992.

Vogel, David. *Fluctuating Fortunes: The Political Power of Business in America.* New York: Basic Books, 1989.

———. "The Power of Business in America: A Re-appraisal." *British Journal of Political Science* 13.1 (1983): 19–43.

Wade, Robert. "Globalization and Its Limits: Reports of the Death of the National Economy are Greatly Exaggerated." *National Diversity and Global Capitalism.* Suzanne Berger and Ronald Dore, eds. Ithaca, N.Y.: Cornell University Press, 1996: 60–88.

Walters, V. "State, Capital, and Labour: The Introduction of Federal-Provincial Insurance for Physician Care in Canada." *Canadian Review of Sociology and Anthropology* 19.2 (1982): 157–72.

Warshawsky, Mark J. *The Uncertain Promise of Retiree Health Benefits: An Evaluation of Corporate Obligations.* Washington, D.C.: The AEI Press, 1992.

Weeks, David A. *Rethinking Employee Benefit Assumptions.* New York: Conference Board, 1978.

Weil, Laurence A. "Organized Labor and Health Reform: Union Interests and the Clinton Plan." *Journal of Public Health Policy* 18.1 (1997): 30–48.

Weinstein, James. *The Corporate Ideal in the Liberal State: 1900–1918.* Boston: Beacon Press, 1968.

Weir, Margaret. *Politics and Jobs: The Boundaries of Employment Policy in the United States.* Princeton, N.J.: Princeton University Press, 1992.

———. "American Politics and the Future of Social Policy." *The Social Divide: Political Parties and the Future of Activist Government.* Margaret Weir, ed. Washington, D.C. and New York: Brookings Institution and Russell Sage Foundation, 1998.

———, ed. *The Social Divide: Political Parties and the Future of Activist Government.* Washington, D.C. and New York: Brookings Institution Press and Russell Sage Foundation, 1998.

Weir, Margaret, Ann Shola Orloff, and Theda Skocpol, eds. *The Politics of Social Policy in the United States.* Princeton, N.J.: Princeton University Press, 1988.

Weir, Margaret, and Theda Skocpol. "State Structures and Social Keynesianism." *International Journal of Comparative Sociology* 24 (1983): 4–29.

Weiss, Linda. "Globalization and the Myth of the Powerless State," *New Left Review* no. 225 (September/October 1997): 3–27.

Weissert, Carol. *Governing Health: The Politics of Health Policy.* Baltimore: The John Hopkins University Press, 1996.

White, Joseph. "Budgeting and Health Policymaking." *Intensive Care: How Congress Shapes Health Policy.* Thomas E. Mann and Norman J. Ornstein, eds. Washington, D.C.: American Enterprise Institute and The Brookings Institution, 1995.

Wiebe, Robert H. *Businessmen and Reform: A Study of the Progressive Movement.* Cambridge: Harvard University Press, 1962.

Wildavsky, Aaron. *The Politics of the Budgetary Process.* Boston: Little Brown, 1984.

Wilks, Stephen. "Government-Industry Relations: A Review Article." *Policy and Politics* 14.4 (1986): 491–505.

Wilsford, David. *Doctors and the State: The Politics of Health Care in France and the United States.* Durham, N.C.: Duke University Press, 1991.

Wilson, Graham K. *Unions in American National Politics.* New York: St. Martin's Press, 1979.

Wilson, Rand. "Winning Lessons from the NAFTA Loss," *Labor Research Review* 13.1 (Fall 1994): 29–37.

Witte, Edwin E. "Organized Labor and Social Security." *Labor and the New Deal.* Milton Derber and Edwin Young, eds. (Madison: University of Wisconsin Press, 1957): 239–74.

Woodward, Bob. *The Agenda: Inside the Clinton White House.* New York: Simon & Schuster, 1994.

Woolhandler, Steffie, and David U. Himmelstein. "A National Health Program: Northern Light at the End of the Tunnel." *Journal of the American Medical Association* 262.15 (1989): 2136.

Yates, Charlotte. "North American Autoworkers' Response to Restructuring." *Bargaining for Change: Union Politics in North America and Europe.* Miriam Golden and Jonas Pontusson, eds. Ithaca, N.Y.: Cornell University Press, 1992.

Zieger, Robert H. *American Workers, American Unions.* 2nd ed. Baltimore: The Johns Hopkins University Press, 1994.

———. *The CIO, 1935–1955.* Chapel Hill: The University of North Carolina Press, 1995.

Zuboff, Shoshana. *In the Age of the Smart Machine: The Future of Work and Power.* New York: Basic Books, 1988.

Index

- Seeks fill hole in understanding of devel of welf state _ argues correlation of 1950s issues

- Argues for broader def of welf state

- shows less divided

Laws, created unlikely partners, have unintended consequences

- Traces twists & turns in various gray positions

- bj's small

- unclear view

unempl oppose too little single p'ger

ed-labor vs early model

1978 Prop 13

- graphical treat in here – highlights disorders

- Possibly too much taken for grant

- Ack but does not show power of opposition

- Seems to assume all thing possible

postwar corporate accord